Handbuch der experimentellen Pharmakologie

Handbook of Experimental Pharmacology

Heffter-Heubner New Series

Vol. XVI/13

Springer-Verlag Berlin Heidelberg GmbH 1966

Erzeugung von Krankheitszuständen durch das Experiment

Teil 13

Tumoren II

Bearbeitet von

W. Dontenwill · F. Squartini

Herausgeber

Oskar Eichler

Mit 72 Abbildungen

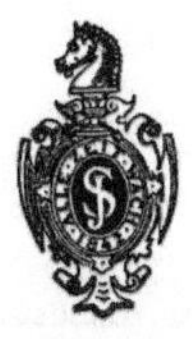

Springer-Verlag Berlin Heidelberg GmbH 1966

ISBN 978-3-662-26801-8 ISBN 978-3-662-26800-1 (eBook)
DOI 10.1007/978-3-662-26800-1

Ursprünglich erschienen bei Springer-Verlag, Berlin · Heidelberg 1966
Softcover reprint of the hardcover 1st edition 1966
Library of Congress Catalog Card Number AGR 25—699

Titel-Nr. 5726

Inhaltsverzeichnis

Erzeugung von Tumoren durch endogenhormonelle Faktoren

Von Walter Dontenwill

Mitarbeiterverzeichnis

DONTENWILL, WALTER, Professor Dr., Wissenschaftliche Forschungsstelle im VdC-Institut, 2000 Hamburg 54, Gazellenkamp 38.

SQUARTINI, FRANCESCO, Dr., Institute of Pathological Anatomy and Division of Cancer Research, Perugia University Medical School, Perugia (Monteluce) Italien.

Tumours arising from vertical transmission*

By

FRANCESCO SQUARTINI

With 25 Figures

I. Introduction

The establishment of the first homozygous strains, many years ago, disclosed unexpected possibilities for specialized investigations in the fields of biological research. Today a large number of inbred strains, specially mouse strains, are available for different purposes. Whoever is familiar with the problems of cancer research knows that there are perhaps no strains at present which are completely free from the development of spontaneous neoplasms. The frequency and site of predilection of these so-called spontaneous tumours in laboratory animals are widely variable according to the animal strain, sex and environmental conditions. The intensive studies devoted, through many years, to some of these spontaneous tumours have decisively shown that they are mainly due to intrinsic causative factors acquired by vertical transmission.

II. The problem

To trace a short outline of this ratherconfused problem a few essential points have to be focused, namely: a definition of tumours arising from vertical transmission, an analysis of what can be acquired by vertical transmission which may lead to tumour formation, a survey of the various types of tumours which may originate through this route, and finally a choice of the best examples to take as models in the study of such a kind of tumours.

1. Definition

The main features of tumours arising from vertical transmission are their apparently spontaneous occurrence and their accumulation in particular animal strains. Thus, although any definition of this matter may fail to be correct in all cases, tumours arising from vertical transmission could be defined as those neoplasms which occur spontaneously, being due to intrinsic transmissible factors, so that, instead of a distribution by chance, they show accumulation in given groups of homogeneous animals and in their descendants, from generation to generation.

2. What can be acquired by vertical transmission

The speculation upon the factors which may be acquired by vertical transmission and may to some extent be responsible for spontaneous tumorigenesis, leads to consider no more than three or four practical possibilities. Whether some of the factors listed below must be regarded as true "causative" factors, or only

* Received for publication August 8th, 1964.

as "permissive" conditions of tumour development, is an open question. It is clear, however, that "factors" transmitted from parents to their offspring may either be chromosomal, *i.e.* inherited through the chromosomes, or extrachromosomal, *i.e.* transmitted through other routes. Briefly, the parents may transmit to offspring:

a) A generic tendency to develop a given type of tumour, in other words, what is called "inherited susceptibility" to tumour formation. This is transmitted through the chromosomes.

b) A particular attitude of the endocrine system, favourable to the development of hormonal inbalances. As it is known, any hormonal imbalance which results in a continuous or umbalanced stimulation of the corresponding target organ or tissue may lead to tumour formation. Also in this case transmission occurs through the chromosomes.

c) A tumour-inducing virus, *i.e.* an extrachromosomal factor which may spread in a vertical epidemic through different routes: the cytoplasm of the ovum, the placenta, the seminal fluid, or the mother's milk.

d) Two or more of these factors together.

The list of heritable factors affecting tumorigenesis will perhaps become longer in the future, because the expression "inherited susceptibility", mentioned under (a), is a confused term in which many different things may be concealed. For instance, the inherited susceptibility to tumour development might act in different cases through a particular tissue sensitivity, or through metabolic deviations, or through immunologic defects, and so on. Also the attitude to develop hormonal imbalances mentioned under (b) may, strictly speaking, be considered as a particular aspect of inherited susceptibility. This emphasizes the limits of present knowledge in the field, limits which in facts permit only the recognition of two fundamental groups of transmissible tumorigenic factors: the chromosomal factors and the extrachromosomal ones.

3. Multiplicity of the chromosomal and extrachromosomal factors

Both chromosomal and extrachromosomal factors are multiple entities. There are no strains of animals susceptible to all types of tumours, as well as there are perhaps no strains entirely resistant to all types. This means that inheritance to neoplasia depends on the action of multiple genetic factors, which are independent of each other and may then be independently transmitted. Likewise, among the extrachromosomal factors, different types of transmissible tumour-inducing agents, or viruses, have been identified so far and others may exist which are unknown at present. Each of these agents has an individual morphology and biological behaviour. Each is responsible for particular types of tumours. There are viruses which induce mammary tumours, and others which induce lymphoid tumours or leukaemias. They may co-exist in the same strain or be independently transmitted in different strains.

4. The types of tumours arising from vertical transmission

The spectrum of tumours which may spontaneously occur in breeding animals is as wide-spread as that of the induced tumours. In most instances spontaneous tumours appear late in the life, and their frequency is low. Therefore, if the animals of a susceptible strain are maintained in good healthy conditions till old age, a certain number of tumours may be expected to occur as a rule in one or different sites. Mammary glands and the haemopoietic tissues are sites of predilection of spontaneous tumour development in inbred mice. Other frequent sites are the lungs, liver, and some endocrine glands. But all the other organs and tissues may sporadically develop spontaneous tumours. The sites of spontaneous tumour development are strictly dependent on the animal strain.

It is generally admitted that tumours can hardly be induced in resistant animals. By contrast, the treatment of susceptible animals with carcinogenic agents results in a high incidence of tumours in one or different sites. The sites of tumour induction in susceptible strains of animals are usually the same which sporadically undergo spontaneous tumorigenesis. In this respect there is good evidence, for certain tumour types, that the rôle of carcinogenic agents might merely be that to accelerate and increase the appearance of those tumours which would spontaneously occur later in the life of the animals. This means that inherited susceptibility is almost an essential condition in tumour induction by carcinogenic agents. Of course, susceptibility should even be more important for the development of spontaneous tumours in each particular strain. The problem is whether the inherited susceptibility, whatever its background will be, is the unique cause of these spontaneous tumours, or whether other factors, *i. e.* environmental factors, are always needed to promote spontaneous tumorigenesis.

Several tumours of the endocrine glands and their end-organs, such as uterus and breasts, are brought about by hormonal imbalances which may occur, usually late in the animal life, on a genetically predetermined basis. However, the highest incidence and the earliest occurrence of spontaneous neoplasms are observed in those strains in which the vertical transmission of an extrachromosomal factor, in form of virus-like tumorigenic particles, takes place.

In conclusion, nearly all the tumours which occur spontaneously in breeding animals appear to be closely related to one or more factors, chromosomal or extrachromosomal, acquired in vertical transmission. Inherited susceptibility causes or co-operates to the development of a certain number of spontaneous tumours. This number may be increased by an excessive release of endogenous hormonal stimuli and, even more, by the presence and transmission of an active, virus-like, tumour-inducing agent.

5. Choice of suitable models for the presentation of this matter

The various types of tumours which spontaneously occur in breeding animals have attracted the interest of the investigators in proportion to their frequency. It was the high incidence of mammary tumours observed in some mouse colonies which, a long time ago, suggested the establishment of inbred strains of mice for the study of the mechanisms of hereditary transmission of those neoplasms. Obviously, the homozygous strains have served later a wider purpose than the original one. Mammary tumours in mice enhanced also the investigations on the rôle of endogenous hormonal factors in the origin of spontaneous neoplasms. In addition, the list of extrachromosomal factors which cause tumour development after spontaneous vertical transmission was initiated by the discovery in 1936 of the mouse mammary tumour virus, or BITTNER milk agent.

Other tumours showing a relatively high spontaneous frequency, which have been extensively studied are the mouse leukaemias. Although to a lesser degree, lung tumours and tumours of the liver in mice have been considered attractive subjects, because of the same reason. Consequently, there has been a large accumulation of papers on some types of tumours, whereas other tumour types have been neglected. As a result, some model tumour-systems have arisen which appear to be particularly suitable for the analysis of factors which cause tumour development in breeding animals. Due to the aims of this presentation and to the specific qualification of the writer, two models, mammary tumours and leukaemias in mice, will be chosen as guides, it being apparent that much more can be learned from the study of single but well known tumour types than from a rapid survey of all the wide-spread family of tumours, occurring in different sites and different animal species, suspected to be caused by vertical transmission. A brief summary of the information concerning the other tumour types will be given.

The reason why mice are preferred is the large availability of inbred mouse strains, in contrast with other animal species. Genetic standardization of the animals is a pre-requisite in studies dealing with vertical transmission of tumorigenic factors. A list of the inbred strains of mice quoted in this review, with explanation of names and incidence of spontaneous tumours, is given in Table 1.

Table 1. *A list of inbred strains of mice in common use for studies on the development of spontaneous tumours, specially mammary tumours and leukaemia* (for detailed information see Heston, 1945; Gross, 1961b)

Original inbred strains[1]		Incidence of spontaneous tumours				Annotations
Derivation of name	Name	Mammary tumours	Leukaemia (lymphatic)	Lung tumours	Liver tumours	
*A*lbino	A	high*	low	high	low	* Only in breeding females; low in virgins
*A*lbino descendants of family *K**	AK or Ak	low	high	low	low	* Selected for leukaemia
AK strain maintained at the *R*ockefeller institute	AKR or RIL*	low	high	low	low	* *R*ockefeller *I*nstitute *L*eukaemia strain
*B*agg *ALB*ino *C*oat colour	BALB/c or C or Balb/C	low	low	medium	low	
*C*oat colour *B*lack *A*gouti	CBA	low*	low	low	medium	* High according to Gardner (1941)
lineal descendants of mouse 8986 named *C3H*	C3H	high	low	low	high	
descendants of female *57* showing *C*oat colour *Black*	C57 Black* or C57b	low	low	low	low	* 10—20% of tumours in various sites, mainly non-epithelial
descendants of female *58* showing *C*oat colour *Black*	C58 Black or C58	low	high	low	low	
*D*ilute *B*rown non-*A*gouti	DBA or dba	high	medium*	low	low	* Reported for subline 212 of this strain
? (Paris albino strain)	RIII	high	low	low	low	

[1] A number of inbred strains have been derived from the original ones by foster-nursing (f). Foster-nursing affects the mammary tumour incidence, but not the incidence of other tumour types. Strains Af, C3Hf or C3Hb, DBAf or DBAb, and RIIIf or RIIIb are low-mammary-tumour strains derived from the corresponding high-mammary-tumour strains (A, C3H, DBA, and RIII) by means of foster-nursing on C57black low-tumour females. Strain BALB/cf is BALB/c foster-nursed by C3H; it is a high mammary tumour strain.

III. The mouse mammary tumours and the mouse mammary tumour virus

The inherited susceptibility, the hormonal stimulation of mammary glands, and a virus-like particle transmitted *via* the mother's milk, or mammary tumour virus, are the essential factors involved in the genesis of spontaneous mammary tumours of the mouse. It is impossible at present to establish an order of importance among these factors. They act synergically producing a complex chain of events, the final result of which is the development of a mammary tumour.

1. Mammary tumour virus (MTV): the Bittner virus

A. Historical

Since the first observations on the spontaneous mouse mammary cancer in stock animals it was apparent that some colonies developed a high incidence of mammary tumours at an early age, whereas other colonies were almost completely free from the disease (Bashford, 1909). When inbred mouse strains became available, some years later, the mechanisms of hereditary transmission of mammary tumours could be studied in detail (Little, 1928). The reciprocal cross between mice of high- and low-mammary-cancer strains led to the detection of a maternal extrachromosomal influence as one of the causative factors of spontaneous mammary tumours in mice (Staff of the Roscoe B. Jackson Memorial Laboratory, 1933). Three years later Bittner (1936) proved that transmission of this extrachromosomal factor from mothers to offspring occurred *via* the milk. After its detection in milk, the mammary tumour-inducing agent of Bittner was found in various other organs, tissues and body fluids of high-cancer-strain mice (see Dmochowski, 1949). Recent studies have shown that this agent has the physical and chemical properties of a virus (Lyons and Moore, 1962).

B. Morphology of particles associated with mammary tumours in mice

The first mention of "virus-like" particles in mouse mammary-tumour cells cultivated *in vitro* was made in 1948 by Porter and Thompson. Successive studies by a number of investigators (Kinosita et al., 1953; Bang and Andervont, 1953; Dmochowski, 1954; Bernhard et al., 1955; Dmochowski, Haagensen and Moore, 1955; Bang, Andervont and Vellisto, 1956; Bang, Vellisto and Libert, 1956; Bernhard, Guérin and Oberling, 1956; Dmochowski, 1956; Suzuki, 1957; Bernhard and Guérin, 1958a; Ichikawa and Amano, 1958; Bernhard, 1958, 1960; de Harven, 1961; Bernhard and Granboulan, 1962; Moore, 1962; Dmochowski et al., 1963a) have shown that different types of particles may be associated with mouse mammary tumours, and have given a detailed description of their fine morphology in thin sections. The location of these particles in or outside the cells and the sites of production have suggested a possible developmental cycle. Finally, by means of correlative biological tests[1], the possible correspondence of one of these particles with the MTV has been proven.

[1] The biological test or bioassay for MTV consists in the inoculation of materials suspected to possess mammary tumour-inducing activity (tissue extracts, tumour extracts, milk or other body fluids) into MTV-free susceptible female mice 1—8 days old. The test animals may be inbred or hybrids. Tissues and tumours to be tested are removed, ground in a mortar with sand, diluted in an equal amount of physiologic saline and centrifuged at about 3,000 r.p.m.; the supernatant is injected. Fluids may be injected directly or after centrifugation and proper dilution. For inoculation the subcutaneous or intraperitoneal routes are used, the latter being preferred. The injected dose is 0.1—0.2 cc. per mouse. After weaning, the test females are mated with males and allowed to deliver 1 to 3 litters as rapidly as possible by removal of newborns and prevention of lactation. Then the test animals are isolated and kept under observation throughout their lives for the occurrence of mammary tumours.

a) Type A and B particles

There are two types of virus-like particles associated with mouse mammary tumours: the type A and the type B particles (BERNHARD, 1958). The type A particles are predominantly intracytoplasmic, measure about 70 mμ in diameter, have a doughnut shape and appear to be composed of an electron translucent center surrounded by a double concentric shell with the inner one more dense (BERNHARD, 1958, 1960). These particles are mainly concentrated in the Golgi area, but occasionally they may also be found outside the cells (BERNHARD and GUÉRIN, 1958a). They form inclusion bodies visible in the light microscope (GUÉRIN, 1955). The significance of type A particles is not yet clearly understood.

The type B particles are mainly extracellular, although they may also be seen within the cytoplasm of the cells. These particles are believed to represent the Bittner milk agent (MOORE et al., 1959; LASFARGUES et al., 1959; MOORE and LYONS, 1963b). They consist of a dense "nucleoid", measuring 30—40 mμ in diameter, contained within a membranous sac of 90—120 mμ in diameter (MOORE, 1962). The nucleoid is eccentric and appears to be composed of coarse granules, or of very close-fitting filaments. The sac membrane consists of an inner dense layer with many spines which protrude from its surface, resembling in this respect other virus-enclosing membranes (see MOORE, 1962). A sac may occasionally contain two or even more nucleoids.

b) Developmental cycle

The synthesis of A particles occurs directly in the cytoplasm from an originally small crescent which rapidly changes into a completed sphere (MOORE, 1962). The intracytoplasmic A particles have been considered as precursors of the extracellular B particles, and a well defined developmental cycle from A to B particles taking place at the cell surface was first suggested (BERNHARD et al., 1955; BERNHARD, 1958). The existence of a close relationship between A and B particles is well established (see BERNHARD and GRANBOULAN, 1962). But it has also been shown (AMANO and ICHIKAWA, 1959; MOORE, 1962) that the release of B particles by means of budding at the cell surface can take place directly without migration of intracellular A particles beyond the cell membrane.

Following the description of MOORE (1962), the steps leading to the development of mature B particles may be summarized as follows. "First, there is a protrusion of the cell membrane with a crescent beneath it consisting of two layers of dense material. The inner layer of the incipient particle is the initial part of a dense inner shell. In some cases the inner shell may represent a pre-assembled A particle which has moved up to the membrane to be included in B particle formation (however at the cell membrane A particles are rarely if ever found). In either case, whether it is laid down at the membrane or pre-assembled as an A particle, the inner shell of the immature B particle is morphologically indistinguishable from the A particle. In the formation process the membrane protrudes further and the proximal side of the sphere is complete. The sphere then breaks away from the membrane. These extracellular immature B particles resemble the cytoplasmic A bodies but are larger and, on close examination, are found to have two additional external membranes. After release from the cell membrane the dense inner shell of the free B particle arranges itself to form the nucleoid of the mature B particles. Particles seem occasionally to form in the same manner in the membrane of cytoplasmic vacuoles. Although many cytoplasmic vacuoles are covered with A particles they seldom seem to bud into the vacuoles to form B particles" (MOORE, 1962). This mode of formation of virus particles at the cell membranes has now been confirmed for various other oncogenic and non-oncogenic viruses (BENEDETTI and BERNHARD, 1958; DE HARVEN and FRIEND, 1960; etc.).

c) Presence of the same particles in normal tissues and other tumours of the mouse

Type A and B particles are not exclusively found in mammary tumour tissues. They have also been observed in prelactating and lactating normal mammary tissue (MOORE, 1962), and in the hyperplastic alveolar nodules which are the recognized precursors of many tumours of the mouse breast (PITELKA et al., 1958; PITELKA, DE OME and BERN, 1960; DE MAN and VAN RIJSSEL, 1961). Particles of type B have been found in the milk (DMOCHOWSKI, 1963a, b). In addition, the biological tests suggest that MTV particles are almost ubiquitously spread in the body of carrying mice. As will be discussed later, type A and B particles have been detected not only in materials from high-cancer-strain mice, but also in the low-mammary-tumour strains which are supposed to be MTV-free.

Apart from mammary tumours, the A particles are present in many other mouse tumours, such as lymphoid and myeloid leukaemias, sarcomas, melanomas, plasmocytomas, Ehrlich ascites tumours, etc. (see BERNHARD and GRANBOULAN, 1962). This suggests that the A particles might represent an early stage or be involved in the production of other tumorigenic viruses of the mouse besides the MTV (BERNHARD, 1958, 1960). A few particles of type B have also been occasionally observed in some mouse leukaemias and salivary gland tumours (BERNHARD, 1960).

C. Size of the particles showing mammary tumour-inducing activity

The biological activity of the milk agent is maintained after passage through Seitz filters and Berkefeld candles (BITTNER, 1942a, c; ANDERVONT and BRYAN, 1944). But, after many studies, the size of particles showing mammary tumour-inducing activity still remains a puzzling question, because of inconsistencies and contrasts in the results obtained by various investigators in different experiments, or even in the same experiment. Approaches towards the determination of the size of particles showing biological activity have been made by various means, including ultracentrifugation, ultrafiltration through calibrated collodion or gradocol membranes, irradiation in a cyclotron with various quantities of 4 mev deuterons, and separation of fractions from a diffusion cell.

a) Ultracentrifugation data

Biological tests of centrifuged samples combined with electron microscope studies have shown that complete sedimentation of tumour-inducing activity occurs when the supernatant does not contain particles of 280 Å average diameter (DMOCHOWSKI and PASSEY, 1952). However, even the sedimentation of milk agent is under question, having been reported either that it is sedimented (VISSCHER et al., 1942; PASSEY et al., 1950b), or that it is not sedimented by ultracentrifugation (BRYAN et al., 1942; GRAFF et al., 1949). In the experiments of GRAFF et al. (1948, 1949) spheric particles ranging from 500 to 1500 Å in diameter (average 980 Å) and showing high tumour-inducing activity were still present in the supernatant of milk obtained from RIII high-cancer-strain females after centrifugation at 120,000 g for 30 minutes. No particles were found in the supernatant of milk obtained from low-cancer-strain C57b mice, which proved to be inactive on biological tests. Experiments of differential centrifugation of tissue extracts (mammary tumours and lactating mammary glands) revealed the highest tumour-inducing activity to be connected with the microsomal fraction containing spherical particles of about 300 Å or even smaller diameter (DMOCHOWSKI and HAAGENSEN, 1955). These data seem to suggest the existence of two active particles with different sizes, one of which, however, is apparently much smaller (approximately 30 mμ of average diameter) than any of the particles seen in the electron microscopic observation of mammary tumour tissue.

b) Ultrafiltration data

The filtrate through Berkefeld candles of trypsinized extracts of normal and neoplastic mammary tissue obtained from high-cancer-strain mice shows spherical particles of 300 Å average diameter (range 300—1200 Å) and possesses tumour inducing activity (PASSEY et al., 1947, 1948, 1950a, b).

Several experiments have been developed to establish the size of particles showing the highest tumour-inducing activity by means of filtration through calibrated membranes. RIII high-cancer-strain clarified milk filtered through collodion membranes of 7,800 Å average pore diameter (APD) under positive pressure showed considerable activity in biological tests, but also the residue left on the membranes still showed high tumour-inducing activity (DMOCHOWSKI, 1956). When the filtrate through membranes of 7,800 Å APD was re-filtered through collodion membranes of smaller APD, such as 1,600, 1,000 and 380 Å, the results obtained in biological tests were also somewhat bizarre. Filtrates through 1,600 Å APD membranes showed only slight tumour-inducing activity; filtrates through 1,000 Å APD membranes were found to be inactive; filtrates through 380 Å APD membranes showed again a moderate activity, which was however a little higher than that of filtrates through membranes of 1,600 Å APD. Finally, a third filtration of the material obtained from the 380 Å APD membrane through a collodion membrane of 70 Å APD still allowed some small tumour-inducing activity of the filtrate (DMOCHOWSKI, 1956). These results are in some contrast to those obtained by ultracentrifugation of mammary tumours, lactating breast tissue and milk, but they again suggest the existence of more active particles with different sizes.

Inconsistencies and curiosities similar to those illustrated above were also found by others in the bioassays of fractions passed through calibrated gradocol membranes, or separated from a diffusion cell (MOORE et al., 1959). Further confirmations of the bizarre results of filtration and centrifugation have been obtained by irradiation of milk with various doses of deuterons, which destroy the particles up to a predetermined minimum size. Samples of irradiated milk containing particles below 30, 100 and 200 mμ induced the following rates of mammary tumours in the bioassays, respectively: 1.5, 18.5 and 15.2%. Non-irradiated milk samples were inactive (MOORE et al., 1959).

c) Assumption of the existence of three particles of different size

In order to explain these conflicting data concerning particle size, MOORE et al. (1959) assume that not one but three particles are involved. The largest one corresponds to the B type particle seen in the electron microscope (90—120 mμ in diameter), which perhaps becomes infective when the sac is discarded. The smallest one, which shows the highest tumour-inducing activity, is the naked nucleoid of B particle (30—40 mμ in diameter), or possibly even other fragments of the particle. The third, not yet identified, is assumed to be an inhibitor which would interfere with the tumour-inducing activity of the small agent and perhaps also of the whole particle (MOORE, 1962).

D. Data which postulate the existence of an inhibitor of MTV

Various data from old and recent experiments support the existence of an inhibitor associated with MTV and interfering with it. These data come from different procedures employed in the analysis of MTV-containing materials, such as serial dilutions, filtration and diffusion, ionizing irradiation, dialysis, treatment with chymotrypsin, EDTA (versene) and extraction with ether.

Extraction of MTV-containing materials with petroleum ether was found to enhance their tumour-inducing activity (BARNUM et al., 1944). The same result was obtained after treatment of milk with trypsin (PASSEY et al., 1950b), chymotrypsin (GRAFF et al., 1949) and EDTA (MOORE et al., 1959). These facts suggest that a labile inhibitor might exist, which is destroyed by the procedures employed. The use of serial dilutions in the bioassay of tumour extracts and milk (BITTNER, 1945a, 1948a, 1960, 1962; BARNUM and HUSEBY, 1950; DMOCHOWSKI, 1956) led to the unexpected observation of a higher mammary tumour incidence associated with the higher rather than with the lower dilutions of the tested materials. Also in this case a satisfactory explanation could be seen in the progressive dilution of an inhibitor associated with MTV. In addition, the assumption of an inhibitor would also help in the explanation of the results, reported above, obtained after diffusion, filtration and irradiation of high-cancer-strain milk (DMOCHOWSKI, 1956; MOORE et al., 1959; MOORE, 1962).

In spite of these supporting data almost nothing is known about the nature of the inhibitor associated with MTV, so that it remains at present a rather vague and mysterious entity. As far as we presently know there may be more than one inhibitor or none. It has been suggested that this inhibitor (or one of them) might be an interfering virus particle of 30—60 mμ in size, as it is postulated from filtration, diffusion and irradiation experiments on milk (MOORE et al., 1959; MOORE, 1963). A particle which could satisfy these requirements has also been observed by means of electron microscopy in a centrifugate (39,000 r.p.m. for 22 h) of mammary tumour extracts from C3Hf (low-tumour-strain) mice (MOORE and LYONS, 1962). But, if this is the case, it must be stated that virus particles other than A and B particles have never been observed either in mammary tumours or in milk from high-cancer-strain mice.

Another suggestion was that the sac membrane of the B particle might itself act as an inhibitor, although this is in contrast with evidence accumulated for other viruses (MOORE, 1962). The viral sac is easily destroyed during ultracentrifugation, freezing and thawing used in the purification of B particles, whereas the biological activity of the product is maintained (MOORE, 1963). This brings up again the question of the infectivity of the naked nucleoid, which appears to be equal to or higher than that of the whole B particle (MOORE, 1962, 1963). The nucleoids might also be composed of several units which could dissociate after various treatments giving rise to a number of infective sub-particles (MOORE, 1963).

In conclusion, various manipulations enhance the tumour-inducing activity of MTV. This is suggestive for the presence of an inhibitor (or inhibitors) in MTV-containing materials. However, the nature of the inhibitor(s) is at present a matter for speculation.

E. Identification, purification and characterization of MTV

Since there are so many lines of evidence that type B particles of BERNHARD (1958) are the MTV (MOORE, 1962), various attempts have been made in recent years towards the purification of these particles as a first step of their biological, chemical and physical characterization. The procedures employed include fluorocarbon extraction, density gradient centrifugation, and electrophoresis of milk by the Tyselius method.

Using the fluorocarbon[1] extraction method for removing host cell components from aqueous suspensions, relatively pure viral particles have been obtained in form of a small pellet after repeated extractions associated with various stages of centrifugation (Stone and Moore, 1959). Analysis of this material in the electron microscope showed typical B particles, but not pure enough to permit chemical investigations. Attempts at further purification of the particles were prevented by their extreme fragility, and the activity shown in bioassays was very poor. Two of three analogous preparations were found to be inactive, whereas the third induced only 4 mammary tumours in 40 test mice. This low tumour-inducing activity was however interpreted as due to viral inactivation by fluorocarbon extraction, in agreement with what is known for other viruses.

The successive approach toward purification of MTV was made by using ultracentrifugation in a rubidium chloride density gradient system (Lyons and Moore, 1962; Moore and Lyons, 1962). In the equilibrium ultracentrifugation the density of the zone containing B particles was 1.22. In the electron microscope the B particles were found to be purer and better preserved than with the previous method. A number of morphologic details could then be clarified, including the presence of surface spines of about 10 mμ in length and the structure of nucleoids which show (at least some) to be composed of large granules. The resemblance of the surface of type B virus particles with that of influenza virus, and the existence of some similarity between the nucleoid of the B particle and that of herpes simplex virus were also noted.

The particles disintegrated after treatment with ether, but were resistant to degradation by trypsin, ribonuclease and desoxyribonuclease. Ultraviolet absorption showed typical nucleoprotein absorption patterns. Nucleic acid extraction associated with chemical tests and ultraviolet absorption indicated the presence of RNA as an integral part of the virus, although low quantities of DNA (possibly contaminants) were also found in the preparations. Staining procedures indicated the presence of nucleic acids within the core of the particles (Lyons and Moore, 1962). The purified B particles obtained by this method have been tested for their tumour-inducing activity, but the results of bioassays have not been published as yet.

Recent experiments have succeeded in the separation of MTV by electrophoresis (Moore and Lyons, 1963a, b). Previous reports had shown that the fractions of tumour homogenates and milk, showing mammary tumour-inducing activity migrated ahead of any visible fraction (Moore, 1952; Moore, Pollard and Haagensen, 1962). Preparation of type B particles has been attempted by the pH gradient electrophoresis. Analysis of the separated B particles in the electron microscope has shown considerable deformation of the particles with the appearance of many tailed forms, which are probably due to the hypertonic salt solutions employed. Nevertheless, the authors state that pH gradient electrophoresis provides a simple means of separating B particles and gives a product that seems morphologically superior to that obtained by the RbCl density gradient method, where osmotic shock also causes considerable damages (Moore and Lyons, 1963a).

To conclude this short outline of the characters of MTV, few other data concerning its physical properties, which are known from earlier reports, will be added.

[1] "Freon 113" or "Genetron 226" ($CF_2Cl-CCl_2F$).

The tumour inducing activity of MTV-containing preparations tolerates variations in pH from 5.5 to 10.2, but activity is lost at pH 4.5 (BITTNER, 1945a). The activity is equally lost after heating at 60—66° C for 1 h (ANDERVONT and BRYAN, 1944; BARNUM et al., 1944), whereas it is preserved for long time by freezing and drying (BITTNER, 1941a, 1942a, 1945a; DMOCHOWSKI, 1946).

F. Some biological properties of MTV

a) Production of MTV in vivo and in vitro

That the MTV actively "multiplies" *in vivo* was hypothesized since 1942 on the basis of its indefinite vertical trasmission and of the increase of its concentration in old female mice (BITTNER, 1942). Data supporting multiplication of the MTV in transplanted mammary tumours were provided later (BITTNER, 1948b). In addition, the occurrence of a rapid production of MTV in lactating mammary glands was suggested by the fact that the tumour-inducing power was found to be the same in milk and lactating breast tissue, being the daily secretion of milk equal to about three times the weight of the producing tissue (HUSEBY, BARNUM and BITTNER, 1950). At that time, however, it was not clear whether "multiplication" of the agent resulted from autoduplication or from neoproduction and release by normal and tumour cells (DMOCHOWSKI, 1953b). Various attempts to cultivate MTV *in vitro* were unable to clarify this point, since it has been reported that MTV can (BITTNER, 1945a; BITTNER, EVANS and GREEN, 1945; PIKOVSKI, 1953), or cannot be cultured in non-murine cells (LASFARGUES, MOORE and MURRAY, 1958; LASFARGUES et al., 1959; LASFARGUES, MURRAY and MOORE, 1960).

Most of the information we now possess on the production of MTV *in vivo* and *in vitro* comes from very recent work by LASFARGUES and FELDMAN (1963). Mammary glands from high- (RIII) and low- (C57b) cancer-strain female mice removed during early pregnancy, late pregnancy, lactation and resting phase, explanted in a modified organ culture method (LASFARGUES and MURRAY, 1959; LASFARGUES, 1963), and maintained in their physiological state (growth, secretion) by the addition to the culture medium of various hormonal combinations, were then examined in the electron microscope for the presence and gross quantification of type B virus particles. The results have shown that the production of B particles in organ cultures of RIII mammary glands is influenced by hormonal stimulation, depending on the physiological status of the explants and on the type of hormones used. Two peaks of higher production of B particles have been observed through the pregnancy-lactation cycle of the glands. The first, in early pregnancy, is induced by a combination of estradiol + progesterone + mammotropin[1] and corresponds to the active stage of epithelial growth and alveolar differentiation. The second, in lactation, is induced by mammotropin + cortisol[1] and corresponds to the period of secretory activity. In both cases formation of the B particles occurs during a phase of high protein synthesis. During late pregnancy, which is an intermediary stage between the end of structural development and the beginning of functional activity, production of B particles could not be detected in organ cultures, neither after addition of ovarian hormones + mammotropin, nor after stimulation by cortisol + mammotropin. In resting breasts, taken one month after weaning, no type B particles were found, unless the organ cultures

[1] The hormones were dissolved in Morgan's synthetic medium 199 routinely enriched with insulin (20 μg/ml). Estradiol 17-β and progesterone in crystalline form were first dissolved in absolute ethanol and then diluted in 199. Prolactin (mammotropin) of ovine origin, 15 i.u. per mg, and cortisol (hydrocortison sodium succinate) were directly added to the medium. The final concentration of each hormone in the medium, expressed in μg/ml, was as follows: Estradiol $= 5 \times 10^{-4}$; Progesterone $= 0.5$; Mammotropin $= 20$; Cortisol $= 20$.

were stimulated by the combination of ovarian hormones + mammotropin which restore the alveolar structure and promote epithelial multiplication. Electron micrographs of the cultured materials showed the B particles to be produced by the epithelial cells and liberated into the lumina where they matured (LASFARGUES and FELDMAN, 1963).

From all these experiments on RIII (high-cancer strain) mammary glands it was also apparent that the absence of hormonal stimulation (control cultures) or the use of an improper combination (for instance: hormones which induce secretion in early pregnancy type explants, or conversely growth-stimulating hormones in lactation type explants) resulted in the inhibition of B particles production. In addition, cultures of MTV-free C57b mammary glands, which show the same morphological reactions of RIII glands under the same hormonal conditions, do not produce however type B particles. This was assumed as further evidence in support of the identity between type B particles and the MTV (LASFARGUES and FELDMAN, 1963).

Various reports from the older literature agree with the findings summarized above. Extracts of mammary tissue from high-cancer-strain mice were found to exert their highest tumour-inducing activity in lactation (HUSEBY, BARNUM and BITTNER, 1950). Cortisol treatment has been reported to increase production of virus particles in mouse mammary tumours (SMOLLER, PITELKA and BERN, 1961). The mammary tumour-inducing activity was observed to disappear from the blood of MTV-carrying mice during late pregnancy and to reappear in lactation (HUMMEL and LITTLE, 1949). These data provide additional support for the existence of a peak of maximum production of the MTV during lactation and, therefore, to the correspondence between B particles released during lactation and MTV.

In summary, production and release of virus particles by the mammary epithelium is a discontinuous process ruled by the physiological state of the cells and by hormonal stimulation. Whether the same pattern may apply to other body tissues is unknown at present, although there is evidence that production of MTV can take place in sites other than the mammary glands (for instance, the secreting epithelium of the male genital tract).

b) Failure to increase MTV concentration or activity by serial passages of tumour extracts

If mammary tumour incidence and tumour age are assumed as parameters of the effectiveness of MTV in bearing animals, the extracts derived from early tumours would be expected to show a higher tumour-inducing activity than those obtained from tumours which develop later in life. Nevertheless, when the tumour-inducing activity of extracts of several mammary tumours has been tested in assay animals, it was observed that the age at onset of tumours in donor females did not relate to the potency of MTV recovered from the tumours, although the range of tumour ages tested was as large as that elapsing between 3 and 23 months (BITTNER, 1960, 1962). In addition, as known from previous reports, the cancer incidence and age in the test animals were not correlated with the dilution of the administered extracts.

These facts raised the question whether or not the concentration or activity of MTV may be influenced by serial passages into suitable hosts. GROSS (1957) demonstrated that if extracts from leukaemias were passed serially in successive generations of day-old mice, the activity of the filtrable agent inducing leukaemia was strongly increased, as shown by the progressively higher incidence and earlier occurrence of the disease in the assay mice. By this method, and after various passages, it was possible to induce leukaemia in 100% of the injected animals after a latency of less than three months (GROSS, 1962).

The same procedure was then applied to the MTV (BITTNER, 1962). Extracts of mammary tumours from virus-carrying mice were injected into MTV-free test animals and some of the resulting neoplasms were used as the donor tissue for the succeeding passage. In this way the MTV was transferred serially for even six consecutive passages. But there was no evidence in the results that the activity or potency of MTV had increased after administration of the tumour extracts in successive generations of test mice. In general, there was a tendency for the tumour-inducing activity of the MTV to decrease with continued passage of tumour extracts (BITTNER, 1962). In addition, the biological tests of tumours observed in successive litters from the same mother showed that the litter when the mice were born had no influence on the results of bioassays (BITTNER, 1962). Here is another example of the peculiar biology of MTV. Accordingly, other data concerning the bioassay of extracts of mammary tumours cultured in eggs have shown that the tumour-inducing activity is maintained but not increased after repeated transfer passages of the tumours in eggs (ARMSTRONG and HAM, 1950). The successful transplantation of mammary tumour cells in eggs had been reported previously by a number of investigators (TAYLOR, THACKER and PENNINGTON, 1942; TAYLOR, HUNGATE and TAYLOR, 1943; BRYAN, KAHLER and RILEY, 1945; HEILMAN, 1945; TAYLOR, CARMICHAEL and NORRIS, 1948).

c) Lack of immunologic response to MTV in mice

Antibodies against MTV have never been demonstrated in mice, regardless of strain and age at infection (BITTNER, 1962). This statement summarizes a number of negative reports (GORER and LAW, 1949; DMOCHOWSKI and PASSEY, 1952), and its importance is obvious in respect to the nature of MTV particles and their relationships with the infected cells. By contrast, other laboratory animals, including rats, rabbits and guinea pigs, react to the introduction of MTV-containing materials with production of antibodies. Antisera obtained by these animals against MTV were found to neutralize or inhibit the tumour-inducing activity of mammary tumour extracts (ANDERVONT and BRYAN, 1944; GREEN, MOOSEY and BITTNER, 1945, 1946; GREEN and BITTNER, 1946; GREEN, 1946). Antisera prepared using normal tissues of MTV-carrying mice were, however, much less effective in this respect. The addition of antisera against MTV to *in vitro* cultures of mammary tumour cells was observed to cause regressive changes and arrest of growth (IMAGAWA, BITTNER and SYVERTON, 1950; IMAGAWA, SYVERTON and BITTNER, 1951, 1954). A precipitin test for antigens present in mouse tissues containing MTV was also developed (IMAGAWA, GREEN and HALVORSON, 1948). Since these antisera have been prepared with materials containing MTV, and not with the pure virus, their specificity still needs to be proved (DMOCHOWSKI and PASSEY, 1952; DMOCHOWSKI, 1953b).

d) MTV in low-mammary-cancer strains and the problem of its latent state

Spontaneous mammary tumours may develop in low-cancer-strain female mice, although with low frequency and very late in life. Animals of these strains are supposed to be free of the MTV. But when their mammary tumours have been observed in the electron microscope, typical A and B virus particles were occasionally detected (BANG, ANDERVONT and VELLISTO, 1956; BANG, VELLISTO and LIBERT, 1956; BERNHARD, GUÉRIN and OBERLING, 1956; DMOCHOWSKI, 1956,

1960; Dmochowski and Grey, 1957). Nevertheless, the bioassays of tumour extracts, tissue extracts and milk from low-tumour-strain mice have long failed to demonstrate the presence of mammary tumour-inducing activity in these materials (Heston, 1958; Pullinger, 1960; Pullinger and Iversen, 1960). These facts gave rise to considerable discussion, and different explanations were suggested: that the virus particles seen in the electron microscope were not the MTV, that they were immature forms of MTV with no biological activity, that they were the active MTV but the biological tests for detecting the virus (present in low concentration) were less sensitive than the morphological method (Bernhard and Granboulan, 1962).

Similar virus particles have recently been found also in the milk of some low-tumour-strain mice (C3Hf, Af: Dmochowski, 1960), but not of others (C57b: Moore and Lyons, 1962). It is perhaps important to note here that the C57b strain is low-tumour since its origin, whereas the C3Hf and Af strains were originally high-tumour strains (C3H, A) from which the milk agent has been removed by means of foster-nursing on low-cancer-strain mothers. Concentrated tumour extracts and high-speed centrifugal pellets from milk of low-tumour C3Hf and Af mice, which were found to contain type B virus particles in the electron microscope, have finally shown some tumour-inducing activity on bioassays (Dmochowski et al., 1963b). This is the first positive test obtained with materials from low-tumour-strain mice after many negative reports and it deserves, therefore, careful consideration. With this result an apparent correlation has been found, for the first time, between presence of characteristic virus particles and tumour-inducing activity on the milk and mammary-tumour extracts of mice from at least some apparently MTV-free strains (Dmochowski, 1963b). Nevertheless, the problems posed by the presence of MTV particles in low-tumour-strain mice still have to be solved: What is the origin of the virus in these mice, and why does it not concentrate after indefinite transmission through succeeding generations of susceptible animals?

Studies with high-cancer-strain mice have shown a lower tumour incidence in early litters then in later litters, supporting the view of an increase of MTV production during the life of the animals (Bittner, 1942b). When C57b low-cancer-strain females have been injected at 3 weeks with virus-containing tumour extracts and then mated, a concentration of mammary tumours in the later litters was observed, supporting the progressive increase of MTV in the recipient hosts (Mühlbock, 1952). In addition, after MTV infection of low-cancer-strain females (C3Hb) by mating them with high-cancer-strain males [BALB/cf (C3H)], the mammary tumour incidence in hybrid descendants was seen to increase progressively from F_1 to F_7, providing further evidence to the opinion of an increase in concentration or activity of MTV through the succeeding generations (Biancifiori, Lotti and Martinez, 1958). In the light of these observations, the strange behaviour of the MTV which appears to be present (though in low quantities) in some low-cancer-strain mice, but does not tend to increase after indefinite transmission through them, is difficult to understand. This leads again to the hypothesis of a latency of MTV in low-tumour-strain mice and demands further investigation.

e) Possible integration of MTV with the infected cells as an explanation for its disappearance and appearance de novo

The MTV may disappear from single mice of a high-cancer-strain and their inbred descendants (Murray and Warner, 1947; Andervont, 1959; Ander-

VONT and DUNN, 1962). Conversely, the MTV has been reported to appear suddenly in mice of a susceptible strain which was deprived of the virus long before by foster-nursing (BITTNER, 1941 b). Since contamination by the environment may practically be excluded in the case of MTV, the latter observation suggests either that the MTV has arisen *de novo* in mice, or that a weak MTV has become activated by as yet unknown factors (DMOCHOWSKI, 1953 b). Even the disappearance of MTV from some high-cancer-strain mice might be explained by opposition as due either to loss or to some change in the activity of the virus which causes it to become "weak".

However, when it became possible to do biological experiments associated with morphological observation in the electron microscope, other important findings have been made. After various transfer generations by subcutaneous transplant of a mammary tumour in low-cancer-strain mice, production of type B particles could not be detected in the electron microscope. But when the tumour was cultured *in vitro* the B particles reappeared (DE BRUYN and BENEDETTI, 1960). Accordingly, the MTV was found to disappear, after many intraperitoneal transfers, from C3H mammary tumour cells cultured *in vivo* as ascites cells into MTV-free C3Hf mice, as shown either by biological tests or by morphological observation in the electron microscope. But when the cells were placed *in vitro* the B particles reappeared (MIROFF and FELDMAN, 1963).

These and several other reports from the previous literature have recently been reviewed by MOORE (1963) in the support of the opinion that the MTV can become integrated with the infected cell and thus disappear from cells which previously showed it, or appear, apparently *de novo*, in cells which did not contain it before. This concept has been accepted for other tumour viruses. Integration of the MTV with cells might explain, among other things, the conflicting results concerning low-tumour-strain mice and the discordant views about the origin of mammary tumours in these animals.

As far as MTV is concerned, it would seem that the production of B particles is partly a function of environment and that the cells can carry under certain conditions the potential to produce the virus without showing detectable production of it (MOORE, 1963). Other facts which, according to the same author, support the hypothesis of a close integration of MTV with the cells are also its production in large quantities by morphologically healthy-looking cells capable of mitosis, and its antigenic similarity to the host cells which prevents them from detectable formation of antibodies. In other words, the MTV seems to be a product of the cell rather than an infectious agent competing with the cell (MOORE, 1963).

f) Effects of MTV on the infected cells

It is impossible to say how many effects the MTV induces in the infected cells. However, there is evidence at present for at least two effects of the virus on the cell: one which causes the cell to produce the virus, another which causes them to become malignant (MOORE, 1962). Whether these effects will be two steps of the same process, or whether they will be independent of each other is unknown at present. Biological and morphological data (MÜHLBOCK, 1950a; MOORE et al., 1963; MOORE, 1963) suggest that in high-cancer-strain male mice production of MTV can take place without any detectable evidence of malignancy during the entire lifespan. On the other hand, in high-cancer-strain females, production of MTV is almost invariably followed by the malignant transformation resulting sooner or later in the development of mammary tumours. There is no doubt, however, that the ability to proliferate the virus precedes, often by months, the appearance of any morphologically detectable change in the mammary epithelium. The compatibility between presence or production of MTV and good healthy conditions of the infected or producing cells has already been mentioned. In addition, it is well known that production of MTV by normal-looking lactating cells can take place even during the first pregnancy, *i.e.* long before the appearance of any of the changes leading to tumour formation. This does not exclude, of course, that the cells liberating the virus may have already been transformed, the development of a tumour being delayed by other factors (MOORE, 1963).

Another interesting fact is that when malignant transformation occurs, abruptly or by steps we do not know, it does not inhibit production and release of virus particles by the cells. Hyperplastic alveolar nodules, which are recognized precursors of mouse mammary carcinoma, when observed in the electron microscope have been found to contain type B particles (DEOME et al., 1959b; PITELKA, DEOME and BERN, 1960). As shown by many biological and morphological data, even the mammary tumour cells produce MTV, although they may lose this property with time or in particular situations (see above). In this respect, the behaviour of MTV seems to be very different from that of other tumour-inducing viruses, for instance the polyoma virus, which disappears after cell transformation (VOGT and DULBECCO, 1962).

g) Possible effects of the MTV on the host metabolism

It has recently been reported that the rate of nail growth in MTV-carrying mice is significantly increased as compared to that found in MTV-free animals of identical genetical background (HAMILTON, HOLLANDER and ANDERVONT, 1958). The investigation was carried out under identical environmental conditions and on inbred animals of two strains, either with or without the MTV [C3H, C3Hf; BALB/cf (C3H), BALB/c], similar in sex, size, age and body weight. A very precise technique was used to ascertain the rate of nail growth and the conclusion was that infection of mice with MTV is associated with sustained increase in elongation rates of nails (HAMILTON, HOLLANDER and ANDERVONT, 1958).

It is known that the structures that proliferate throughout the lifespan can be used to evaluate the rate of formation of body protoplasm. Nails were selected for quantitative studies of regenerative rates, that might serve as an index of the growth and replacement of tissues, because of methodological advantages and of their proved sensitivity to various physiological, pathological and pharmacological situations, such as ageing, starvation, administration of antimitotic drugs, Mongolism, and genetic differences (see HAMILTON, HOLLANDER and ANDERVONT, 1958). The importance of the peculiar result observed in mice carrying MTV is apparent. Here is a suggestion that the MTV may affect the general metabolism of the host animals increasing the rate of formation of body protoplasm.

h) Mutant forms of MTV

BLAIR (1958, 1960) has reported the occurrence in A strain female mice of a mutant of MTV showing distinct biological properties. In breeding females of this inbred strain followed for over 85 generations the average age at onset of mammary tumours has consistently been about 12 months. At a certain time it was noted that, in one branch of the strain, breeding females were developing mammary tumours at about 8 months of age. The latter group was separated out and maintained as a subline. Reciprocal crosses and foster-nursing experiments between the two lines of animals ensured that the difference in mean age of tumour development was not the result of a change in the genotype of the host, being evidently mediated by factors carried in the milk. The two types of MTV were found to retain their difference in activity through successive generations of identical animals

(Blair, 1958, 1960). These facts seem to suggest that the MTV, though maintained in the same environment, may undergo mutations which become detectable by the acquisition of new biological properties. Of somewhat different significance are the data reported below concerning the observation of strain differences in the behaviour of MTV.

i) Strain differences in the behaviour of MTV

The possibility that the MTV carried by different strains may not be identical was first suggested by the considerable differences in mammary tumour incidence and average tumour age found among various high-cancer strains. Reciprocal crosses between two of these strains showed that such differences in tumour parameters were transmitted through the mother's milk and not carried by the genotype (Bittner, 1948a). But there was no mention in the literature that strain variations occurred in the biological and morphological behaviour of neoplasms until some recent investigations showed that the histological origin, rate and type of growth, hormone dependence, and morphological picture are also variable characters, in some way related to the mouse strain (Squartini and Rossi, 1959a, b, 1960; Squartini, 1961, 1962a, b; Squartini et al., 1964). These investigations were on three high-cancer strains: C3H, BALB/c foster nursed by C3H [BALB/cf (C3H)], and RIII.

Analysis of mammary tumours occurring in these strains led to the detection of the existence of strain differences in the characters of neoplasms. Under the same conditions, C3H and BALB/cf (C3H) mice show a nearly parallel behaviour, whereas in the RIII mice the behaviour of tumours is peculiar enough to make this strain not comparable with the others. In the two former strains most of the tumours have a short clinical duration, possess a high growth rate, rarely undergo partial regressions, show regular types of growth (mainly a sigmoidal curve), are unresponsive to pregnancies, originate in hyperplastic alveolar nodules, and present pure morphological pictures. By contrast, in the RIII strain most of the tumours have a long clinical duration, possess a slow growth rate, frequently undergo partial regressions, show irregular and unpredictable types of growth, are responsive to pregnancies, originate in plaques, and present varied pictures. These differences were found to be statistically significant (Squartini and Severi, 1962).

The results observed raised the question of what causes the difference found in tumour behaviour in different strains, and various investigations were carried out in order to show whether there were genetic, hormonal, viral, or other causes. Attempts to modify the behaviour of mammary tumours in the RIII strain by increased hormonal stimulation gave negative results. Neither the type nor the frequency of endogenous hormonal stimuli showed any definite influence on the behaviour of mammary tumours in mice of this strain (Squartini et al., 1960; Squartini and Rossi, 1961a, b). Attempts to transfer the behaviour of mammary tumours from mice of one strain to another by foster-nursing were successful. Two new lines of inbred mice were established by reciprocal foster-nursing: RIII foster-nursed by BALB/cf (C3H) (or RIIIf) and BALB/c foster nursed by RIII [or BALB/cf (RIII)]. The behaviour of mammary tumours which developed in RIII mice foster-nursed by BALB/cf (C3H) closely resembled that of BALB/cf (C3H) tumours. Conversely, the behaviour of mammary tumours which developed in BALB/c mice foster-nursed by RIII was quite similar to that of RIII mammary tumours (Squartini, 1962b; Squartini and Severi, 1962; Squartini and Rossi, 1962; Squartini, Rossi and Paoletti, 1962a, b, 1963). The characters of tumours acquired by foster-nursing have been maintained by mice of the fostered lines, raised as inbred substrains, in the course of the first 10 generations.

These results have led to assume that MTV particles may be the carriers of certain specific tumour properties in each strain (SQUARTINI and SEVERI, 1962). This is specially emphasized by the fact that a striking difference has been observed in behaviour between mammary tumours which develop in the same strain (BALB/c) following foster-nursing by mothers from different strains, such as C3H and RIII (SQUARTINI, ROSSI and PAOLETTI, 1963).

Data obtained by other investigators support these findings and views. Mammary tumours showing the same behaviour as that of RIII tumours have been observed by Foulds in (RIII × C57b)F_1 and reciprocal hybrids, which bear the same MTV as their RIII strain parent (FOULDS, 1949a, b, 1956b). ANDERVONT (1959) noticed that the MTV may be lost in mice of some sublines of the RIII strain, and irregularities in the propagation of MTV through the same strain have also been reported (SQUARTINI and RIBACCHI, 1960). In addition, the existence of some differences in potency or behaviour between the RIII MTV and that carried by mice of other strains has recently been confirmed from various sources, on the basis of foster-nursing experiments (HUMMEL and LITTLE, 1959; ANDERVONT and DUNN, 1962) and of comparative studies of the mammary gland structure and tumorigenesis (RICHARDSON and HUMMEL, 1959; RICHARDSON and HALL, 1960). Whether the difference in behaviour between the MTV of RIII strain and that of other mouse strains is due to differences in the concentration or in the structure and activity of the virus is unknown at present, although the former hypothesis seems to be more realistic.

In this respect, an unexpected result observed during the experiments of crossed foster-nursing summarized above deserves particular attention. When BALB/c mice were foster-nursed on RIII mothers an unexpectedly high incidence of lymphatic leukaemia, increasing with the generations, was observed. Data are shown in Table 2. Thus, the BALB/cf (RIII) substrain, which has reached the 10th inbred generation, is a high-mammary-tumour strain (82.1% in females) with a medium incidence of lymphatic leukaemia (40.3% in males) (SQUARTINI and ROSSI, 1964a). Since both the strains which contributed to the establishment of this new inbred line, BALB/c and RIII, are low-leukaemic strains, the suggestion was made that a latent leukaemia virus carried by mice of the RIII strain and transmitted *via* the milk together with MTV had become active after transfer into BALB/c mice. This is at present only a working hypothesis. However, if it is true, the low malignancy of mammary tumours occurring in RIII mice and in BALB/c mice foster-nursed by RIII might also conceivably be interpreted as the result of an interaction between two different viruses growing in the same host: the MTV and a leukaemia virus (SQUARTINI and ROSSI, 1964a). Although any further discussion of these facts would not be justified at this time, the existence of at least some linkage between the reported observation and the question of the inhibitor of MTV in RIII milk (MOORE, 1962) is apparent and it should be kept in mind.

G. Vertical transmission of MTV

Embryos obtained by mating high-cancer-strain mice do not harbour MTV (DMOCHOWSKI, 1949; HUMMEL and LITTLE, 1949). The contagion occurs only after birth and is generally direct, from the carrier animal to the non carrier one without mediation of the environmental medium. Epidemiological studies have shown that the MTV does not propagate from carrier to non carrier mice following cohabitation within the same cage (ANDERVONT, SHIMKIN and BRYAN,

1942). Urines and faeces from infected animals do not contain MTV (Dmochowski and Passey, 1951; Mühlbock, 1950b). Apart from milk, the only other secretion material which has been found rich in infective MTV is the sperm of carrying males (Andervont and Dunn, 1948a, b; Mühlbock, 1950a). Therefore, in spite of its wide distribution within the body of adult mice, the virus leaves the host only through two routes: the mammary gland in females and the spermatic tract in males. This means that MTV transmission occurs only periodically during the host life, being closely related to the reproductive activity of the animals, and is controlled by various hormones. Due to the peculiar routes of contagion the epidemic spreads vertically, from parents to offspring, and both mother and father may infect the litters.

Table 2. *Frequency of mammary tumours and lymphatic leukaemia in BALB/c mice foster-nursed by RIII, in the strain of origin (BALB/c) and in the strain of the milk donor (RIII)*

	Strain and sex	No.	Mammary tumours			Lymphatic leukaemia			Without tumours	
			No.	%	Age (onset)	No.	%	Age (death)	No.	Age (death)
Original	BALB/c strain									
	— males	30	—	—	—	1	3.3	633	29	639
	— females[1]	33	10	30.3	582	1	3.0	484	22	648
Milk donor	RIII strain									
	— males	58	—	—	—	4	6.9	597	54	547
	— females	37	31	83.7	292	—	—	—	6	532
Derived	BALB/cf (RIII)									
	— males	77	—	—	—	31	40.3	303	46	496
	— females	106	87	82.1	291	13[2]	12.3	344	8	408

[1] Normally bred females.
[2] In two females leukaemia coexisted with mammary tumours.
After Squartini and Rossi (1964a).

a) Transmission by the female parent

MTV is present in the mother's milk throughout the entire suckling period (Andervont and McEleney, 1939; Bittner, 1939a). Although a single nursing may be enough to induce some mammary tumours in the offspring (Andervont and McEleney, 1941; Shimkin and Andervont, 1942), a rather close relationship has been found between quantity of ingested milk and mammary tumour incidence and age (Andervont and McEleney, 1939; Bittner, 1940; Andervont, Shimkin and Bryan, 1942). The concentration of MTV in the mother's milk seems to increase with age (Bittner, 1942b). Milk removed from the stomach of suckling newborns still shows a high tumour-inducing activity (Dmochowski, 1949; Hummel and Little, 1949).

The ability to transmit MTV may be very different in female mice of different strains. When MTV is introduced into a resistant strain, the virus may not be transmitted from mothers to offspring (Andervont, 1945), or it may be transmitted but for a single generation, or for several generations (Dmochowski, 1948). Even if these females carry and transmit MTV, they may often fail to develop mammary tumours (Bittner, 1942c). By contrast, when MTV is introduced into susceptible low-tumour strains, the females show a high incidence of mammary tumours and a high ability to transmit the virus through an indefinite number of successive generations (Andervont, 1940, 1949; Miller and Pybus, 1945). Therefore, either the susceptibility to develop mammary tumours after MTV infection, or the ability to transmit MTV are controlled by chromosomal factors. Some experiments suggested that the sets of genes controlling susceptibility to the virus and transmission of the virus might be different (Heston, Deringer and Andervont, 1945; Heston, 1946); but other experiments showed that this was questionable (Bittner, 1946). Generally, in females the ability to transmit MTV runs parallel with their susceptibility to the virus (Dmochowski, 1953b).

b) Transmission by the male parent

Several investigations have shown that mating high-cancer-strain males to low-cancer-strain females the MTV present in the sperm of the father can occasionally be transmitted to the offspring (Foulds, 1949a; Bittner, 1950, 1952a; Mühlbock, 1952; Dmochowski, 1953a; Severi et al., 1958). The tumours occurring in hybrid progeny infected by the male parent have a variable frequency, according to the strains used, and an erratic distribution, being usually accumulated only in the later litters of some of the females mated (Mühlbock, 1952). Biological tests show the presence of mammary tumour-inducing activity in these tumours.

Transmission of MTV from males to offspring occurs after birth and is usually indirect. In this case the females are infected at coitus and re-transmit the paternal MTV to newborns *via* the milk (Severi et al., 1958). When the litters are born in presence of the father, there is, however, a little possibility for direct infection through contamination of the environment (Peacock, 1953). Data recently published by Andervont (1963) indicate that direct transmission *in utero* of the paternal MTV could take place in particular cases. But it is too early to discuss this isolate report, which contrasts with many previous results.

Various data suggest that the transmission of MTV from the male parent is closely ruled by genetic factors. The receptivity to infection from male is greatly different in females of different low-cancer strains (Foulds, 1949a; Bittner, 1952a). Conversely, males of different high-cancer strains show significant differences in the ability to transmit their MTV and to infect the females and/or the offspring (Foulds, 1949a; Bittner, 1952a; Bittner and Frantz, 1954). However, it must be reported here that in males the ability to transmit the MTV does not correlate with their susceptibility to the virus. Male mice of different susceptible high-cancer strains, all of which show a high mammary tumour incidence when treated with estrogens, behave differently in regard to virus transmission to descendants (Squartini, 1958, 1960).

Recent investigations have shown that the transmission of MTV from males to offspring is significantly influenced by at least three factors, namely: the presence of males in the cages when the litters are born ($P < 0.05$), the type of females used for hybridization ($P < 0.01$), and the type of males used for hybridization ($P < 0.001$) (Squartini and Severi, 1963). However, the different ability shown by males of different high-cancer strains to transmit their MTV to the offspring is not due to strain differences in the amount of MTV present in the sperm (Bianciflori and Squartini, 1958).

H. Distribution in the host

The fate of MTV in the first periods after introduction into susceptible hosts is not entirely known. An investigation along this line showed that the virus inoculated intraperitoneally in susceptible adult female mice reaches high concentrations in the circulating blood serum within a few hours, and that in this stage it can be eliminated in small amounts with urine (SQUARTINI, 1958; SQUARTINI and BIANCIFIORI, 1958). The whole blood of adult high-cancer-strain mice still contains MTV (WOOLLEY, LAW and LITTLE, 1941), though in minimal quantities according to some investigators (GRAFF et al., 1946). However, variations in the blood rate of MTV in relation to age, reproductive activity of the host and development of mammary tumours have been observed (BITTNER, 1945b; HUMMEL and LITTLE, 1949).

After infection the MTV spreads to many organs and tissues both in males and females. Using biological tests it has been demonstrated in the brain (BITTNER, 1939b), thymus (BITTNER, 1939b, 1940), spleen (BITTNER, 1937; ANDERVONT, SHIMKIN and BRYAN, 1942; PREHN, 1952), heart, lungs, kidneys (DMOCHOWSKI, 1949), mammary glands and tumours (BITTNER, 1939b, 1940, 1941a; ANDERVONT, SHIMKIN and BRYAN, 1942; HUSEBY, BARNUM and BITTNER, 1950), male genital tract (ANDERVONT and DUNN, 1948a; MÜHLBOCK, 1950a), etc. It is still unknown whether in some of these organs the virus is present by virtue of their blood content or whether it is specifically propagated into them (DMOCHOWSKI, 1953b). The presence of MTV in the liver is doubtful (BITTNER, 1941c, 1947). The placenta contains either no MTV (HUMMEL and LITTLE, 1949) or only small amounts of MTV (DMOCHOWSKI, 1949). In addition, the placental tissue was found to neutralize *in vitro* the tumour-inducing activity of mammary tumour extracts (HUMMEL, LITTLE and HEDDY, 1949). This may perhaps explain the lack of transplacental transmission of MTV from mothers to their embryos *in utero*.

I. Summary of present knowledge and opinions

Present opinions concerning the MTV may roughly be divided into two sets. According to some investigators the MTV must be regarded as an essential factor in carcinogenesis of the mouse breast (MOORE, 1963). By contrast, other investigators recognize the importance of this agent but still consider it as a non essential factor in mammary carcinogenesis, where only the hormonal factors would have a primary rôle (MÜHLBOCK, 1955a, 1956; MÜHLBOCK and BOOT, 1959, 1960). These two different opinions will be shortly summarized here.

a) The five statements of MOORE

Recently MOORE (1963) has presented five basic statements, with the supporting reasons for making them, which summarize previous data and opinions concerning the MTV. These statements are reported below [statements 4—5 are discussed under (b)].

Statement 1. BERNHARD's type B particle, which has the physical and chemical properties of a virus, represents one form of the MTV. A smaller particle, possibly fragments of the virus, can also carry MTV activity.

Statement 2. There are associated with the MTV interfering substances, suppressors or inhibitors.

Statement 3. The MTV can become integrated with the infected cell and thus appear: (a) to be heritable; (b) to arise *de novo*.

Statement 4. Hormones can influence the mammary tumour incidence in families that harbour the MTV but not in established virus-free families.

Statement 5. The occurrence of spontaneous mammary adenocarcinomas is usually (chemicals and other viruses, for example, polyoma, seem to be exceptions) dependent on the presence of MTV, whether acquired through the milk, through the ovum or through the seminal fluid. As in other diseases, genetics can influence the susceptibility of the animal to the virus. Susceptibility to the virus, not tumour, is inherited. Genetic factors, whether acting on the virus directly or through control of hormones and also possibly inhibitors, account for the observed resistance of some mice (MOORE, 1963).

b) The criticism of MÜHLBOCK

MÜHLBOCK (1956, 1957, 1958b; MÜHLBOCK and BOOT, 1959, 1960) has repeatedly emphasized the fact that mammary tumours can develop in mice even in the absence of MTV. Female mice of the so-called low-mammary-tumour strains, which are supposed to be MTV-free, may develop spontaneous mammary tumours. The mammary tumour incidence is very low in virgin females of these strains (0–9%), but it may be increased by normal or forced breeding up to 38–56%. In either case, however, the average tumour age is high, ranging between 19 and 22 months (see MÜHLBOCK, 1956). Comparison of these data with those observed in high-cancer strains, where the mammary tumour incidence approaches 100% and the average tumour age is usually below 10 months, indeed justifies the opinion that MTV acts as an accelerator and intensifier of spontaneous mammary tumorigenesis, being a non essential factor (MÜHLBOCK, 1956).

Biological evidence for the absence of MTV in low-tumour-strain mice, on which the previous conclusion is mainly based, is convincing. Various strains were obtained by foster-nursing litters of MTV-carrying mothers on MTV-free females, a method which had been shown to be successful since 1936 (BITTNER, 1936). To prevent any possibility of infection either before or after birth, that method was improved: the young mice were removed from the uterus by caesarean section, or even fertilized ova from a high-cancer-strain mother were transferred to a low-cancer-strain mother (FEKETE and LITTLE, 1942). Nevertheless, a certain percentage of mammary tumours was still found. The possibility that MTV might have arisen *de novo* in some low-tumour strains was also kept in mind and tested. But a number of bioassays performed with tumour extracts, tissue extracts and milk failed to demonstrate the virus in low-tumour-strain mice (MÜHLBOCK, 1956).

In spite of these convincing data, we presently know that MTV particles have been found in mammary tumours and milk of some low-cancer-strain mice, and that some tumour extracts and milk preparations from low-cancer-strain mice have also shown tumour-inducing activity (DMOCHOWSKI et al., 1963a, b). In the light of these new facts, the whole problem of mammary tumours in low-cancer strains will perhaps be reviewed. However, some recent examples of mouse mammary carcinogenesis in the absence of MTV appear to be unquestionable. In some sublines of the C57b strain the MTV has never been detected either in tissues or milk (MOORE and LYONS, 1962). Accordingly, the females of these sublines do not develop mammary tumours (MOORE and LYONS, 1963b; HESTON, 1964), even when their mammary tissue is strongly stimulated with appropriate hormones by means of forced breeding (LITTLE and PEARSON, 1940), a procedure which is known to increase the mammary-tumour incidence in mice. Males of the same strain also fail to develop mammary tumours after suitable hormonal stimulation (see SHIMKIN, 1945). Nevertheless, when virus-free C57b mice have been submitted to repeated subcutaneous implants of hypophyses a few mammary tumours were obtained (MÜHLBOCK and BOOT, 1959). Although negative results with the same procedure on the same strain of animals have also been reported (JESSE and HAAGENSEN, 1963), the induction of mammary tumours in highly resistant and MTV-free C57b virgin female mice by subcutaneous isografts of hypophyses has recently been confirmed by HESTON (1964). These results strongly re-emphasize the primary importance of hormonal stimulation in mammary carcinogenesis.

2. Hormonal factors

A. Endogenous and exogenous hormones

Hormonal stimulation of the breast is essential for the development of mammary tumours in the mouse. Administered estrogens, as well as the endogenous hormones involved in the development of normal breast structures, are both able to cause tumours in the mammary glands. Susceptible male mice of high-cancer strains, which do not develop spontaneous tumours despite the presence of MTV, develop mammary cancer when an adequate estrogenic stimulation is supplied[1] (see SHIMKIN, 1945). Virgin females usually show a lower tumour incidence than pseudopregnant and breeding females (LATHROP and LOEB, 1913; MÜHLBOCK, 1950c, 1956). Forced breeding (removing the newborn soon after delivery and breeding as rapidly as possible) furthermore increases the mammary tumour rate (BAGG, 1936a, b; MÜHLBOCK, 1950c). On the other hand, lactation has an antitumorigenic action on the mouse breast (FEKETE, 1940; MÜHLBOCK, 1956), as it has been shown for women (SEVERI and SQUARTINI, 1958, 1962). A great deal of information has been accumulated during the last half century on the hormonal factors (the first to be detected) involved in mouse mammary carcinogenesis (see SHIMKIN, 1945; GARDNER, 1953; GARDNER et al., 1953; MÜHLBOCK, 1956; SQUARTINI, 1958). Only recent or essential data will be reported here.

B. Strain differences in the production and excretion of hormones

Much work has been done on the mouse to find out whether there are differences in the production or in the excretion of hormones between strains susceptible and resistant[2] to mammary cancer. Results have been negative as regards to excretion (AUB, KARNOFSKI and TOWNE, 1941), whereas differences in the hormone production have been shown by morphological studies of the endocrine glands.

The ovaries of adult susceptible females show, at each estrum, a higher number of follicles under maturation and of corpora lutea as compared with those of females resistant to mammary cancer (TAYLOR and WALTMAN, 1940; FEKETE, 1946). In the latter, a lower fertility is observed (BARBIERI and OLIVI, 1958). Also the adrenals and hypophysis behave differently in the two series of animals, as demonstrated by castration or by administration of estrogen (SQUARTINI, BOLLI and ROSSI, 1958). In spite of these facts the behaviour of estrous cycles, observed on vaginal smears, is not significantly different in susceptible and resistant strains (BRUNSCHWIG and BISSEL, 1936; TAYLOR and WALTMAN, 1940; DERINGER, HESTON and ANDERVONT, 1945). This may be due to the fact that the susceptibility to hormones of the female genital tract is different in these animals (GARDNER and ALLEN, 1939; VAN GULIK and KORTEWEG, 1940a; SHIMKIN and ANDERVONT, 1941; MÜHLBOCK, 1947; TRENTIN, 1950). Strain differences in hormone production and

[1] The effect depends on the type of estrogen, dose, solvent, frequency and duration of treatment. Estradiol benzoate, estradiol dipropionate and diethylstilbestrol are the synthetic compounds more commonly used. Usually the hormones are dissolved in oil and administered by subcutaneous injections at weekly or fortnightly intervals for several weeks (variable). The weekly dose of injected estrogen varies between 10 and 50 γ. Lower doses are ineffective. Higher doses have a stunting effect on mammary glands and tumours.

[2] Low-mammary-tumour strain is not synonymous to resistant strain. Many low-mammary-tumour strains are susceptible to the development of mammary tumours. Some are resistant.

tissue sensitivity to hormones are controlled by genes (Trentin, 1950). The inherited susceptibility to mammary cancer behaves as a dominant character. Another type of "inherited hormonal influence" controls the mammary tumour incidence in virgin females of high-breast-cancer strains (Bittner, 1939c; Bittner et al., 1944, 1951, 1952b; Heston and Andervont, 1944; Huseby and Bittner, 1948).

C. Endocrine glands involved in mammary carcinogenesis

The secretion of the ovary, suprarenal an d hypophysis are the most important in breast carcinogenesis. Early castration can prevent the appearance of tumours in the mouse (Loeb, 1919; Cori, 1926, 1927; Murray, 1927, 1928). Nevertheless, in spayed animals the adrenals sometimes assume a vicarious function and secrete sexual hormones capable of causing the development of mammary tumours (Woolley, Fekete and Little, 1939, 1940, 1941a, b; Smith, 1945, 1946, 1948; Smith and Bittner, 1945). In hypophysectomized animals, female sex hormones either produced or administered are inactive on the mammary glands; hyperplastic alveolar nodules and tumours do not develop in such experimental conditions (Gardner, 1940). This fact, and the successful induction of mammary tumours in susceptible or even in resistant strains by subcutaneous isografts of pituitary glands (Loeb and Kirtz, 1939; Mühlbock and Boot, 1959; Boot et al., 1962; Heston, 1964), indicate that the hypophysis is a key organ in all the processes of mammary carcinogenesis.

D. Hormones involved in mammary carcinogenesis

It is assumed that the hormones necessary for the development of mammary cancer are the same which control the physiological growth of the breast, that is estrogen, progesterone, prolactin (mammotropin) and/or somatotropin. Of these, progesterone and the pituitary hormones deserve special mention. Experimental data suggest the existence of a close relationship between the number, size and duration of corpora lutea and tumour incidence in animals (Fekete, 1946; Huseby and Bittner, 1948). In the mouse, where during the estrous cycle an efficient luteal phase is lacking (Pullinger, 1947; Mühlbock, 1956), mammary tumours hardly develop in MTV-free virgins; even if the virus is present the tumour incidence in virgins is usually lower than in the breeders, especially in certain strains, *e.g.* strain A (Bittner, 1939c). An exception to this rule is represented by C3H virgin females (Bittner et al., 1944).

The difference in tumour incidence in virgins and breeders may mean that the placental hormones are involved in mammary carcinogenesis. It is interesting to note, however, that pseudopregnancy has the same effect as pregnancy in the causation of tumours (Law, 1941; Mühlbock, 1956). The only difference between normal estrus and pseudopregnancy is the development in the latter of larger corpora lutea which function well and which stimulate the mammary glands to a hyperplasia comparable with that attained at the middle of pregnancy. Thus, it may be concluded that luteostimulation of the mammary glands is essential for the development of mammary tumours in mice with and without MTV (Mühlbock, 1956, 1958).

Despite its apparently great importance in spontaneous mammary carcinogenesis, injected progesterone does not induce tumours (Gardner, 1939) and does not increase the tumorigenic activity of estrogens (Lacassagne, 1937; Burrows and Hoch-Ligeti, 1946), but may diminish it (Heiman, 1945). However, when administered in strain A virgin females and related hybrids, progesterone accelerates and increases the appearance of mammary tumours (TRENTIN, 1953). Another interesting finding is that transplant of hypophyses from various high-cancer-strain mice into virgin females of the A strain induces both an increase in number and size of their corpora lutea and an increase in mammary tumour incidence (LOEB and KIRTZ, 1939). This brings out again the primary rôle of pituitary hormones in mammary carcinogenesis (GARDNER et al., 1953). Recent investigations on the development and malignant transformation of hyperplastic alveolar nodules in the mammary glands of high- and low-cancer-strain virgin female mice have provided confirmatory evidence that mammotropin or somatotropin are essential hormones in some steps of breast carcinogenesis (NANDI, BERN and DEOME, 1960b; NANDI and BERN, 1960; DEOME et al., 1962; BERN, 1963).

E. Relations between MTV and hormones

In spite of the high mammary tumour incidence which MTV causes, the virus does not itself possess any growth stimulating action on the mamma. In MTV-carrying males the mammary glands remain in a rudimentary state and do not develop tumours. Therefore, an adequate hormonal stimulation is necessary for the development of breast tumours when MTV is concerned.

It is known that in female mice of the same strain, with and without MTV, the mammary glands show morphological differences a few months after birth. In the MTV-carrying females the glandular tree is more extended and shows a larger development of the lobuloalveolar system, usually in form of alveolar hyperplastic nodules (FEKETE, 1938; STRONG, 1938; GARDNER, STRONG and SMITH, 1939; VAN GULIK and KORTEWEG, 1940b; HUSEBY and BITTNER, 1946). Therefore, the question arises as to whether MTV acts by stimulating some endocrine glands to a greater production of hormones, or by diminishing the destruction or the elimination of those hormones, or by increasing the breast susceptibility to hormones.

The first two hypotheses are still under question. RANADIVE (1956) found more corpora lutea in the ovaries of MTV-carrying virgin mice than in those of MTV-free mice of the same strain. However, the age at onset, frequency and duration of estrous cycles are not significantly different in mice genetically identical with and without MTV (SHIMKIN, 1943; ARMSTRONG, 1948; BITTNER, 1948a), strain A being perhaps an exception in this respect (HUSEBY and BITTNER, 1947). Even the minimal dose of estrogen required to induce an estrous cycle is the same in MTV-carrying and MTV-free mice (SHIMKIN and ANDERVONT, 1941; TRENTIN, 1950). On the other hand, no differences have been found in the destruction or inactivation rates of hormones between identical mice with and without MTV (TWOMBLY and TAYLOR, 1942), although the fecal excretion of 17-ketosteroids was found to be lower in mice carrying MTV (SAMUELS, BITTNER and SAMUELS, 1947; BITTNER, 1948a).

The mammary hyperplasia induced by small, identical doses of estradiol benzoate reaches approximately the same level in susceptible MTV-carrying and MTV-free mice (MÜHLBOCK, 1949; TRENTIN, 1951; SQUARTINI, 1956a), but in the former it occurs earlier (SHIMKIN, 1943), is sometimes slightly higher (SILBERBERG, SILBERBERG and BITTNER, 1951) and shows to be persistent (SQUARTINI, 1956a). Recent investigations performed with new methods have shown that MTV increases the hormone sensitivity of normal mammary tissues before hyperplastic alveolar nodules are formed. The specific hormone sensitivity increased by the MTV can be determined by the genetic constitution of the host and is expressed at the level of the mammary tissue itself (DEOME,1963).

3. Inherited factors

A. The role of heredity in mammary carcinogenesis

Even if inherited susceptibility cannot be considered as a true etiological factor, it is a condition in the absence of which spontaneous mammary tumours do not develop in the mouse. The induction of breast cancer by various means is also difficult to achieve in resistant strains. The influence of hereditary factors on mammary carcinogenesis is exerted through the control of hormonal production by the endocrine system and of the susceptibility of mammary glands to hormones and MTV.

B. Mammary susceptibility to MTV

The tumorigenic activity of MTV after introduction into different hosts depends on the type of genes to which it is associated (HESTON, 1946). The action of genes controlling the susceptibility of mice to mammary cancer seems to be located in the breast tissue (HESTON, DERINGER and ANDERVONT, 1945; HESTON, 1948, 1954), although the mammary tumour incidence in different strains is to a large extent determined through the genetic control of hormonal secretions by the endocrine glands (HESTON, 1945). Genetic factors may also influence production of MTV through the same hormonal mechanism. As mentioned above, even the ability to transmit the MTV from male or female parents to offspring is controlled by inherited factors (HESTON, DERINGER and ANDERVONT, 1945; SEVERI et al., 1958). It has been shown that MTV derived from different genetic sources presents differences in behaviour or activity (DMOCHOWSKI, 1945; BITTNER, 1948a; SQUARTINI and SEVERI, 1962). These too may be, at least in part, genetically determined (MURRAY and LITTLE, 1939; MURRAY, 1941a, b; HESTON, DERINGER and ANDERVONT, 1945). In conclusion, genetic factors influence, through various routes, the susceptibility or resistance of mice to the MTV, the production of MTV and its vertical transmission (DMOCHOWSKI, 1953b).

C. Mammary susceptibility to hormones

The mammary hyperplasia induced by small identical doses of female sex hormones is much more intense in susceptible than in resistant mice (GARDNER, SMITH and STRONG, 1935; BONSER, 1936; MÜHLBOCK, 1948; TRENTIN, 1951; SILBERBERG and SILBERBERG, 1951). In susceptible mice treated with estradiol benzoate, the mammary glands rapidly undergo a massive hyperplasia both in animals with and without MTV, whereas in resistant mice a very small or even negative response may be observed (SQUARTINI, 1956a, b, c; SQUARTINI, BOLLI and ROSSI, 1958). Increasing the estrogen dose or adding progesterone, results are unmodified.

Under exogenous hormonal stimulation (estradiol benzoate), the breasts of susceptible (BALB/c) and resistant (C57b) virgin females behave in opposite ways. On the other hand, under endogenous hormonal stimulation (pregnancy) mammary glands undergo hyperplasia of the same type and extent in both series of animals (see Table 3). In other words, in the BALB/c females mammary glands are as much susceptible to endogenous hormonal stimuli as to those administered in this experiment, while in the C57b females glands are only susceptible to endogenous hormonal stimuli (SQUARTINI, BOLLI and ROSSI, 1958; SQUARTINI, 1960). The question arises as to whether the breast susceptibility to exogenous hormones is a condition connected with the mammary tissue only or rather with the whole endocrine apparatus, of which mammary glands are end organs.

D. Vaginal susceptibility to hormones

Also the vaginal epithelium, like that of mammary glands, shows a different degree of sensitivity to injected estrogens in susceptible and resistant mice (GARDNER and ALLEN, 1939; VAN GULIK and KORTEWEG, 1940a; SHIMKIN and ANDERVONT, 1941; MÜHLBOCK, 1947). However, an inverse relationship exists between vaginal and mammary susceptibility to administered estrogens, that is to say that the hereditary transmission of the two characters is independent and crossed. The sensitivity of the genital tract is minimal in strains susceptible to mammary tumours (SILBERBERG and SILBERBERG, 1951); the contrary is seen in resistant strains. This dissociation in sensitivity to the same administered hormone of two different tissues in the same animal suggests the existence of inherited differences in the susceptibility of various tissues to hormones (TRENTIN, 1950). This would explain why mice showing a great tendency to mammary cancer seldom develop genital cancer.

Table 3. *Response of the mammary glandular tree to exogenous and endogenous hormonal stimuli in susceptible (BALB/c) and resistant (C57b) female mice*

Exogenous hormonal stimulation (estradiol benzoate)[1]							
BALB/c virgin females				C57b virgin females			
N. of mice	Age in days	Total dosis (mgs.)	Surface area of the glandular tree in section (mm²)[2]	N. of mice	Age in days	Total doses (mgs)	Surface area of the glandular tree in section (mm²)
5	94	—	5.3	5	56	—	5.3
5	102	0.2	12.3	4	76	0.2	4.4
5	117	0.3	15.3	2	93	0.3	3.8
3	150	0.5	16.5	2	119	0.5	3.5
5	229	—	6.3	2	365	—	4.8

Endogenous hormonal stimulation (pregnancy)							
BALB/c breeding females				C57b breeding females			
N. of mice	Age in days	Days of pregnancy	Surface area of the glandular tree in section (mm²)	N. of mice	Age in days	Days of pregnancy	Surface area of the glandular tree in section (mm²)
5	94	—	5.3	5	56	—	5.3
3	150	10	19.9	2	95	10	27.0
1	153	delivery	56.6	3	95	delivery	48.1
3	162	20 after delivery	6.5	3	115	20 after delivery	7.3
3	176	40 after delivery	6.2	3	117	40 after delivery	5.5

[1] 0.05 mgs in olive oil by weekly subcutaneous injections.
[2] For method see SQUARTINI (1957).
After SQUARTINI (1960).

Nevertheless, as in the case of the breast, the response of the vagina to endogenous hormonal stimulations (estrus) is the same in susceptible and resistant mice. The estrous cycles, as revealed by vaginal smears, do not show any significant difference in both series of animals (BRUNSCHWIG and BISSEL, 1936; TAYLOR and WALTMAN, 1940; DERINGER, HESTON and ANDERVONT, 1945). On the basis of these observations it has been suggested that the development of mammary tumours in susceptible animals might be the result of both a higher susceptibility of their mammary glands to hormones and a greater production of hormones, which is required to overcome the lower sensitivity of their genital tract to estrogens (Korteweg, 1948).

E. Endocrine-gland susceptibility to hormones

Mice of resistant strains are prone to develop pituitary adenomas in response to estrogenic stimulation, whereas susceptible mice seem to be refractory (Gardner, 1941; Mühlbock, 1955b, 1956). In virgin females of the BALB/c and C57b strains, when estradiol benzoate is given, not only the breasts, but also some endocrine glands of the mammary constellation behave in a remarkably different way. In the BALB/c strain, in which mammary glands undergo a marked hyperplasia, ovaries and adrenals become atrophic, and the hypophysis fails to develop adenomas. In the C57b strain, in which mammary glands remain normal, ovaries and adrenals undergo hyperplasia and the hypophysis may develop adenomas. By contrast, during the course of pregnancy, not only the breasts but also endocrine glands behave similarly in both susceptible and resistant animals (Squartini, Bolli and Rossi, 1958).

As it is known, the administered hormones act on the breasts through the mediation of the endocrine glands (Leonard and Reece, 1942; Mixner and Turner, 1942; Gardner, 1953). Hence, the sensitivity of the mammary glands to administered hormones does not seem to be a character connected with the mammary cells only, but it may partly be dependent on the structure and behaviour of some endocrine glands (Squartini, 1960). A similar suggestion could be advanced for the vaginal epithelium.

F. Inherited control on endocrine glands and on hormonal production

The endocrine glands of susceptible- and resistant-cancer-strain mice display structural differences which become apparent along with age. Therefore, the hormonal production too is different. In adult susceptible females, ovaries and adrenals are larger than in the resistant ones (Fekete, 1946; Squartini, Bolli and Rossi, 1958). In several susceptible strains castration induces hyperplasia of the adrenals which substitutes for the function of the absent gonads (Woolley, Fekete and Little, 1939, 1940, 1941a, b; Smith, 1945, 1946, 1948). Differences have been found, between susceptible and resistant mice, even in the disposition of the pituitary gland to develop adenomas (see above). These data suggest that the differences in structure and behaviour of endocrine glands and relative end organs, observed in susceptible and resistant strains, are mostly dependent on the hypophysis, which is responsible for a higher production of gonadotropic and mammotropic hormones in susceptible animals as compared to resistant ones. Thus, a particular structure of the hypophysis, inherited, could be at the origin of mammary susceptibility to hormones and cancer.

4. Environmental factors

Factors such as changes in temperature, crowding of the animals in the cages and diet play some rôle in the origin of mouse mammary cancer. After the casual observation that white mice kept at 18–24° C developed some mammary tumours though in low percentage (10–15%), whereas no tumours were observed in the same animals kept in a warm, moist environment (Fuller, Brown and Mills,

1941), detailed investigations were carried out. Three equal groups of DBA mice were kept for 18 months in a hot room at 32° C and 60–70% humidity, in a cold room at 18° C, and in a control room where the temperature varied from 21° C in winter up to 34° C in summer. The animals developed mammary tumours in the following percentages respectively: 6.0, 19.7 and 20.9%. In addition, tumours occurring in mice kept in the hot room showed a lower rate of growth and a higher duration (FULLER, BROWN and MILLS, 1941). The same experiment was repeated using C3H virgin females, and the results obtained were slightly different. The 32° C group and the control group developed the same incidence of mammary tumours (50%) at the same age, whereas more tumours were observed in the 18° C group (72%) at a comparable age. Mammary tumours occurring in the latter group were often multiple and showed a higher rate of growth (WALLACE, WALLACE and MILLS, 1944). In C3H spayed females the stimulating effect of low temperature on mammary tumorigenesis was confirmed (WALLACE, WALLACE and MILLS, 1945).

Very little is known about the effect of light on mouse breast tumorigenesis. The exposure to artificial light and darkness are known to influence the estrous cycle and sexual behaviour of mice (MORRIS, 1945a). Another factor which affects estrous cycles is represented by crowding and isolation of animals in the cages. ANDERVONT (1944) observed that C3H mice developed more mammary tumours when maintained in individual boxes. Among 58 segregated virgin females there was an incidence of mammary tumours equal to 98.3% at an average age of 9.6 months, whereas among 56 nonsegregated animals the mammary tumour incidence was 80.4% and the tumour age 11.9 months. These observations were extended later by MÜHLBOCK (1955a) with similar results.

Extensive investigations have been developed in past years concerning the influence of dietary factors on mouse mammary carcinogenesis (for review see MORRIS, 1945a; TANNENBAUM and SILVERSTONE, 1953). Underfeeding, caloric restriction (TANNENBAUM, 1945a, b), or deficiency of proteins in the diet (TANNENBAUM and SILVERSTONE, 1949a; WHITE and WHITE, 1944) result in a decrease of spontaneous mammary tumours in mice. The proportion of dietary fat has less importance in respect to mammary tumorigenesis (TANNENBAUM and SILVERSTONE, 1949b). The same factors are known to influence the growth rate of established mammary tumours. Dietary factors have also a remarkable effect on the estrous cycle and sexual behaviour of mice (MORRIS, 1945a, b).

Environmental factors are not primary causative factors in mouse mammary tumorigenesis (MÜHLBOCK, 1956), but they can increase or decrease the tumour incidence and growth by acting on the endocrine system of the animals (TRENTIN and TURNER, 1941; HUSEBY, BALL and VISSCHER, 1945; MORRIS, 1945a, b; MÜHLBOCK, 1956).

5. Mammogenesis and carcinogenesis

A. Mammogenesis as a detector of hormonal production in mice

Normal growth of the mammary glandular tree is caused by the female sex hormones. It is accepted that estrogens promote the development of the duct system and progesterone that of the lobulo-alveolar system (PULLINGER, 1947). Estrogens and progesterone act on the breasts only in presence of the hypophysis (GOMEZ and TURNER, 1937). Mammogenic activity of the hypophysis seems to be carried out by prolactin since estrogens, progesterone and prolactin are able to induce development of the mammary glandular tree with lobulo-alveolar differentiation in ovariectomized, adrenalectomized and hypophysectomized animals.

However, when growth hormone is added to this hormonal triad, the mammary response is enhanced (COWIE and FOLLEY, 1958).

In female mice, after the onset of sexual cycles, a rhythmic and progressive development of the mammary-duct system occurs. During proestrus the ducts are thin and show a few solid, lightly stained buds. At estrus the buds develop new ducts and other buds appear. At metestrus the glands undergo slight retrogressive changes. However, ductal growth resumes during the next estrous cycle. Therefore, with each succeeding estrus the growth of the ducts is slightly extended, until the complete development is approached (TURNER and GOMEZ, 1933; COLE, 1933; SQUARTINI and LOTTI, 1955). The lack of a rhythmic development of alveoli at metestrus, that is the time in which estral corpora lutea are formed in the ovaries, has led some investigators to suppose that the sexual cycle of mice is characterized by a defect in luteal hormone production (PULLINGER, 1947), or that the estral corpora lutea do not function in mice (MÜHLBOCK, 1956). Therefore, it has been postulated that only corpora lutea of pregnancy and pseudopregnancy are able to induce lobulo-alveolar proliferations in the mammary glands of mice.

However, an investigation on the development of mammary glands in susceptible, virgin females of the BALB/cf (C3H) strain, with the MTV, has shown the presence of alveoli from the end of the third month of life until the regression which affects end pieces of the glandular tree early in the second year (Table 4: SQUARTINI, 1959). Mammogenesis proceeds from the buds; each bud develops branches; terminal branches grow alveoli; when the alveolar development is advanced, in the distal ends of the branches rudimentary lobules appear. End and lateral buds are frequently seen in the first months of life up to the 7—8th month, but disappear later. The small terminal branches, recognizable from the third month onwards, undergo variations in number and size from animal to animal, until they progressively decrease in old mice. The earliest alveoli appear at the end of the third month. They also undergo quantitative variations from case to case. Usually they increase in number showing a direct relationship with the animal's age. In several instances they are grouped to compose clusters of a lobular aspect. The presence of alveoli should mean that progesterone and prolactin stimulate the breast tissue (SQUARTINI and CASCHERA, 1958). The question whether or not cyclic variations in the number of alveoli take place with the recurring estrous cycles remains unanswered. It is however interesting to note that the first estrous cycles occur in the BALB/cf (C3H) virgin females at the beginning of the second month (PASSARETTI and CASCHERA, 1956), while the first alveoli occur in the breasts at the end of the third month. Therefore, several estrous cycles occur in the early life without any alveolar development in the mammary glands (SQUARTINI, 1959).

Early in the second year the breast tissue undergoes senile involutive changes. These affect mainly the alveoli and small terminal branches, while the gross duct system is unaffected. Morphologically, the breast involution appears as a fragmentation of the glandular structures, which lose their colour and then disappear into the surrounding fat tissue. The picture resembles that visible after pregnancy and lactation. This leads to suppose that the senile involutive changes are due to a critical reduction of the hormonal stimuli on the breasts (SQUARTINI and CASCHERA, 1958). As a result of the involution, the mammary glandular tree of old BALB/cf (C3H) virgin females is almost constantly of pure ductal type (BARBIERI, CASCHERA and OLIVI, 1958b). Nevertheless, estrous cycles are still present in old animals of this (CASCHERA, 1960a; CASCHERA and MALTZEFF, 1960), as well as of all the other strains of mice investigated till now, though the cycles show irregularities and interruptions (THUNG et al., 1956; CASCHERA, 1959).

Table 4. *Proliferative and regressive physiological changes and number of hyperplastic alveolar nodules in the mammary glands of BALB/cf (C3H) virgin female mice*[1] *of scalar ages*

Age (months)	1	1	2	3	3	4	4	4	4	5	5	5	5	5
Buds	+ – –	+ – –	+ – –	+ – –	+ + –	+ + –	+ + –	+ + –	+ – –	+ – –	+ – –	+ + –	+ + –	+ – –
Branches	– – –	– – –	– – –	+ + –	+ – –	+ – –	+ – –	+ – –	+ + –	+ – –	+ – –	+ – –	+ – –	+ + –
Alveoli	– – –	– – –	– – –	+ – –	– – –	+ – –	+ – –	– – –	+ + –	+ – –	+ – –	+ – –	– – –	– – –
Nodules[2]	0	0	0	0	0	0	0	0	0	0	0	0	0	0
Age (months)	5	6	6	7	7	7	7	7	7	7	7	8	8	8
Buds	+ – –	+ + +	+ + –	+ + –	+ – –	+ + –	– – –	+ – –	+ – –	+ – –	+ – –	– – –	+ – –	– – –
Branches	+ – –	+ + –	+ + –	+ – –	+ + +	+ – –	+ + –	+ – –	+ + –	+ + –	+ – –	+ + –	+ + –	+ + –
Alveoli	– – –	+ + +	+ + +	+ + +	+ + +	+ + –	+ + +	+ – –	+ + –	+ – –	+ – –	+ – –	+ + –	+ – –
Nodules	0	1	3	0	8	0	2	0	0	0	0	1	0	0
Age (months)	8	8	9	9	9	9	9	9	9	10	10	10	11	11
Buds	– – –	+ – –	– – –	– – –	– – –	– – –	– – –	– – –	– – –	– – –	– – –	– – –	– – –	– – –
Branches	+ + –	+ + –	+ + +	+ + +	+ – –	+ + –	+ + –	+ + –	+ + +	+ + +	+ + –	+ + –	+ + –	+ + +
Alveoli	+ + +	+ + +	+ + +	+ + +	+ – –	+ – –	+ – –	+ + –	+ + +	+ + +	+ + –	+ + –	+ + –	+ + +
Nodules	1	0	0	3	0	1	0	0	6	27	1	4	3	17
Age (months)	13	13	14	14	14	14	14	15	15	15	16	16	16	16
Buds	R[3]	R	R	R	– – –	– – –	– – –	– – –	– – –	– – –	– – –	– – –	– – –	– – –
Branches	R	R	R	R	+ – –	– – –	– – –	– – –	– – –	– – –	+ + –	+ – –	+ – –	+ – –
Alveoli	R	R	R	R	– – –	– – –	– – –	– – –	– – –	– – –	+ – –	– – –	– – –	– – –
Nodules	3	23	9	5	0	0	0	0	0	0	1	0	0	0
Age (months)	17	17	17	17	18	18	18	19	19	19	20			
Buds	– – –	– – –	R	– – –	R	– – –	– – –	R	– – –	– – –	– – –			
Branches	+ + –	+ – –	R	– – –	R	– – –	+ – –	R	+ + –	– – –	+ – –			
Alveoli	+ – –	– – –	R	– – –	R	– – –	+ – –	R	+ – –	– – –	– – –			
Nodules	0	0	0	0	0	0	0	0	1	0	0			

[1] 67 virgin females; thoracic mammary glands of the 2nd pair; whole mount.
[2] Mean diameter > 0.4 mm.
[3] R = In regression.
After SQUARTINI (1959).

The preceding data lead to the conclusion that in virgin females of the BALB/cf (C3H) strain there is a deficient liberation of progesterone and prolactin in the first and in the last months of life, while during the middle ages these hormones are produced in sufficient quantities to induce lobolo-alveolar development in the breasts. Obviously, mice of different strains may show a different behaviour of their mammary glandular tree, as a consequence of different endocrine situations.

B. Carcinogenesis, with an analysis of the sources of endogenous progesterone and prolactin

In the breasts of female mice carrying the MTV circumscribed proliferations of alveoli occur some months after birth: the hyperplastic alveolar nodules, which are precancerous. Nodules are clusters of alveoli indistinguishable morphologically, histochemically and biochemically from the lobules of pregnancy (DeOme et al., 1956; Harkness et al., 1957; Severi, Olivi and Biancifiori, 1958). Therefore, the luteal hormone seems to be an important factor in the etiology of nodules, as well as of tumours arising in nodules by progression. Production of progesterone is ruled by the pituitary hormones and causes, in turn, release of mammotropic hormones by the hypophysis. Hence, analysis of the sources of endogenous progesterone provides also useful information to evaluate the functional activity of the hypophysis.

The endogenous sources of progesterone needed for the development of mammary nodules and tumours, the mechanisms inducing progesterone release and the amounts of progesterone produced are different, being influenced by the animal strain and, in the same strain, by the endocrine state of mice, such as virgins, pseudopregnant, breeding females or estrogenized females and males.

a) Virgin females

Virgin females of the BALB/cf (C3H) strain show a tumour incidence (37%) which is about half that of the breeders (81.2%). Also the average tumour age is considerably higher (Squartini, 1960). Therefore, in this as in other strains, pregnancy doubles the percentage of tumours and lowers tumour age.

Tumour incidence in virgins of the high-mammary-cancer strains is controlled by the "inherited hormonal influence". In the strains that possess the hormonal influence, *e.g.* the C3H strain, virgin females have a high mammary tumour incidence; they also show more and larger corpora lutea in the ovaries (Huseby and Bittner, 1948), and, when gonadectomized, usually undergo adrenal hypertrophy. The hypertrophic adrenals may also assume a vicarious ovarian function and cause hyperplastic nodules and tumours in the breasts (Smith, 1948). By contrast, in the strains that do not possess the hormonal influence, *e.g.* the A strain, virgin mice have a very low mammary tumour incidence, they show less and smaller corpora lutea, and do not undergo adrenal hypertrophy when gonadectomized. These data lead to suppose that the inherited hormonal influence acts by increasing the production and/or the release of gonadotropic hormones by the pituitary (Gardner et al., 1953).

The above considerations lead to the conclusion that ovaries and adrenals are a good source of progesterone in virgin females which possess the inherited hormonal influence. However, strain differences in progesterone production may exist among these, which would explain the different tumour incidence in C3H virgins, as high as that of breeders (Andervont, 1941), when compared with BALB/cf (C3H) virgins. On the other hand, in virgin animals which do not possess any inherited hormonal influence, the endogenous production of progesterone probably remains inadequate over the whole life period. In this way the very low tumour incidence in virgin females of the A strain could be explained. Therefore, the assumption of an inadequate progesterone stimulation in virgin female mice cannot be generalized.

Pseudopregnancy has been suspected to occur in mice, independently of sterile coitus, following coabitation of females in the cages or even for other reasons. Therefore, it cannot be excluded that the presence of alveoli and lobules and/or alveolar hyperplastic nodules in the breasts of susceptible virgin females is due to the occurrence of spontaneous pseudopregnancies. However, an investigation on the behaviour of estrous cycles in BALB/cf (C3H) virgin females, varying in number from 2 to 5 in each cage, failed to demonstrate spontaneous pseudopregnancies (SQUARTINI and CASCHERA, 1958), although further investigations showed the occasional occurrence of rare pseudopregnancies (4% of the cycles examined) in virgin animals kept 5 per cage (CASCHERA, 1960a, b). This frequency is too low to explain noduligenesis in BALB/cf (C3H) virgin mice. Hence, alveolar nodules occurring in the breasts of these animals are mainly independent of pseudopregnancies.

b) Breeding females

In mated females the hormones necessary for the development of hyperplastic alveolar nodules and mammary tumours, may be supplied by the gravidic corpora lutea and by placenta or decidua. The genesis of nodules occurring in pluriparous or pseudopregnant females is usually referred to subinvoluted areas of the gravidic or pseudo-gravidic physiological hyperplasia (FEKETE, 1938; BARBIERI, CASCHERA and OLIVI, 1958a).

Breeding females of the BALB/cf (C3H) strain, with an average of 3 to 4 pregnancies, show a high mammary tumour incidence (81,2%) (SQUARTINI, 1959). A study of the relationship between incidence of tumours and number of deliveries has shown that after a single pregnancy the mammary tumour incidence rises from the mean values of the virgins to the high one characteristic of the breeders (SQUARTINI, 1955). A high tumour incidence would be related to a high number of hyperplastic alveolar nodules in the breasts. However, it has often been observed that after the first pregnancy the regression of glandular hyperplasia is complete, that is no nodules persist due to lobular subinvolution (FEKETE, 1938; OLIVI, CASCHERA and BARBIERI, 1958a, b). On the other hand, it has recently been demonstrated that in breasts of uniparous females, some time after postgravidic regression, a considerable number of hyperplastic alveolar nodules occurs. Therefore, in the breeders, as well as in virgins, nodules would not always be due to subinvolution of a previously hyperplastic parenchyma, but also to direct proliferation of the mammary cells during the resting phase (OLIVI, CASCHERA and BARBIERI, 1958a, b).

c) Estrogenized females and males

The tumour incidence induced by administration of estradiol benzoate in virgin females or intact males of the BALB/cf (C3H) strain is as high as, or higher than, that of the breeders (OLIVI and CONSOLANDI, 1955). In other words the administered estrogens may well replace pregnancy (MÜHLBOCK, 1956). BALB/cf (C3H) virgin females injected with 0.05 mg of estradiol benzoate in olive oil at weekly intervals develop a rapid mammary hyperplasia with marked lobulo-alveolar differentiation. This means that the estrogen administration increases the release of endogenous progesterone and prolactin. When treatment is discontinued after a short time, the mammary hyperplasia regresses completely (SQUARTINI, 1958). When treatment is protracted the hyperplasia is followed by tumour growth at an earlier time than in breeders (OLIVI and CONSOLANDI, 1955).

6. Changes preceding the development of mouse mammary tumours

A. Alveolar premalignant changes (hyperplastic alveolar nodules)

Although it is not to be excluded that mammary tumours may exceptionally arise in normal glands (FOULDS, 1956b), usually they develop from preexisting hyperplastic lesions. These may be alveolar, ductular or ductal in origin. Their distinction according to the involved segment of glandular tree is important in view of the different hormonal control and of the different site of attack of carcinogenic agents on the breasts (SQUARTINI, 1960). The simplest and most frequent precancerous lesions of the mouse mammary gland are the alveolar ones, or hyperplastic alveolar nodules.

a) Definition

The hyperplastic alveolar nodules are composed of grouped alveoli, ranging from few to some hundreds, usually not cystic and surrounded by a moderately increased layer of connective tissue without any appreciable evidence of inflammatory reaction (Plate 1) (HUSEBY and BITTNER, 1946). On the basis of this definition it appears difficult to recognize a "nodule" from a mammary lobule. Histologic, cytologic and cytochemical tests have not revealed characteristic differences between nodules and normal lobules, except for the presence of MTV particles in the former (BERN et al., 1958a; DEOME et al., 1959a, b; HARKNESS et al., 1957; PITELKA et al., 1958; PITELKA, DEOME and BERN, 1960). In addition, there is no mention about what size a cluster of alveoli should have to be considered as a nodule.

b) Small and large nodules

In an investigation by means of the whole mount procedure on mammary glands of BALB/cf (C3H) virgin female mice, alveolar clusters have been measured in the two largest diameters and recorded when their mean diameter was higher than 0.1 mm. Over this diameter the term "nodule" has been used, regardless of the size of the clusters. Measured, nodules have been grouped into classes of size and then divided according to animal age (Table 5). Nodules larger than 0.4 mm have also been separately recorded for each animal (see Table 4). With this procedure, differences in the behaviour of small and large nodules have been observed (SQUARTINI, 1959).

Small nodules are recognizable at the fourth month, then progressively increase in number, reach a peak at the 10th month, and thereafter disappear

---

Plate 1

No. 1. BALB/c virgin female aged 205 days; left thoracic breast; whole mount method; × 6. Typical aspect of the mouse mammary gland by the whole mount method. Thin ducts without alveoli in a low-mammary-tumour virgin female. After OLIVI and CASCHERA (1960)

No. 2. RIII virgin female aged 197 days; left thoracic breast; whole mount method; × 6. Ducts with alveoli and hyperplastic alveolar nodules in a high-mammary-tumour virgin female. After BARBIERI, CASCHERA and OLIVI (1958a)

No. 3. RIII breeding female aged 331 days; left thoracic breast; whole mount method; × 6. Several hyperplastic alveolar nodules. After BARBIERI, CASCHERA and OLIVI (1958a)

No. 4. RIII virgin female aged 288 days; left thoracic breast; whole mount method; × 26. A nodule with alveoli distended by secretion. After BARBIERI, CASCHERA and OLIVI (1958a)

No. 5. RIII breeding female, 43 days after weaning of a litter; right abdominal breast; histological method; × 33. Small hyperplastic alveolar nodule as it appears in histological section. After OLIVI, CASCHERA and BUCCIARELLI (1961)

No. 6. BALB/cf (C3H) breeding female, 54 days after weaning of a litter; right thoracic breast; × 36. Hyperplastic alveolar nodule with secretion. After OLIVI, CASCHERA and BUCCIARELLI (1961)

By courtesy of Dr. MARIA OLIVI

Plate 1

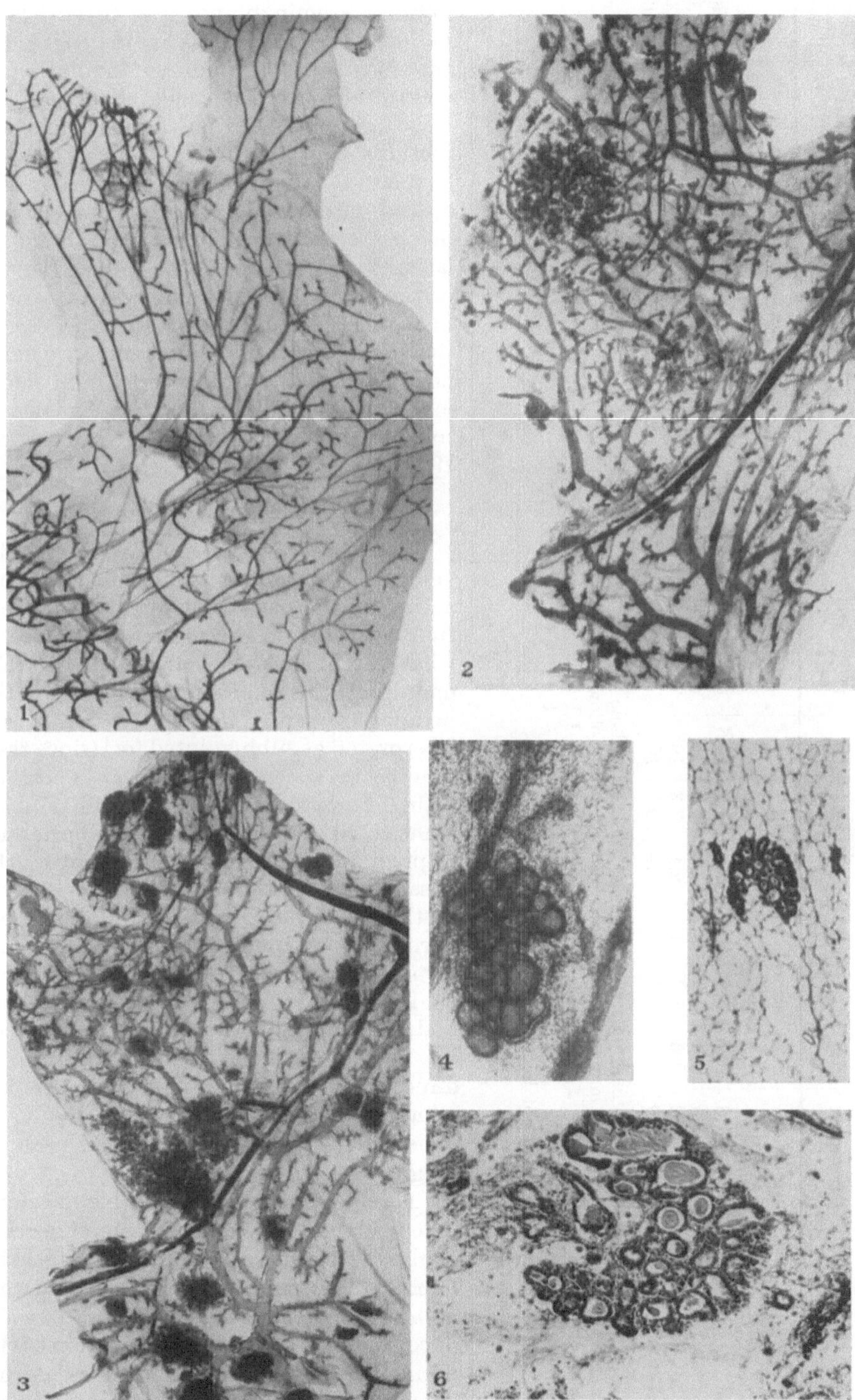

Table 5. *Average number of "nodules" per mammary gland according to their diameter and animal age in BALB/cf (C3H) virgin female mice*[1]

Animal age (months)	4	5	6	7	8	9	10	11	12[3]	13	14	15	16	17	18	19	20	Total of averages	Total of counted nodules
Average diameter of «nodules»:																			
> 0.1 ≤ 0.2 mm	3.5	1.8	10.5	5.4	10.2	18	44.7	16.5	=	4.5	3.8	.0	2.5	1.7	2	1	.0	126.1	486
> 0.2 ≤ 0.3 mm	2.5	1.5	11.5	7.6	5.2	9	45.7	31	=	13.5	7.8	.0	1.5	.0	1.7	1	.0	139.5	475
> 0.3 ≤ 0.4 mm	.2	.2	1.5	1.2	1	2.1	7.3	16	=	8.5	1.4	.0	.2	.0	.0	.0	.0	39.6	114
> 0.4 mm[2]	.0	.0	2	1.2	.4	1.4	10.7	10	=	13	2.8	.0	.2	.0	.0	.3	.0	42.0	120

[1] 67 virgin females; thoracic mammary glands of the 2nd pair; whole mount.

[2] «Nodules» of more than 0.4 mm in diamter were grouped in the following classes of sizes:

Average diameter:	≤ .5	≤ .6	≤ .7	≤ .8	≤ .9	≤ 1.	≤ 1.1	≤ 1.2	≤ 1.3	≤ 1.4	≤ 1.5	≤ 1.6	= 3.5	= 4 mm
Total nodules counted:	61	16	15	8	5	4	1	4	3	0	0	1	1	1

[3] Animals of this age have not been examined.

After SQUARTINI (1959).

almost completely. Some of the small nodules seemingly progress toward large nodules by an increase in their size, but the mostly they undergo involution in connection with the senile changes of the breast, as evidenced by the morphological pictures (SQUARTINI and CASCHERA, 1958; SQUARTINI, 1959). Large nodules, which appear later and then disappear, show a moderate numerical increase in direct relationship to the age of the animal. Several of the largest nodules progress to cancer, but some of them do not seem to escape the senile involution since only two large nodules have been discovered in 21 mammary glands of different virgin females 14 to 20 months old (see Table 4: SQUARTINI, 1959).

c) *Hormone dependence of nodules*

The hyperplastic alveolar nodules develop as a response to hormonal stimuli acting on the mammary glands of susceptible hosts. However, it is still obscure to what extent hormones are needed for the nodules to be maintained. Some of the nodules occurring in breeders, which are interpreted as subinvoluted foci (since they survive to the postgravidic and postlactating regression of the glandular tree) seem to be independent of the hormones of pregnancy and lactation; however, the possibility that they are still under control of the ovarian, adrenal and hypophyseal hormones continuously released during intermissions of gestation, cannot be excluded. This applies still more to those nodules, developing in virgins and breeders, which are considered to be due to direct proliferation in response to hormonal stimulations acting on the mammary glands independently of pregnancy and pseudopregnancy.

Therefore, to test the possible hormone independence of nodules, the endocrine glands secreting sex hormones must be removed. Hypophysectomy, carried out in breeding females of high-cancer-strain mice, induces a complete regression of the normal mammary tissue, but does not influence the large hyperplastic nodules, which do not regress, and does not prevent the appearance of tumours (GARDNER, 1942). This finding has been interpreted as demonstrative of a large hormone independence of hyperplastic nodules in their late stages (MÜHLBOCK, 1958a).

In BALB/cf (C3H) virgin females most of the small nodules persist for a long time but disappear during the senile involution of mammary glands. Therefore, they behave as hormone dependent structures. Some of them, however, undergo a progression towards large nodules by an increase in their size. At the same time their hormone independence seems to increase, since large nodules, though partially showing regression, are still numerous in the breasts when the small ones are disappearing (see Table 5). The above data lead us to suppose that the hormone dependence of nodules is a function of their size, but also that not all the large nodules reach a state of complete independence from the hormonal stimuli before they undergo malignant degeneration by progression (SQUARTINI, 1959).

d) Influences of MTV in the genesis of nodules

The hyperplastic alveolar nodules are not exclusive of MTV-bearing female mice. They may also be observed in susceptible animals deprived of MTV by foster-nursing (JONES, 1951; MÜHLBOCK, VAN EGGENHORST TENGBERGEN and VAN RIJSSEL, 1952). In this case they are fewer and occur much later. Therefore, as well as for mammary tumours, MTV accelerates and intensifies the appearance of nodules.

e) The fate of nodules

In virgin females of the BALB/cf (C3H) strain only a small number of large nodules may be found in the breasts some time after senile involution (see Tables 4 and 5). This is because many of them have previously progressed towards palpable mammary tumours and some others have regressed during senile changes of the glands (SQUARTINI, 1959). Also in RIII virgin females the breasts undergo senile involution. However, along a glandular tree of "wintry" type, several hyperplastic nodules are still present in aged animals from 400 to 600 days (BARBIERI, CASCHERA and OLIVI, 1958b). The number of nodules found in the breasts beyond the time of senile involution is, therefore, different in different strains. The BALB/cf (C3H) virgin females exhibit a tumour incidence lower than RIII virgin females. In both strains tumours do not develop beyond the 15th and 19th month respectively. In other words, nodules persisting in mammary glands beyond this time do not grow tumours. The causes of that are still unknown. It has been supposed, however, that also the nodules of aged animals require a further hormonal stimulation to evolve towards cancer (BARBIERI, CASCHERA and OLIVI, 1958b).

The above data lead us to conclude that hyperplastic alveolar nodules partly develop into palpable mammary tumours, partly undergo regression, and partly remain unaltered along the involuted senile breasts, being unable either to regress or to progress towards cancer (SQUARTINI, 1960).

f) Recent advances in nodule research by means of a new transplantation technique: A summary of papers by DEOME *et al.*

Remarkable progress about the causes, significance and behaviour of the hyperplastic alveolar nodules of the mouse breast have been achieved recently following the development of two technical procedures. The first permitted the identification and removal of nodules from living mice (DEOME et al., 1956), the second permitted the transplantation of nodules into gland-free mammary fat pads of suitable host mice and thus made possible the study of such structures under a variety of host conditions (DeOme et al., 1959b). The present status of knowledge promoted by these techniques and collateral studies will be summarized here in form of short statements.

Nodules are preneoplastic changes. When nodules and samples of normal mammary tissue, removed from the same donor, are transplanted, mammary tumours arise more frequently and in less time from the nodule transplants than from the normal transplants (DeOme et al., 1959b). Normal transplants may undergo nodular transformation after some time, and the tumours which they grow are supposed to develop after this transformation (DeOme et al., 1962).

Nodules are non homogeneous cell populations. Individual nodules differ from one another with regard to growth rate, secretory status, hormone dependence and cancer-producing capability (Blair, DeOme and Nandi, 1961; DeOme, Blair and Faulkin, 1961). The characteristics shown by individual nodules are remarkably stable in transplant-lines, and are independent of each other. In particular, the cancer-producing capability of nodules is independent of the growth rate and the secretory pattern (DeOme et al., 1962).

Nodules are hormone dependent structures. The various hormonal combinations necessary for lobulo-alveolar development (mammogenesis), lactogenesis, noduligenesis, nodule maintenance, and progression (tumorigenesis) have been determined in hypophysectomized-ovariectomized-adrenalectomized C3H mice. Estradiol + a C-21 steroid (luteoid or corticoid) + somatotropin (STH) and/or mammotropin (MH) are the minimum hormone combinations required for the induction of either lobulo-alveolar mammogenesis or noduligenesis. Lobules and nodules can be stimulated to secrete milk by cortisol + MH and/or STH. The majority of nodules are dependent on pituitary hormones for their maintenance. In endocrinectomized mice they can be maintainend by corticoids + MH or + STH. While nodule formation requires estrogenic stimulation, nodule maintenance appears to be independent from estrogen. Neoplastic transformation of transplanted nodules requires pituitary and ovarian or adrenocortical hormones; estrogen can enhance the effect of the other hormones but it is not essential. Corticoids are interchangeable with progesterone in lobulo-alveolar development, nodule formation and nodule maintenance. STH and MH are interchangeable in all steps of mammary growth, including tumorigenesis (Nandi, 1958, 1959; Nandi and Bern, 1961; Nandi, Bern and DeOme, 1960a, b; Bern and Nandi, 1961; DeOme et al., 1962).

Strain differences exist in the hormonal requirement for nodule formation. In mice of the strain A hormonal combinations containing STH are ineffective, whereas only MH-containing combinations are effective. In C3Hf mice, without MTV, MH-containing combinations are more effective than STH-containing combinations. In C3H mice, with MTV, both STH- and MH-containing combinations are equally effective. In spite of these strain differences concerning nodule formation, no differences were found with regard to the hormones required for nodule maintenance and progression (Blair et al., 1960; Nandi, 1961a, b, c; Bern and Nandi, 1961; DeOme et al., 1962).

MTV is concerned with noduligenesis, not with neoplastic transformation of nodules. The tumour-producing capability of nodules is determined at the time of nodule formation. Nodules from MTV-free mice, possessing low tumour-producing capability, are not changed into high tumour-producing nodules after *in vivo* exposure to MTV. Therefore, the MTV seems to be concerned with the normal mammary tissue alterations preceding nodule formation, but not with the neoplastic changes within the cell population of nodules (Blair and DeOme, 1961; DeOme, 1963).

MTV increases hormone sensitivity of normal mammary tissues before nodules are formed. Normal C3Hf (MTV-free) mammary tissue transplanted into young C3H (MTV-carrying) females develops nodules which possess high tumour-producing capability. The specific hormone sensitivity increased by the MTV can be determined by the genetic constitution of the host (DEOME, 1963).

MTV may be responsible for a variety of abnormal cell types. This is suggested by the observation of nodule cell populations which possess stable and heritable variant characteristics, in addition to tumour-producing capability (DEOME, 1963; BERN, 1963).

As is apparent, many previous results have been confirmed, clarified or solved by these recent observations, which provide a valuable background for the future understanding of the whole process of mammary tumorigenesis.

B. Ductular premalignant changes

With the term "ductules" we refer to the thin prealveolar tubules of the mammary tree. Morphologically, they look like ducts, but, due to the absence of an elastic coat, their structure resembles more alveoli than large ducts. Also from the functional standpoint, ductules behave like alveoli, conspicuous ductular proliferations having been observed only during pregnancies. Therefore, alveoli as well as ductules belong to the functioning section of mammary parenchyma and seem to be controlled by progesterone and pituitary mammotropic hormones. Precancerous duotular hyperplasias have been infrequently observed. To this group belong the "plaques" and, if they exist, the hyperplastic nodules of small ducts.

a) Plaques

In some hybrids and their inbred descendants precancerous lesions susceptible of reaching palpable sizes, have been occasionally observed; owing to their shape, they are referred to as plaques (FOULDS, 1956b). Plaques have been recently discovered also in breeding females of some inbred strains, such as RIII (SQUARTINI and ROSSI, 1959a; SQUARTINI et al., 1960), BALB/cf (C3H) (SEVERI, OLIVI and BIANCIFIORI, 1958; SQUARTINI and ROSSI, 1960, 1962), and DD (HESTON, VLAHAKIS and TSUBURA, 1964).

MTV seems to be involved in the etiology of plaques, as these have been usually observed in virus-bearing females. Pregnancy, or better the hormones of pregnancy, are essential causative factors, since plaques have never been observed in non gestative periods. Another important factor would be the hybrid vigor (FOULDS, 1956b), since plaques were first detected in hybrids (RIII $\times$ C57b)F_1.

Histologically, plaques comprise a central portion or "medulla" of loose, fatty connective tissue in which normal-looking tubules are scattered, and a more compact "cortex" of radially disposed branching tubules (Plate 2) (FOULDS, 1956b). Plaques are composed of ductules, showing a duct-like picture but lacking, like the alveoli, an elastic coat (SEVERI and SQUARTINI, 1959; SEVERI et al., 1959). Plaques are supposed to have the same significance as hyperplastic alveolar nodules, of which they represent alternative and non-consecutive steps in the development of mammary tumours. Further information on the biological behaviour of plaques will be given later.

b) Hyperplastic nodules of small ducts

The hyperplastic nodules of small ducts, which presumably belong to the ductular preneoplastic lesions of the mouse breast, are very uncommon, having been observed only few times (GARDNER, 1942; HUSEBY and BITTNER, 1946), so

Plate 2

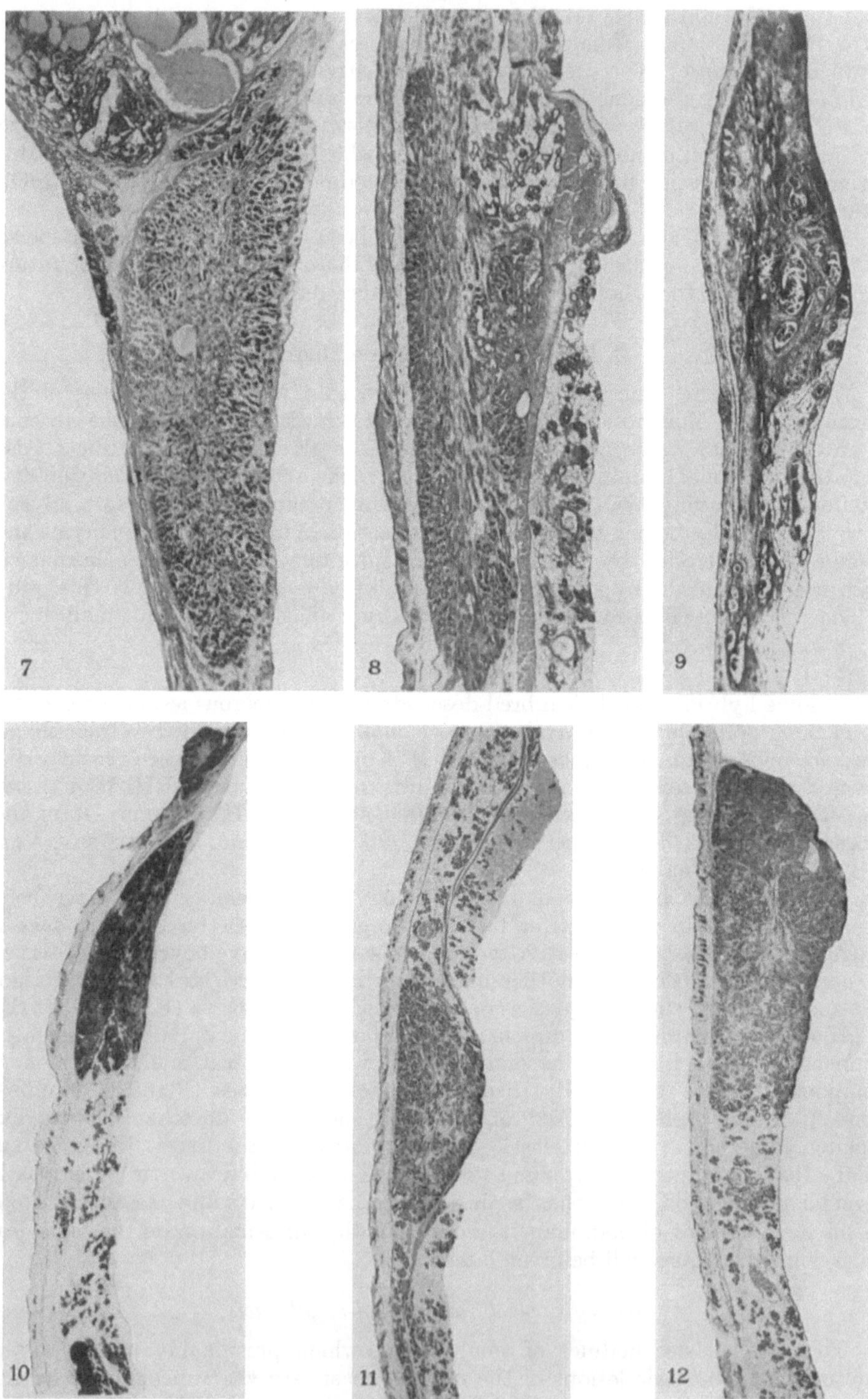

that some doubt is advanced about their existence. In breasts examined by the whole mount procedure they appear as an extensive proliferation of very fine ducts. These radiate from a relatively small locus, so that the lesion simulates a many pointed star of which the branches are smooth, as neither ducts nor alveoli develop along them (HUSEBY and BITTNER, 1946). The histological picture is unknown. Therefore, the question of a possible identity between nodules of small ducts and plaques, both of which affect breeding females, though suggestive, remains unanswered.

C. Ductal premalignant changes

Excretory ducts of the mammary gland seem to be dependent on hormones different from those which control the secreting parenchyma, as they do not undergo any noticeable reduction during the resting state of the gland. It is generally supposed that the development of the duct system is controlled and promoted mainly by estrogens. This suggests that the genesis of premalignant changes occurring in ducts may be different from that in ductules and alveoli. Precancerous changes within the ducts have been infrequently observed in mice and are, therefore, still scarcely known. They may sometimes be referred to as papillomas of the ducts (ORR, 1956). These compose fine intraductal pictures, the evolution of which is towards sepimentation of the lumina by epithelial projections. Usually they lead to the formation of carcinomas of the "comedo" type (FOULDS, 1956b).

7. Mammary tumours

A. Age distribution of tumours in relation to the problem of "menopause" in mice

Tumour incidence, tumour age and the singleness or multiplicity of tumours in the same host are useful elements to evaluate the degree of inherited susceptibility in animals, as well as the number, type and intensity of causative factors involved in tumorigenesis. When, in controlled experiments, the intensity of one single etiological factor is varied, *e.g.* the hormonal factor, tumour incidence and tumour age have revealed to be reliable detectors of that variation. Therefore, the age distribution of tumours in homogeneous group of mice may be assumed to be a detector of the variations that have occurred in the degree of endogenous hormonal stimulations during the life of the animal. The study, by vaginal smears, of estrous cycles in aged female mice of several strains has led to the conclusion that a true menopause does not exist in mice (MÜHLBOCK, 1958b). Although with irregularities and prolonged interruptions, cycles still continue until the oldest ages, or the death of the animal (THUNG, BOOT and MÜHLBOCK, 1956; CASCHERA, 1959, 1960b; CASCHERA and MALTZEFF, 1960). Also the histological examination of the ovaries in old mice suggests that hormonal production gradually decreases with age, but without stopping completely.

Plate 2

No. 7. RIII breeding female aged 181 days, in the course of 5th pregnancy; left thoracic breast; × 30. Typical plaque. After SQUARTINI and ROSSI (1959b)

No. 8. RIII breeding female aged 354 days, soon after 7th delivery; left thoracic breast; × 17. Plaque in initial regression. After SQUARTINI and ROSSI (1959b)

No. 9. RIII breeding female aged 369 days, some days after 4th delivery; right abdominal breast, × 30. Regressed plaque. After SQUARTINI and ROSSI (1959b)

No. 10. BALB/cf (C3H) breeding female aged 322 days, in the course of 5th pregnancy; right abdominal breast; × 17. Incomplete plaque near to the nipple. After SQUARTINI and ROSSI (1960)

No. 11. BALB/cf (C3H) breeding female aged 279 days, in the course of 4th pregnancy; left thoracic breast; × 17. Small plaque. After SQUARTINI and ROSSI (1960)

No. 12. BALB/cf (C3H) breeding female aged 279 days, in the course of 4th pregnancy; right abdominal breast; × 17. Plaque (in another breast of the same animal of Fig. 11). After SQUARTINI and ROSSI (1960)

Nevertheless, an analysis of the age distribution of tumours in virgin females of the BALB/cf (C3H) strain has revealed that no tumours develop after the 15th month. This fact does not seem due to chance (SQUARTINI and CASCHERA, 1958). This suggests that after the 15th month the factors which promote the development of palpable mammary tumours are ineffective in BALB/cf (C3H) virgin females. An analogous behaviour is observed in RIII virgin females which do not develop tumours beyond the 19th month of life (BARBIERI, CASCHERA and OLIVI, 1958b).

As previously stated the involuted senile breasts of BALB/cf (C3H) virgin females do not contain hyperplastic alveolar nodules which are the habitual sources of tumour development, and this may be the cause of the non occurrence of tumours in old ages. On the other hand, the breasts of RIII virgin females still contain nodules, even beyond the latest cancer ages. This suggests that in the latter animals the failed progression of nodules towards palpable tumours might depend on a deficient hormonal stimulation (BARBIERI, CASCHERA and OLIVI, 1958b). Therefore, it may be supposed that, even if a true menopause does not exist in mice, hormones produced during the irregular estrous cycles of aged females are ineffective on the mammary glands.

B. Histological origins of tumours

The direct origin of tumours from normal breast structures is rare in inbred mice. In several high-cancer strains [including C3H, BALB/cf (C3H), DBA, etc.], as well as in low-cancer strains, mammary tumours usually originate in hyperplastic alveolar nodules (Plate 4). By contrast, in the RIII strain and related hybrids most of the tumours were seen to originate in plaques (Plate 3, No. 13, 14, 16) (FOULDS, 1956b; SQUARTINI and ROSSI, 1959b). As previously stated, the origin of mammary tumours from plaques has been occasionally observed also in mice of those strains which have a predilection for nodule tumorigenesis (SQUARTINI and ROSSI, 1960). Nodules and plaques are alternating, not consecutive, steps in mammary carcinogenesis, and correspond with similar biological stages of development (FOULDS, 1956b). However, apart from the structural differences, they are greatly different because of their size. Nodules are microscopic lesions and therefore cannot be explored clinically, whereas plaques which attain palpable sizes do not escape clinical investigation and are, therefore, more suitable for revealing responsiveness and progression occurring in early stages of mammary neoplasia.

C. Responsiveness and progression of tumours

a) Responsiveness

Most of the mammary tumours which develop in high- and low-cancer-strain mice have been reported to be hormone independent when palpable (MÜHLBOCK, 1958a). However, tumours showing responsiveness to hormones during their early stages of development have also been observed in mice, specially in the RIII strain and related hybrids. The word "responsiveness", although covering a wider range, will be used here only to indicate tumours which modify their growth in relation to pregnancy and puerperium. Most of the recent information concerning responsive mammary tumours in mice derives from FOULDS (1947, 1949b, c, 1954, 1956a, b, c, d, 1958), and refers to hybrid force-bred female mice (RIII × C57b and reciprocal). With few exceptions, these animals possess the milk agent, having derived it from their RIII high-cancer parents (FOULDS, 1949a), and they develop a high percentage of mammary tumours. The tumours are often influenced during their growth by pregnancies occurring in the hosts. A similar behaviour of mammary tumours was later observed in the RIII strain (SQUARTINI and ROSSI, 1959a, b; SQUARTINI, 1962; SQUARTINI and SEVERI, 1962).

Responsiveness to pregnancies may be of three different types (Fig. 1). Responsive tumours of type I grow only during pregnancy and regress completely after parturition. Responsive tumours of type II undergo only a partial regression after delivery and grow to a higher peak during the next pregnancy. Responsive tumours of type III are stationary or slow-growing for long periods of time and show slight waves in their trends at each pregnancy. The tumours which do not modify their growth curves during pregnancy are called unresponsive.

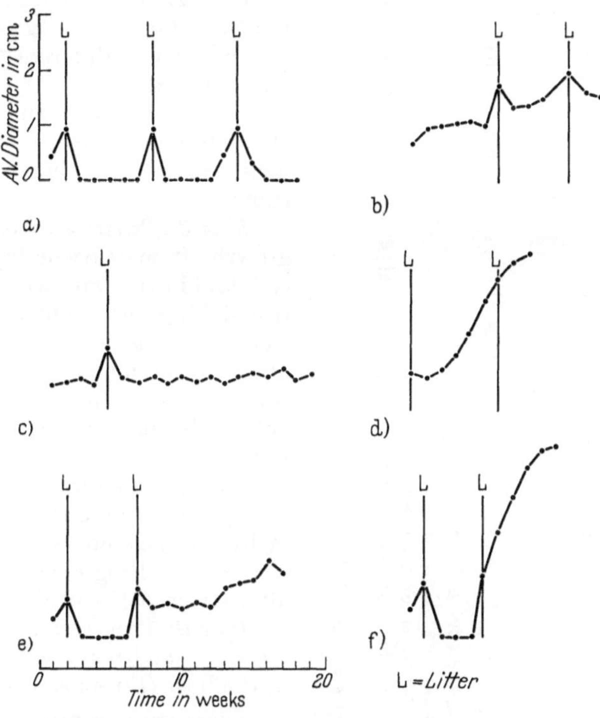

Figure 1. Responsiveness and progression of mammary tumours in inbred mice. (a) RIII breeding female no. 1651; tumour of the left thoracic region. Responsive tumour of type I. (b) RIII breeding female no. 1574; tumour of the left thoracic region. Responsive tumour of type II. (c) RIII breeding female no. 1088; tumour of the right thoracic region. Responsive tumour of type III. (d) BALB/cf (C3H) breeding female no. 1975; tumour of the left groin region. Unresponsive tumour. (e) RIII breeding female no. 1972; tumour of the right groin region. Responsive tumour changing the type of responsiveness during growth. (f) RIII breeding female no. 2060; tumour of the left groin region. Responsive tumour becoming unresponsive during growth. After SQUARTINI and SEVERI (1962)

During their clinical course the responsive tumours may either change the type of responsiveness, from type I to type II or III but not *vice versa*, or they may become unresponsive by progression, which means evolution of neoplasms towards increased autonomy. When transplanted, the responsive tumours maintain their dependence on hormones until autonomy results from progression (FOULDS, 1947, 1949c). Apart from the RIII strain and related hybrids, tumour responsiveness to pregnancy has been occasionally observed in other inbred strains, where it appears to be an unusual event (Table 6: SQUARTINI, 1962; SQUARTINI et al., 1964).

b) Progression: the six rules of FOULDS

Progression may be referred to as the occurrence of stable, heritable and irreversible changes in one or more characteristics of a developing tumour (FOULDS,

Table 6. *Responsiveness to pregnancy of mammary tumours in breeding female mice of three high-cancer strains: C3H, BALB/cf (C3H) and RIII*

Strain	Number of tumour-bearing mice[1]	Number of pregnancies[2]	Number of palpable mammary tumours[3]	Responsive tumours[4]								Unresponsive tumours	
				Type I		Type II		Type III		Total			
				No.	%	No.	%	No.	%	No.	%	No.	%
C3H	23	25	23	1	4.3	3	13.0	—	—	4	17.3	19	82.7
BALB/cf (C3H)	44	48	63	4	6.3	6	9.5	2	3.2	12	19.0	51	81.0
RIII	50	85	66	26	39.4	15	22.7	12	18.2	53	80.3	13	19.7
Total	117	158	152	31	20.4	24	15.8	14	9.2	69	45.4	83	54.6

[1] Only the animals that delivered litters during the clinical course of neoplasms.
[2] Only the pregnancies that occurred after tumour detection.
[3] Only the tumours, during the growth of which pregnancy occurred.
[4] The tumours were classified according to their behaviour during first pregnancy. Several of them changed the type of responsiveness or later became unresponsive.

After SQUARTINI (1962) and SQUARTINI et al. (1964); modified.

1949b, 1954). Such changes may result in an increased growth rate, decreased visible signs of differentiation, increased independence of hormonal influences, a broadening range of transplantability, etc. (KLEIN and KLEIN, 1958b). After careful analysis of hundreds of mouse mammary tumours FOULDS (1949b) proposed the following rules of progression.

Rule 1. Independent progression of multiple tumours: progression occurs independently in different tumours in the same animal.

Rule 2. Independent progression of characters: progression occurs independently in different characters in the same tumour.

Rule 3. Progression is independent of growth: it may occur in latent tumour cells and in tumours whose growth is arrested. Two important corollaries of this rule are: (a) at its first clinical manifestation a tumour may be at any stage of progression; (b) progression is independent of the size or clinical duration of a tumour.

Rule 4. Progression may be continuous or discontinuous, by gradual change or by abrupt steps.

Rule 5. Progression follows one of alternative paths of development.

Rule 6. Progression does not always reach an end-point within the life-time of the host (FOULDS, 1949b).

These rules of progression come from the analysis of the clinical and morphological behaviour of spontaneous mammary tumours in hybrid mice. However, they are general rules, being largely applicable to a number of other tumours, in animals and human beings (FOULDS, 1954).

c) *Histology of responsiveness and progression*

Responsive tumours of type I are pure ductular growths with an organoid structure, or plaques. Near the end of pregnancy the plaques attain full development and show the typical picture recorded above (Plate 2, No. 7, 11, 12). However, slight deviations from the model structure may occur in plaques (Plate 2, No. 10). After delivery the connective tissue overcomes the epithelial structures and plaques regress (Plate 2, No. 8), being replaced by a small, plaque-shaped mass of sclerotic stroma (Plate 2, No. 9). During the next pregnancy plaques resume their growth, and so on, until they modify the type of responsiveness or become unresponsive by progression (FOULDS, 1956b; SQUARTINI and ROSSI, 1959b).

When progression occurs in plaques, it may be focal or diffuse. Focal progression is the most frequent and appears as a small, round-shaped area of varied structure within a plaque (Plate 3, No. 13, 14). Multifocal progression may also occur (Plate 3, No. 16). After each delivery the remnant plaque regresses, but not the central area(s) of focal progression (Plate 3, No. 13–16). Therefore, the clinical course of the tumour is irrevocably changed, depending now on the growth potential and on the level of cellular differentiation of the progressing focus. Diffuse progression is rare and more difficult to recognize.

The partially responsive tumours of types II and III are in part tumours in progression having a slow intrinsic growth rate around which remnant plaques, or new plaques, or plaque-like responsive proliferations occur during pregnancy (Plate 3, No. 13, 14), and in part tumours in progression having a well-differentiated epithelium which undergoes milky secretion in relation to the reproductive activity of host mice (Plate 3, No. 17). Frequently, both conditions are mixed within the same tumour. In the absence of these conditions, the tumours that have arisen in plaques by focal or diffuse progression, behave as unresponsive ones and grow steadily until the death of the animal (FOULDS, 1956b; SQUARTINI and ROSSI, 1959b).

d) Mechanisms of tumour progression

Progression of premalignant changes to malignancy and of responsive tumours towards increased autonomy is the result of subsequent cell changes. It is supposed that these changes do not always follow a single route; in other words, the malignant change may travel along a number of different pathways leading to the same end result, neoplasia, but differing as to its detailed cytological mechanism (KLEIN and KLEIN, 1958a).

It seems to be clear that spontaneous mutations occur continuously in populations of tumour cells. Therefore, a premalignant or malignant cell population does not usually show genetical homogeneity. This results in a competitive proliferation of different cell strains within the same population. If one of these is provided with a greater resistance to environmental stimuli or with a higher reproductive rate, it may overcome the others. In this way the independence of a tumour cell population may progressively increase following successive selections on a mutational basis (KLEIN and KLEIN, 1958b).

Sometimes progression of hormone dependent mammary tumours towards hormone independence might be the result of an acquired ability of neoplastic cells to produce and utilize endogenous substances capable of substituting the exogenous hormonal stimuli previously needed. This assumption comes from having observed that mammary tumours, which had already acquired hormone independence through several successive transplantations, can regress to hormone dependence when the inoculum used is very small. With a small cell number the hormone substituting products elaborated by the transplanted cells may become too much diluted and unable to promote reproduction and "taking", thereby making the cells once more dependent on the exogenous hormonal stimulation. These observations suggest that progression might sometimes depend on cell proliferation *per se*. The population of proliferated cells would depend on an

Plate 3

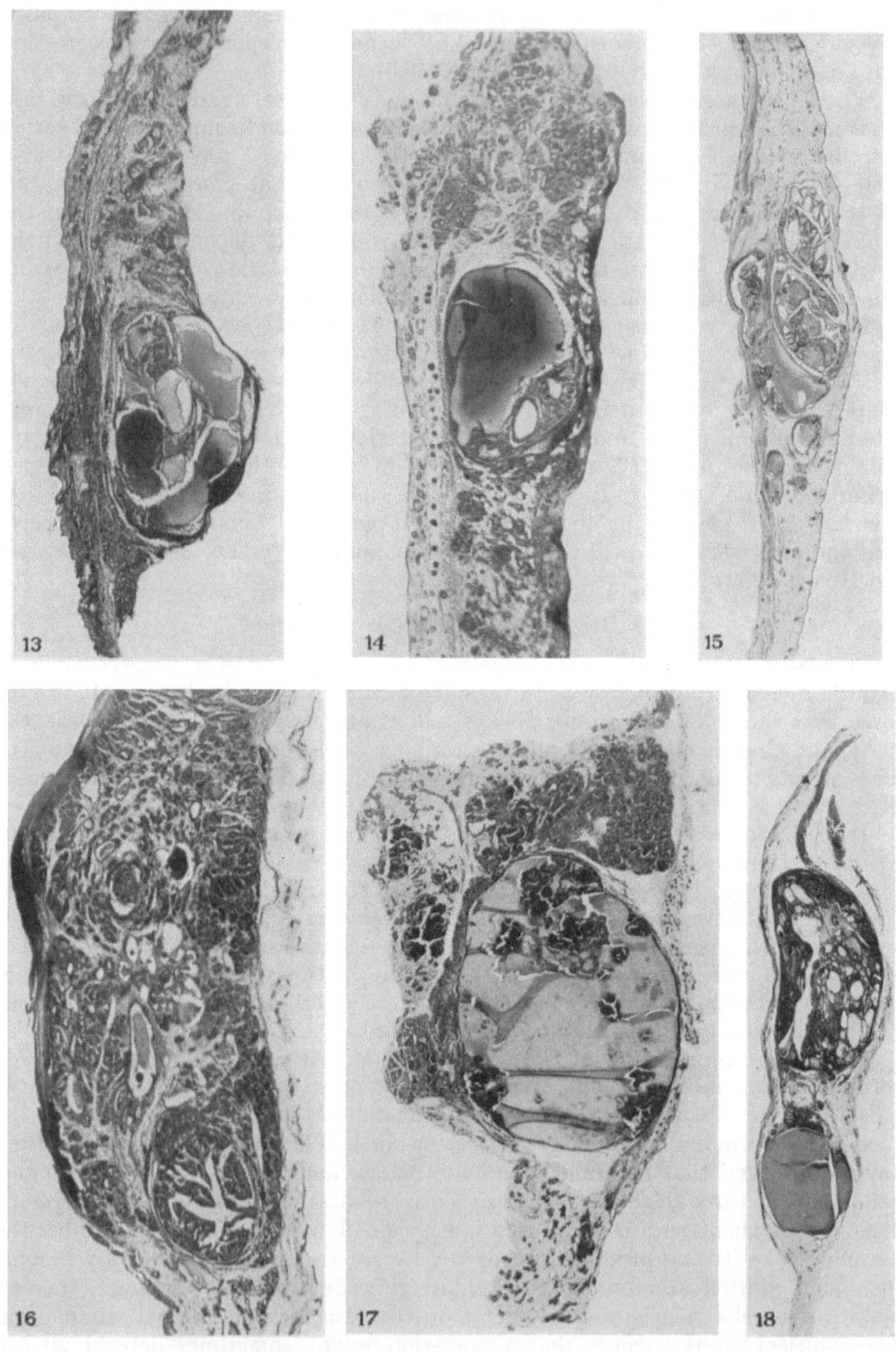

exogenous stimulus for initial growth, until it has reached a certain size, whereafter substances produced by the tumour cells themselves would assume this function, making the tumour more independent (KLEIN and KLEIN, 1958b). However, this interpretation contrasts with the postulated irreversibility of tumour progression.

In other cases tumour progression might be due to either loss of some isoantigens or acquired resistance of tumour cells against the action of some specific isoantibodies (KLEIN and KLEIN, 1958b).

D. Growth rate of tumours

The rates of mammary tumour growth are variable in mice of different strains or even of the same strain. In addition, a change in growth rate may be observed during the clinical course of a tumour as result of progression. However, strain differences in the average mammary tumour growth were found to be significant in some cases (Table 7: SQUARTINI, 1961). Mammary tumours of the C3H strain grow at an average rate of 0.238 cm per week; they are highly malignant. Tumours of the RIII strain show a lower growth rate, 0.135 cm per week and are less malignant in behaviour. Accordingly, even the clinical duration of tumours is different in different strains.

E. Types of tumour growth

Useful information can be derived from the growth curves of tumours in regard to the degree of differentiation, homogeny and independence on extrinsic stimuli of the tumour cell populations. Mammary tumours occurring in high-cancer-strain mice show a variety of types of growth, such as sigmoidal, linear, parabolic and exponential. However, a number of tumours fall into none of those categories of recognizable model curves, because of recurring stops and regressions which make their trends irregular. As for the rate of growth, strain differences have been found even in the predilected type of tumour development (Table 8: SQUARTINI, 1961; for review see SQUARTINI and SEVERI, 1962).

F. Morphology of tumours

The morphological features of mammary tumours in mice are so variable as to discourage any serious attempt at classification based on histology. Nevertheless, at various times different classifications have been suggested (HAALAND, 1911; NICOD, 1936; BONSER, 1946, 1954; DUNN, 1953; CLOUDMAN, 1956; FOULDS, 1956a, c; for review see SEVERI, OLIVI and BIANCIFIORI, 1958). The classification more commonly used today, for its simplicity, is that of DUNN (1953), which is reported below.

The most important morphological feature of mammary tumours in inbred mice with and without MTV is their adenocarcinomatous form. The picture,

---

Plate 3

No. 13. RIII breeding female aged 354 days, 4 days after 4th delivery; left thoracic breast; × 17. Area of focal progression (varied carcinoma) within a regressing plaque. After SQUARTINI and ROSSI (1959b)

No. 14. RIII breeding female aged 354 days, soon after 7th delivery; left thoracic breast, × 17. Multilobular plaque in focal progression (partial reproduction). After SQUARTINI and ROSSI (1959b)

No. 15. RIII breeding female aged 381 days, 51 days after 6th delivery; right thoracic breast; × 15. Varied (cystic-haemorrhagic) carcinoma surrounded by sclerotic stroma. After SQUARTINI and ROSSI (1959b)

No. 16. RIII breeding female aged 218 days, 24 days after 4th delivery; right thoracic breast; × 20. Multifocal progression within the remnants of a plaque. After SQUARTINI and ROSSI (1959b)

No. 17. RIII breeding female aged 283 days, in the course of 2nd pregnancy; left inguinal breast; × 17. Cystic carcinoma with secretion surrounded by multilobular areas of glandular proliferation. After SQUARTINI and ROSSI (1959b)

No. 18. RIII breeding female aged 351 days, 104 days after 3rd delivery; left thoracic breast; × 6. Varied carcinomas: the peculiar aspect of mammary tumours in the RIII strain. After SQUARTINI and ROSSI (1959b)

Plate 4

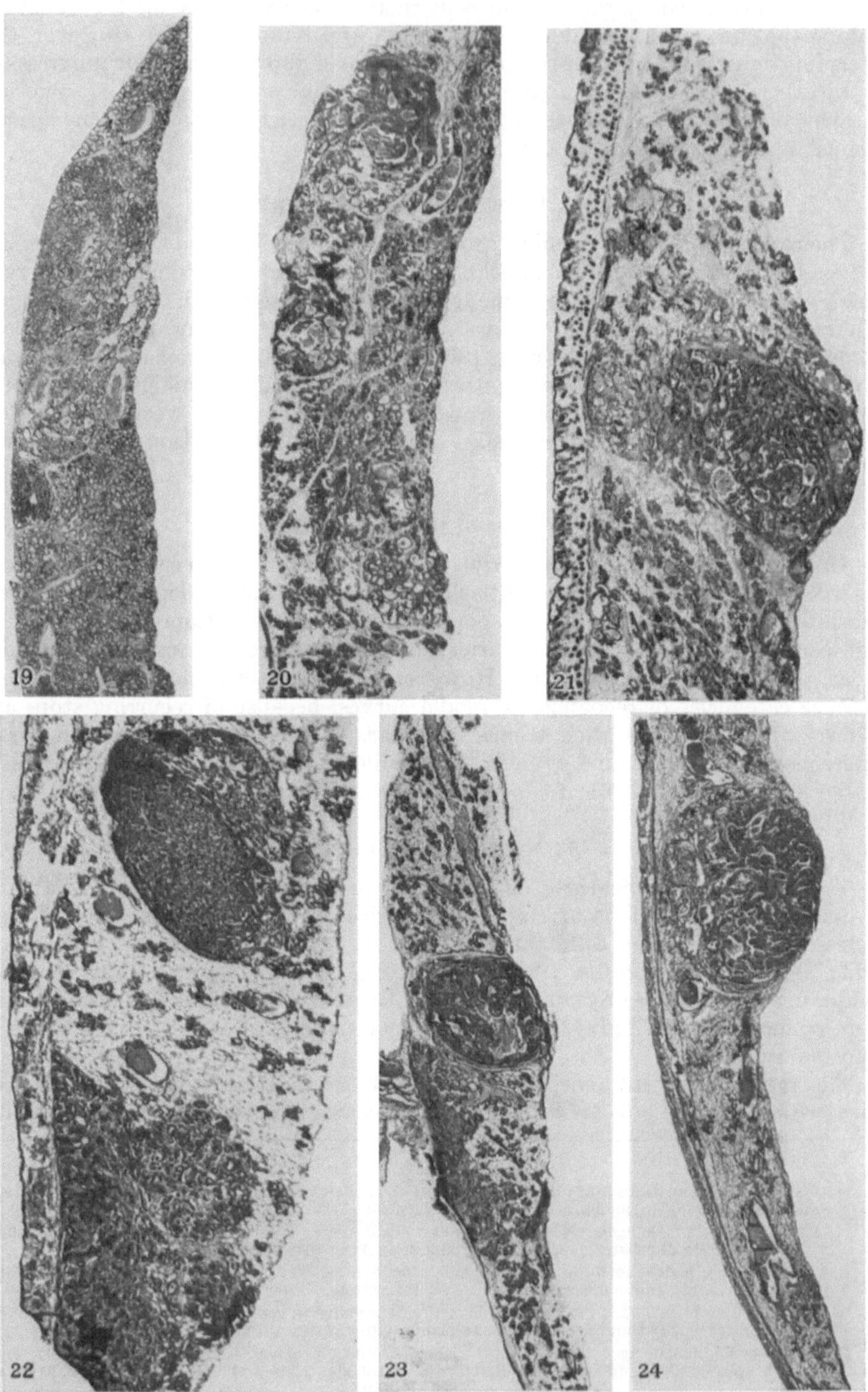

however, is not always the same, as, together with adenocarcinomas of pure alveolar structure (A type: see Plate 4), also papillary-cystic adenocarcinomas showing sometimes areas of solid proliferation and haemorrhages (B type: see Plate 3), micro-cystic adenocarcinomas (C type), mucous adenocarcinomas (M type), adenoacanthomas, and carcinosarcomas can be observed (DUNN, 1953; OLIVI, BIANCIFIORI and BARBIERI, 1955). It must also be remembered that the histology of mammary tumours may be influenced by the causative agents.

G. Metastatic spread of tumours

In various strains of mice most of the mammary tumours show a typical sigmoidal curve. There is an initial phase of slow growth, followed by a rapid growth phase and ending with a further slow phase. This is considered the model curve of independent tumours. Usually, metastases appear during the rapid growth phase of the tumour (MARTINEZ, 1957). Therefore, they do not occur in the preclinical stage nor in the early clinical stage. The autonomy of neoplastic cells seems to increase with time. This is another example of progression occurring in the cancer-cell populations.

Usually, mammary tumours of mice do not metastasize by lymphatic channels. As they spread by the blood stream, they are frequently found in the lungs, but very rarely elsewhere. Lymphatic channels are very small in the mouse and this could explain the absence of lymphatic metastases. Moreover, the early sclerosis associated with tumour formation might cause their occlusion. Another reason may be the short duration of the primary tumour, which might also explain the absence of metastases by the blood stream in organs other than the lungs, usually representing the first step in metastatic spread of mammary cancer. In addition, there is no direct venous connection between the mammary and vertebral circulations in mice, as it is present in woman, which is responsible for many skeletal metastases (CONSOLANDI and VERONESI, 1957, 1958).

8. Comment

Spontaneous mammary tumours of mice are still an inexhaustible source of information for the whole cancer problem. Here is the reason for some recent definitions. Breast has been defined as the fountain of cancer lore (HADDOW, 1958), and mammary tumours of mice as a model in studies on carcinogenesis (SQUARTINI, 1960). The co-existence and interaction, in this particular type of tumours, of all the factors which are known to support spontaneous tumorigenesis (viruses, hormones, genetic factors), make mammary tumours of mice the most valuable material even for an approach to the problems posed by those neoplasms arising in breeding animals from vertical transmission. In the succeeding chapters brief

---

Plate 4

No. 19. BALB/cf (C3H) breeding female aged 342 days, in the course of 5th pregnancy; left thoracic breast; × 17. Gravidic breast with a small area of alveolar carcinoma (dark). After SQUARTINI and ROSSI (1960)

No. 20. BALB/cf (C3H) breeding female aged 288 days, in the course of 2nd pregnancy; right inguinal breast; × 17. Gravidic breast with multiple foci of carcinomatous progression. After SQUARTINI and ROSSI (1960)

No. 21. BALB/cf (C3H) breeding female aged 308 days, in the course of 4th pregnancy; left thoracic breast; × 17. Hyperplastic alveolar nodule in diffuse progression. After SQUARTINI and ROSSI (1960)

No. 22. BALB/cf (C3H) breeding female aged 235 days, in the course of 5th pragnancy; left abdominal breast; × 34. Homogeneous glandular carcinoma (top) and diffuse alveolar proliferation (bottom). After SQUARTINI and ROSSI (1960)

No. 23. BALB/cf (C3H) breeding female aged 308 days, in the course of 4th pregnancy; right inguinal breast; × 17. Microscopic carcinoma arising from a nodule. After SQUARTINI and ROSSI (1960)

No. 24. BALB/cf (C3H) breeding female aged 263 days, 14 days after 5th delivery; right abdominal breast; × 17. Microtubular fissured carcinoma surrounded by the vestigial structures of a nodule. After SQUARTINI and ROSSI (1960)

Table 7. *Rates of mammary tumour growth in breeding female mice of the C3H, BALB/cf (C3H) and RIII strains*

Strain	Number of tumour-bearing mice[1]	Number of palpable mammary tumours[2]	Average initial tumour size (cm)	Tumours divided according to their average growth in cm per week																Average tumour growth per week (cm)	Standard deviation	t
				Stationary or regressing		Progressing																
						0.001 to 0.100		0.101 to 0.200		0.201 to 0.300		0.301 to 0.400		0.401 to 0.500		0.501 to 0.600		0.601 to 0.700				
				No.	%	No.	%	No.	%	No.	%	No.	%	No.	%	No.	%	No.	%			
C3H	50	76	0.6	1	1.3	5	6.7	25	33.8	24	32.4	12	16.2	5	6.7	1	1.3	1	1.3	0.238	0.123	—
BALB/cf (C3H)	133	254	0.7	4	1.6	26	10.5	73	29.5	84	34.0	37	15.0	17	6.9	6	2.4	—	—	0.231	0.121	1.16[3]
RIII	58	75	0.6	4	5.4	29	39.2	23	31.1	10	13.5	8	10.8	—	—	—	—	—	—	0.135	0.108	10.3[4]
Total	241	405	0.7	9	2.3	60	15.2	121	30.6	118	29.9	57	14.4	22	5.6	7	1.8	1	0.2	0.214	0.125	

[1] Only the animals which did not deliver litters during the clinical course of neoplasms.

[2] Ten of these tumours: 2 of the C3H strain, 7 of the BALB/cf (C3H) strain, and 1 of the RIII strain, were discarded, having been measured once only.

[3] $0.3 > P > 0.2$. [4] $P < 0.001$.

After SQUARTINI (1961).

Table 8. *Types of mammary tumour growth in breeding female mice[1] of the C3H, BALB/cf (C3H) and RIII strains*

Strain	Number of palpable mammary tumours	Tumours discarded[2]	Tumours divided according to type of growth												Chi square
			Regular types of growth										Irregular growths		
			Sigmoidal		Linear		Parabolic		Exponential		Total				
			No.	%	No.	%	No.	%	No.	%	No.	%	No.	%	
C3H	76	20	22	39.3	6	10.7	7	12.5	1	1.8	36	64.3	20	35.7	—
BALB/c_f (C3H)	254	72	41	22.5	42	23.1	20	11.0	9	4.9	112	61.5	70	38.5	0.137[3]
RIII	75	15	4	6.7	9	15.0	4	6.7	1	1.6	18	30.0	42	70.0	13.68[4]
Total	405	107	67	22.5	57	19.1	31	10.4	11	3.7	166	55.7	132	44.3	

[1] Only the animals which did not deliver litters during the clinical course of neoplasms have been considered here.

[2] All tumours measured less than 4 times and some tumours measured 4 or 5 times in which the type of growth was not recognizable.

[3] $0.8 > P > 0.7$. [4] $P < 0.001$.

After SQUARTINI (1961).

information will be given on the other types of tumours occurring spontaneously in breeding animals. It will be apparent that the general problems are the same, irrespective of the type and site of tumour development.

IV. The mouse leukaemia and the mouse leukaemia viruses

Studies on mouse leukaemia have received a great impulse after the discovery of a leukaemogenic virus as one of the primary causative factors (Gross, 1951 a, b). A short survey of the main facts concerned with the spontaneous occurrence of leukaemia in inbred mice will be given here. Complete reviews on the etiology and pathogenesis of mouse leukaemia have been published recently (Gross, 1961 a, b; Miller, 1961) and may be consulted for detailed information.

1. High- and low-leukaemic strains

Some strains of mice, such as C58 and AK, exhibit a high incidence of leukaemia. In other strains the incidence of leukaemia is moderately high, whereas in most of the available inbred strains the incidence is low. The latter include A, BALB/c, C3Hf, C57b, CBA, and others. Many of the low-leukaemic strains are susceptible to leukaemia and may develop it when appropriate factors are given. In this respect the situation is analogous to that of mammary tumours in mice, with the difference that high-mammary-tumour strains are usually low-leukaemic strains and *vice versa.*

2. Detection of a leukaemogenic virus in mice: the Gross virus

In 1951 Gross demonstrated that filtrates prepared from spontaneous lymphatic mouse leukaemia reproduce the disease after inoculation into newborn mice of the susceptible C3Hf strain (Gross, 1951 b). In this first experiment the filtrates showed a very low leukaemogenic potency. But after a number of serial passages of leukaemia filtrates into suitable newborn mice the potency of the filtrable agent was greatly increased, as shown by the progressively higher incidence and earlier occurrence of the disease in assay mice (Gross, 1957). As previously stated, the behaviour of MTV is different in this respect (Bittner, 1962). Another difference between leukaemogenic agent and MTV is in the progressive decrease of activity of the former after serial dilutions. When the filtrable agent of leukaemia was analyzed it showed the usual characteristics of a virus (Gross, 1961 a, b).

A. Structure and properties of the leukaemia virus

Leukaemic tissues from high-leukaemic strains and virus-induced leukaemias usually show the presence of extracytoplasmic virus-like particles. These particles have been designated as type C particles (Bernhard and Guérin, 1958 b; Bernhard, 1960). They show a spherical shape, a size around 90 mμ of average diameter (range 60–150 mμ), have a double membrane and an internal electron dense nucleoid. Intracytoplasmic type A particles have also been found in leukaemia, and even type B particles, *i.e.* the MTV, have been seen on occasion in some types of mouse leukaemia (Bernhard and Granboulan, 1962). There is little doubt at present that the C type particle is involved in the leukaemogenic process. The A particles might be the precursors of C particles, in some manner like that suggested for the development of type B particles.

The leukaemia virus is relatively susceptible to heat and is promptly destroyed *in vitro* by ethyl ether. It is well preserved at low temperatures or by lyophilization. Ultracentrifugation and filtration experiments with gradocol membranes suggest that particles which possess leukaemia-inducing activity have a diameter of 70–100 mμ, in contrast with the sizes observed in the electron microscope. The biological activity of leukaemia extracts may be sedimented in about 30 min by ultracentrifugation at 125,000 × g. The virus is moderately antigenic (Gross, 1961a, 1962).

B. Variant strains of leukaemia viruses[1]

After the demonstration of the viral etiology of leukaemia in mice (Gross, 1951b), various investigators attempted to reproduce the original pattern following inoculation of newborn mice with cell-free extracts prepared from various mouse tumours. By this method a number of leukaemia-inducing viruses were detected. Graffi (1957) inoculated newborn mice of the Agnes-Bluhm strain with filtrates of several transplantable tumours of the mouse (Ehrlich ascites carcinoma, Landschutz sarcoma I and II, sarcoma 37); leukaemia developed in 34 to 75% of the test animals, and it was usually of the myelogenous type. Friend (1957), using cell-free extracts prepared from Ehrlich ascites carcinoma and newborn mice of the Swiss stock for bioassay, isolated a viral agent which produces a disease characterized by proliferation of reticulum cells associated with erythroblastosis and lymphocytosis. There is little doubt that this disease belongs to the broad group of leukaemias (Gross, 1961a). Moloney (1960) recovered a leukaemogenic agent from a transplantable mouse sarcoma (sarcoma 37). This agent, like the Gross virus, induces lymphoid leukaemia. Rauscher (1962) isolated a potent leukaemogenic virus from BALB/c mice, which induces a disease characterized by rapid and extreme proliferation of erythrocytic and leukocytic elements. Leukaemia-inducing viruses have also been isolated from radiation-induced leukaemias (Lieberman and Kaplan, 1959), but not from leukaemias induced by chemical carcinogens (Miller, 1961). In addition, a number of other leukaemogenic agents, recovered from different sources, have been reported recently by various investigators (see Sinkovics, Shullenberger and Clifton, 1964).

All these viruses show similar characters and properties, though differing from each other in some property. Electron microscopic studies seem to confirm that they belong to the same family or group (Bernhard and Granboulan, 1962). As stated above, the cytological and morphological characters of the diseases induced by each of these viruses may be considerably different. It has been shown, however, that the morphology of virus-induced leukaemias is at least in part dependent on host factors, being influenced by various treatments of the recipient hosts, such as removal of the thymus, spleen, etc. (see Fiore-Donati and Chieco-Bianchi, 1964).

C. Natural transmission of leukaemia virus and distribution in the host

In the first experiments concerned with the transmission of leukaemia in high-leukaemic strains the hypothesis of an extrachromosomal transmission of the disease, like that demonstrated for mouse mammary tumours, was tested, but with negative results since foster-nursing of high-leukaemic litters by low-leukaemic mothers did not prevent the occurrence of the disease (Barnes and Cole, 1941). Many years later this fact could be explained. Embryos removed from normal healthy mice of the high-leukaemic AK strain proved to contain the leukaemogenic virus on bioassay (Gross, 1951a). This means that in certain mouse strains the virus of leukaemia is transmitted from generation to generation through

[1] Further details, see Graffi, Vol. I: Erzeugung von Tumoren durch Virus.

the embryos (GROSS, 1951a). However, recent experiments with potent leukaemia viruses have shown that infected mothers transmit the disease, whereas infected fathers do not (GROSS, 1962), and that vertical transmission of the virus through the maternal line may occur by the following natural routes: (a) infection of the embryo prior to placenta formation, (b) infection of the foetus across the placental barrier, and (c) infection of the newborn through the milk (MOLONEY, 1962).

There is little information about the fate of leukaemia virus after its introduction into susceptible hosts. Preliminary experiments have shown the presence of the virus in blood plasma, leukaemic liver, thymus, spleen, mesenteric and peripheral lymphnodes (GROSS, 1961a).

3. Other factors involved in the etiology of mouse leukaemia

Apart from viruses, other factors are important in the causation of leukaemia. These include genetic and hormonal factors, the thymic factor, and some minor ones such as the environmental factors.

A. Genetic factors

The rôle of genetic factors in the occurrence of spontaneous leukaemia was early investigated by means of crosses between high- and low-leukaemic strains. At that time the viral etiology of leukaemia was unknown. In addition, no strains are available entirely free from leukaemia. These facts made extremely difficult both planning and interpretation of the experiments. The incidence of leukaemia in the F_1 hybrids obtained by mating high- to low-leukaemic animals was found to be intermediate and it was usually the same for reciprocal crosses, whereas the frequency of leukaemia in the successive generations appeared to be a function of the total heredity contributed by the high-leukaemic strain. Backcross of F_1 hybrids, leukaemic and non leukaemic, to the low-leukaemic parent gave rise to the same incidence of the disease in offspring, but results obtained by mating backcross males to low-leukaemic females suggested that segregation was occurring for genes influencing susceptibility to leukaemia (MACDOWELL, POTTER and TAYLOR, 1945; see LAW, 1954; see MILLER, 1961). The importance of genetic factors in the development of leukaemia is also shown by the strain specificity of various leukaemogenic agents (physical, chemical, hormonal agents and viruses), and by the practical impossibility to eliminate leukaemia from high-leukaemic strains even after transfer of fertilized ova (FEKETE and OTIS, 1954), or to establish it in low-leukaemic strains. All these facts have been recently summarized and discussed by MILLER (1961), who suggests that the genetic constitution could determine the degree of tissue susceptibility to leukaemia virus and control the mechanisms of virus transmission from parents to offspring.

B. Hormonal factors

A number of endocrine factors may affect leukaemogenesis in mice, either spontaneous or induced. The activity of these factors may result in an increase, acceleration, decrease, delay, or inhibition of the development of spontaneous leukaemia. The same factors are known to influence the behaviour of normal lymphatic tissue. Although consistent strain differences have been detected in the response of lymphatic organs to hormones, present knowledge in this field may be shortly summarized as follows.

The incidence of spontaneous lymphomas or lymphoid leukaemias is usually higher in females than in males (LAW, 1947). Virgin females are more prone to develop leukaemia than breeding females (Squartini and Rossi, 1964b). Ovariectomy may inhibit or decrease the incidence of lymphomas (McEndy, Boon and Furth, 1944), or even be without effect (Law, 1947). Estrogens are leukaemogenic for some low-leukaemic strains and increase leukaemia incidence in high-leukaemic strains (Murphy and Sturm, 1949), their activity depending on the dosage. In addition, estrogens enhance the leukaemogenic activity of chemical and physical (X-rays) carcinogens (Kirschbaum, Saphiro and Mixer, 1953). Orchidectomy either increases or accelerates the occurrence of spontaneous leukaemia (Law, 1947). Accordingly, the administration of testosterone greatly reduces leukaemia incidence in AKR high-leukaemic mice (Murphy, 1944).

Adrenal corticoids have a great influence on both normal lymphatic tissues and leukaemogenesis. Adrenalectomy is followed by hypertrophy of the lymphoid tissues, and significantly enhances spontaneous development of lymphomas (Law, 1947). The state of adrenal hypofunction detected in AKR mice might therefore account for their high leukaemia incidence (Metcalf, 1960). Injection of cortisol, which causes acute involution of the normal lymphoid tissue, also inhibits the induction of leukaemia by various agents and delays the development of spontaneous lymphomas (Upton and Furth, 1954). In contrast with these facts, prolonged administration of ACTH increases the incidence of spontaneous lymphomas in C57b mice (Silberberg and Silberberg, 1955). Thyroid hormones are also involved in leukaemogenesis, although it is not clear whether their influence is direct, or whether it is dependent on the general effects of these hormones on the host metabolism and body weight (Grad, 1957). The pituitary does not appear to be essential for the development of lymphomas in mice (Miller, 1961). Hypophysectomy does not prevent nor reduces the occurrence of spontaneous and induced leukaemia (Law, 1957; Nagareda and Kaplan, 1955). Accordingly, there is no evidence for any effect of the growth hormone on the genesis of lymphomas in mice (Kaplan, Nagareda and Brown, 1954; Miller, 1961).

With the only exception of estrogens, hormones causing thymus involution were found to inhibit leukaemogenesis. By contrast, endocrine treatments resulting in thymus hypertrophy were found to increase leukaemia incidence (Kaplan, Nagareda and Brown, 1954; for review see Miller, 1961).

C. The thymic factor

The thymus is an essential organ for the development of spontaneous leukaemia in mice. Total thymectomy almost completely prevents the occurrence of lymphatic leukaemia. Conversely, the subcutaneous implant of thymuses in thymectomized mice restores leukaemia development (see Miller, 1961). However, mice injected with Gross leukaemia virus and then thymectomized may sometimes develop myelogenous leukaemia later in life, a form which is never observed in virus-injected, intact hosts (Gross, 1962). The rôle of the thymus in mouse leukaemogenesis is obscure, although several hypotheses have been suggested. To explain the drastic effect of thymectomy on the occurrence of spontaneous leukaemia, the thymus was supposed to be: (a) the source of leukaemogenic virus, (b) the site of multiplication of such a virus, (c) the tissue most susceptible to leukaemia transformation, (d) the source of a humoral factor involved in leukaemogenesis (Miller, 1961). The first three hypotheses were found to be inconsistent, whereas the fourth has received some experimental evidence (see Miller, 1961).

Lymphopoietic activity of the thymus greatly exceeds that of other lymphoid tissues, and extracts of this organ were found to produce a temporary lymphocytosis when injected (METCALF, 1956, 1957). These results have not been confirmed as yet. In addition, the relations of this thymic lymphocytosis stimulating factor to leukaemogenesis have to be clarified. Recent data, which are indicative for the possible existence of a lymphocytosis stimulating factor liberated by thymic transplants but not present or active in thymic extracts, have also led to the conclusion that something more than a mere diffusible humoral thymic factor is required to determine neoplastic change in lymphocytes when all the other known factors are effective (MILLER, 1962).

D. Environmental factors

Like many other experimental tumours, even the mouse leukaemia is influenced by nutritional factors. Caloric restriction of the diet, or reduction in the amount of sulphur-containing aminoacids in the diet, strongly reduce the incidence of spontaneous or induced leukaemia (WHITE and MIDER, 1943; WHITE et al., 1944). The mechanisms of this action of nutritional factors are unknown, although mediation through the endocrine glands may be supposed. The effects of other environmental factors on mouse leukaemia have not been investigated so far.

V. Hepatomas in mice

Various sublines of the C3H strain (C3H/He[1], C3Hf/He, C3He/De[2]), either with or without MTV have recently shown a high and increasing incidence of spontaneous hepatomas. Since its establishment the C3H strain has been considered to be the highest hepatoma strain available. But early reports on the spontaneous occurrence of liver tumours in this strain described incidences much lower than those observed in recent studies. ANDERVONT in 1941, for his C3H substrain raised at the National Cancer Institute (NCI), published an incidence of 27% in males and 10% in females. DERINGER in 1959, for her C3He/De substrain also raised at the NCI, has reported incidences of hepatomas ranging from 30% in breeding females to 90.5% in males. In 1960 HESTON, VLAHAKIS and DERINGER have reported the following incidences of hepatomas for males of the three C3H substrains mentioned above (all raised at the NCI): C3H/He = 85%; C3Hf/He = 72%; C3He/De = 78%.

A search for the causes of this increased incidence of hepatomas among C3H mice raised at the NCI showed that a part of the increase was undoubtedly due to the diet of NCI pellets. When the animals were fed with a different diet (Purina laboratory chow), the incidence of hepatomas was significantly lower (HESTON, VLAHAKIS and DERINGER, 1960). However, the 57% incidence of hepatomas found in males fed Purina laboratory chow was still considerably higher than the 27% incidence reported by ANDERVONT (1941) in males fed Purina dog chow. This fact suggests the possibility of some genetic change affecting the incidence of hepatomas in C3H strain (HESTON, VLAHAKIS and DERINGER, 1960). The MTV present in one of the substrains examined but not in the others, is apparently not involved in the development of hepatomas.

Apart from the higher incidence of hepatomas in males than in females of the C3H strain, other data suggest the importance of hormonal factors in the development of liver tumours. Hypophysectomy was found to prevent completely the development of spontaneous hepatomas in highly susceptible $(C3H \times YBR)F_1$ hybrid male mice (HESTON, 1963). The adrenal glands have been reported to be involved in liver carcinogenesis, since adrenalectomy may inhibit the occurrence

[1] He = maintained by HESTON.
[2] De = maintained by DERINGER.

of hepatomas by azo-dyes in rats (EVERSOLE, 1957, 1958). In conclusion, at least three factors seem to be involved in the development of spontaneous hepatomas in rodents: genetic, hormonal, and nutritional factors. To date, a virus has not been searched in high-hepatoma lines of the C3H strain.

VI. Tumours of the lung

Spontaneous development of pulmonary tumours is frequent in inbred mice. As for the other tumour types, there are however pronounced strain differences in the incidence of lung tumours. The highest incidence of pulmonary tumours has been reported for mice of strain A, the figure being from 80 to 90% in animals living 18 months or longer (BITTNER, 1939c). When dibenzanthracene is given by subcutaneous injection, practically all young mice of this strain develop multiple tumours of the lungs within two months, showing that a close relationship exists between development of spontaneous tumours and susceptibility to induced neoplasms (ANDERVONT, 1937). Moderate incidences of spontaneous lung tumours were also found in other strains of mice. In the BALB/c strain spontaneous tumours of the lung were observed in 24% of the animals autopsied at an average age of 21 months (ANDERVONT and DUNN, 1948b). In various sublines of the C3H strain, either with or without MTV, the incidence of pulmonary tumours ranges from 4.6 to 12.7% (HESTON, VLAHAKIS and DERINGER, 1960). Mice of strain L rarely develop this neoplasm (HESTON, 1942a). Pulmonary tumours of mice are adenomatous and almost always identical in appearance (STEWART, 1958). They may undergo malignant transformation by progression (BIANCIFIORI et al., 1963).

Studies on the genetics of mouse pulmonary tumours, by means of crosses between high- (A) and low-pulmonary-tumour (L) strains and analysis of F_1, F_2 and backcross hybrid generations, have shown that genetic factors are involved in the susceptibility to induced tumours, as well as in the development of spontaneous neoplasms (HESTON, 1942a, b). The genetic factors influencing susceptibility to lung tumours are multiple, and the site of gene action seems to be directly localized in the lung tissue (HESTON and DUNN, 1951). HESTON (1942a, b) also estimated that 86% of the susceptibility to pulmonary tumours depended upon genetic factors, and 14% upon non genetic factors, the latter being environmental factors (see STEWART, 1958). Among these, the diet was shown to have some importance (HESTON, VLAHAKIS and DERINGER, 1960). Possible influences of hormones and viruses in the causation of spontaneous lung tumours of mice have not been demonstrated. However, a form of infectious pulmonary adenomatosis, which is related to lung cancer and supposed to be virus-induced, has been described in the sheep (see DURAN-REYNALS, 1958).

VII. Other tumours

A group of miscellaneous tumours may be occasionally observed in old inbred mice or in other laboratory rodents. It is perhaps surprising that tumours of the stomach and digestive tract in general, which represent the commonest malignant growths in man, are extremely rare in the animals. This probably means that exogenous factors, specially chemical carcinogens in the diet, play an essential rôle in their causation. However, gastric cancer may be induced in mice by various carcinogenic treatments (see STEWART, 1953a). The same considerations may apply, with due changes, to tumours of the skin, urinary tract and kidneys in mice and other laboratory animals.

With few exceptions, spontaneous tumours of the endocrine glands and related end organs (other than breasts), are also rare in laboratory animals, in spite of their easy induction by a number of experimental means. Spontaneous pituitary adenomas, ovarian, testicular, and adrenal tumours have been sometimes observed. Spontaneous, prolactin-secreting pituitary adenomas have been reported to occur in females of a new strain, NZY, where 81% of virgins and 91% of breeders undergo spontaneous hyperplasia of the pituitary mainly supported by prolactin-secreting cells (BIELSCHOWSKY, BIELSCHOWSKY and LINDSAY, 1956). Females of this strain show also hyperplastic breasts and have a high incidence of mammary tumours ranging from 33% in virgins to 65% in breeders. By contrast, uterus undergoes marked atrophy. Ovariectomy prevents pituitary enlargement, pituitary adenomas and mammary cancer, but induces a high incidence of adrenal tumours (BIELSCHOWSKY, 1958). The spontaneous development of some complex hormonal imbalance in animals of this strain is apparent, although it has still to be elucidated.

SLYE, HOLMES and WELLS (1920) found only 44 cases of ovarian tumours among 22,000 mice autopsied, 38 of which were benign. A very low incidence of spontaneous ovarian tumours has also been reported for rats (IGLESIAS, STERNBERG and SEGALOFF, 1950). Leydig-cell tumours of the testis are also rare in mice and rats (GARDNER et al., 1953). However, an exceptional strain of mice has been described, the H strain, in which males develop spontaneous testicular tumours of the Leydig-cell type, and also mammary tumours (FURTADO-DIAS, 1958). Also the adrenal tumours, either cortical or medullary, are rare to occur in rodents as spontaneous neoplasms, the only exception being phaeochromocytomata which occur in aged rats of several colonies and both sexes with variable and sometimes high frequency (GILLMAN, GILBERT and SPENCE, 1953). Prostatic cancer does not arise spontaneously in laboratory animals, except the dog, although benign enlargement of the gland may be caused to develop by administration of estrogens (BURROWS, 1949). Estrogens have also an inexplicable carcinogenic action on the hamster kidney (see BIELSCHOWSKY and HORNING, 1958).

Spontaneous uterine tumours have rarely been found in very old female mice and rats, but rabbits are exceptional in this respect. Endometrial carcinoma is a common spontaneous tumour in rabbits, accounting for 50% of the neoplasms observed in this species (STEWART, 1953b). The total incidence in a large female population two or more years of age was found to be 17%, but it raised up to 80% in animals of five or six years (GREENE and SAXTON, 1938; GREENE, 1941). Genetic factors and hormonal disorders are involved in the causation of these malignant tumours. Usually these animals undergo severe toxemia during pregnancy which causes liver damage. The subsequent impairment of the estrogen-inactivating function of the liver, resulting in an increase of estrogen level in the blood stream, is believed to play an important rôle in the development of uterine neoplasms (GREENE, 1937, 1938, 1941; GREENE and SAXTON, 1938; GREENE and NEWTON, 1948; see STEWART, 1953b).

Malignant tumours of the bones, though rare, may sporadically be observed in inbred mice (PYBUS and MILLER, 1940; LIPPINCOTT et al., 1942). There is, however, a report in the older literature which deserves particular mention. PYBUS and MILLER (1938, 1940) established an inbred strain of mice with a high incidence of spontaneous bone tumours, greater in females (77.3%) than in males (29.6%). Bone tumours were osteogenic sarcomas. Treatment with estrogen reduced the latent period of tumour development in males, causing also a kind of benign bone lesions which regressed after removal of the hormone. Conversely, ovariectomy considerably delayed the appearance of palpable tumours in females (MILLER,

Orr and Pybus, 1943). The relation of these tumours to hormonal and genetic factors was apparent. Unfortunately, the strain showing high-bone-tumour incidence suddenly failed to develop further tumours for unknown reasons, thus causing the loss of an extremely valuable experimental material (see Bielschowsky and Horning, 1958).

VIII. Conclusive comment

The model problems of mammary tumours in mice, including the relations of these tumours to the MTV, have been reviewed and discussed in detail. A shorter survey has been dedicated to mouse leukaemia and the related viruses. Additional information concerning mouse hepatomas, lung tumours, and other spontaneous tumours of the laboratory animals have been given. Comparison of all these materials leads to the conclusion that, though the mechanisms may be remarkably different, the factors involved in spontaneous tumorigenesis are invariably the same. Four different groups of causative factors may be recognized at present, which include genetic factors, hormonal factors, tumour-inducing viruses and, to a lesser extent, environmental factors.

Genetic factors may act through many different routes: increasing the susceptibility of particular tissues to a tumour-inducing virus or to hormonal stimuli, controlling the vertical transmission of viruses, increasing the production and release of hormones by some endocrine glands, favouring endocrine imbalances, affecting the metabolism of the animals, etc. Also the hormonal factors may display different activities in tumorigenesis: their growth-stimulating activity has long been considered and still appears to be the most important in relation to tumour development; but recently hormones were also shown to increase the production and release of particular tumour-inducing viruses by some normal cells. The mechanism of action of viruses as tumour-inducing agents is still obscure, although there is evidence that some of them might act by increasing the sensitivity of particular tissues to hormones. This and the previous sentence clearly indicate the close linkage which should exist between hormones and viruses in tumorigenesis. The environmental factors, including diet, are marginal factors in spontaneous tumorigenesis; they usually act through the endocrine system. With the exception of the last, marginal factors all the other factors involved in spontaneous tumorigenesis are acquired by vertical transmission, from generation to generation.

None of these factors is able to cause spontaneous tumour development when acting alone. This means that at least two causative factors are involved in any example of spontaneous tumorigenesis, one of these being a genetic factor. When three or more factors are effective, the tumour incidence is remarkably increased.

One of the most outstanding aspects connected with the analysis of spontaneous tumorigenesis in inbred mice is the almost ubiquitous diffusion of some tumour-inducing viruses. Although considerable progress has recently been achieved, many problems have still to be solved along this line. First of all, the difference which seems to exist in this respect between mouse and man. Laboratory animals are an incredible source of spontaneous tumorigenesis. The reasons for this fact have in part to be explained. Inbreeding is certainly important in this respect, although we do not know to what extent. Spontaneous tumours in animals are the closest to human neoplasms that we presently know. This makes their study important. In reviewing the results of more than half century the impression was that this study has just begun.

References

AMANO, S., and Y. ICHIKAWA: Electron microscopical aspects of developing modes of the cancer virus and the problem of "pseudovirus particles". Acta Path. Japan 9, 455—479 (1959).

ANDERVONT, H. B.: Pulmonary tumors in mice. I. The susceptibility of the lungs of albino mice to the carcinogenic action of 1,2,5,6-dibenzanthracene. Publ. Hlth Rep. Wash. 52, 212—221(1937).

— The influence of foster nursing upon the incidence of spontaneous mammary cancer in resistant and susceptible mice. J. nat. Cancer Inst. 1, 147—153 (1940).

— Spontaneous tumors in a subline of strain C3H mice. J. nat. Cancer Inst. 1, 737—744 (1941).

— Influence of environment on mammary cancer in mice. J. nat. Cancer Inst. 4, 579—581 (1944).

— Fate of the C3H milk influence in mice of strains C and C57 black. J. nat. Cancer Inst. 5, 383—390 (1945).

— The incidence of mammary tumors in mice of strains C3H and in descendants of fostered strain C. J. nat. Cancer Inst. 10, 193—200 (1949).

— Disappearance of the mammary tumor agent from RIII mice. Acta Un. int. Cancr. 15, 124—127 (1959).

— *In utero* transmission of the mouse mammary tumor agent. J. nat. Cancer Inst. 31, 261—272 (1963).

—, and W. R. BRYAN: Properties of the mouse mammary tumor agent. J. nat. Cancer Inst. 5, 143—149 (1944).

—, and T. B. DUNN: Mammary tumours in mice presumably free of the mammary tumor agent. J. nat. Cancer Inst. 8, 227—233 (1948a).

— — Efforts to detect a mammary-tumor agent in strain C mice. J. nat. Cancer Inst. 8, 235—240 (1948b).

— — Studies on the mammary-tumor agent of strain RIII mice. J. nat. Cancer Inst. 28, 159—185 (1962).

—, and W. J. MCELENEY: The influence of foster nursing upon the incidence of spontaneous breast cancer in strain C3H mice. Publ. Hlth Rep. (Wash.) 54, 1597—1603 (1939).

— — Effect of ingestion of strain C3H milk in the production of mammary tumors in strain C3H mice of different ages. J. nat. Cancer Inst. 2, 13—16 (1941).

— M. B. SHIMKIN, and W. R. BRYAN: Technique suitable for quantitative studies on the mammary tumor inciter of mice. J. nat. Cancer Inst. 3, 309—318 (1942).

ARMSTRONG, E. C.: Observations on the nature of the oestrous cycle and on the effect upon it of the milk factor, in mice of two inbred strains, differing in mammary cancer incidence. Brit. J. Cancer 2, 59—69 (1948).

ARMSTRONG, M. I., and A. W. HAM: Demonstration of milk factor in a C3H mouse mammary tumor after the tumor had been transferred 31 times in fertile eggs. Cancer Res. 10, 201—202 (1950).

AUB, J. C., D. KARNOFSKI, and L. E. TOWNE: Sex hormone excretion rates in high and low tumor strains of mice. Cancer Res. 1, 737—741 (1941).

BAGG, H. J.: Functional activity of the mammary gland in relation to extrachromosomal influence in the incidence of mammary tumors. Science 83, 374—375 (1936a).

— Further studies on the relation of functional activity to mammary carcinoma in mice. Amer. J. Cancer 27, 542—550 (1936b).

BANG, F. B., and H. B. ANDERVONT: Detection of the mammary tumor inciter (M.T.I.) in thin sections of spontaneous mouse tumors. J. appl. Physics 24, 1418 (1953).

— —, and I. VELLISTO: Electron microscopic evidence concerning the mammary tumor inciter (virus). II. An electron microscopic study of the spntaneous and induced mammary tumors of mice. Bull. Johns Hopk. Hosp. 98, 287—308 (1956).

— I. VELLISTO, and R. LIBERT: Electron microscopic evidence concerning the mammary tumor inciter (virus). I. A study of normal and malignant cells from the mammary gland of mice. Bull. Johns Hopk. Hosp. 98, 255—285 (1956).

BARBIERI, G., F. CASCHERA e M. OLIVI: La fase precancerosa morfologica: i noduli di iperplasia alveolare nella mammella del topo (RIII/Dm/Se substrain). Lav. Ist. Anat. Univ. Perugia 18, 89—106 (1958a).

— — — I noduli di iperplasia alveolare della mammella nelle femmine del topo, vecchie e vergini (RIII/Dm/Se e BALB/cf C3H/Cb/Se). Lav. Ist. Anat. Univ. Perugia 18, 125—135 (1958b).

— e M. OLIVI: Il numero dei parti nelle femmine del topo appartenenti a "inbred strains" con diversa incidenza di cancro mammario, sottoposte al "forced breeding". Lav. Ist. Anat. Univ. Perugia 18, 149—153 (1958).

BARNES, W. A., and R. K. COLE: The effect of nursing on the incidence of spontaneous leukemia and tumors in mice. Cancer Res. 1, 99—101 (1941).

BARNUM, C. P., Z. B. BALL, J. J. BITTNER, and M. B. VISSCHER: The milk agent in spontaneous mammary carcinoma. Science **100**, 575—576 (1944).

—, and R. A. HUSEBY: The chemical and physical characteristics of preparations containing the milk agent virus: A review. Cancer Res. **10**, 523—529 (1950).

BASHFORD, R. F.: The incidence of cancer of the mamma in female mice of known age. Proc. Roy. Soc. B **81**, 310—323 (1909).

BENEDETTI, E. L., and W. BERNHARD: Recherches ultrastructurales sur le virus de la léucemie érythroblastique du poulét. J. Ultrastr. Res. **1**, 309—336 (1958).

BERN, H. A.: Relation between sensitivity to lactogenic hormones and tumorigenesis in hyperplastic mammary nodules in C3H/Crgl mice. Proc. Soc. exp. Biol. (N. Y.) **112**, 864—866 (1963).

— K. B. DEOME, M. ALFERT, and D. R. PITELKA: Morphologic and physiologic characterization of hyperplastic nodules in the mammary glands of the C3H/He Crgl mouse. In: Proceedings of the II International Symposium on Mammary Cancer, pp. 565—573, L. Severi ed., Division of Cancer Research, Perugia 1958.

—, and S. NANDI: Recent studies of the hormonal influence in mouse mammary tumorigenesis. In: Progress in Tumor Research, Vol. 2, pp. 90—144. F. Homburger ed. New York: S. Karger 1961.

BERNHARD, W.: Electron microscopy of tumor cells and tumor viruses. A review. Cancer Res. **18**, 491—509 (1958).

— The detection and study of tumor viruses with the electron microscope. Cancer Res. **20**, 712—727 (1960).

— A. BAUER, M. GUÉRIN et C. OBERLING: Etude au microscope électronique de corpuscules d'aspect virusal dans des épithéliomas mammaires de la souris. Bull. Cancer **42**, 163—178 (1955).

—, and N. GRANBOULAN: Morphology of oncogenic and non-oncogenic mouse viruses. In: A Ciba Foundation Symposium on Tumour Viruses of Murine Origin, pp. 6—55, G. E. W. WOLSTENHOLME and M. O'CONNOR eds., London: J. & A. Churchill Ltd. 1962.

—, et M. GUÉRIN: Evaluation quantitative du virus dans les tumeurs mammaires spontanées ou graffées de différentes souches de souris et étude de ses rapports avec l'appareil de Golgi. In: Proceedings of the II International Symposium on Mammary Cancer, pp. 627—639, L. SEVERI ed., Division of Cancer Research, Perugia 1958a.

— — Présence de particules d'aspect virusal dans les tissus tumoraux de souris atteintes de leucémie spontanée. C. R. Acad. Sci. (Paris) **247**, 1802—1805 (1958b).

— — et C. OBERLING: Mise en évidence de corpuscules d'aspet virusal dans différentes souches de cancers mammaires de la souris. Acta Un. int. Cancr. **12**, 544—557 (1956).

BIANCIFIORI, C., E. BUCCIARELLI, F. E. SANTILLI e R. RIBACCHI: Cancerogenesi polmonare da idrazide dell'acido isonicotinico (INI) e suoi metaboliti in topi CBA/Cb/Se substrain. Lav. Ist. Anat. Univ. Perugia **23**, 209—220 (1963).

— G. LOTTI, and C. MARTINEZ: Incidence of spontaneous mammary carcinoma in hybrid mice (C3H/Cb/Se × BALB/c_fC/Cb/Se) from the 1st to the 7th generation. In: Proceedings of the II International Symposium on Mammary Cancer, pp. 419—422, L. SEVERI ed., Division of Cancer Research, Perugia 1958.

—, e F. SQUARTINI: Tumori mammari in ibridi suscettibili trattati con sperma di maschi ad alta incidenza. Lav. Ist. Anat. Univ. Perugia **18**, 137—140 (1958).

BIELSCHOWSKY, F.: Breast cancer and hyperplasia of the prolactin-secreting cells of the adenohypophysis in NZY mice. In: Proceedings of the II International Symposium on Mammary Cancer, pp. 481—489, L. SEVERI ed., Division of Cancer Research, Perugia 1958.

— and E. S. HORNING: Aspects of endocrine carcinogenesis. Brit. med. Bull. **14**, 106—115 (1958).

BIELSCHOWSKY, M., F. BIELSCHOWSKY, and D. LINDSAY: A new strain of mice with a high incidence of mammary cancers and enlargement of the pituitary. Brit. J. Cancer **10**, 688—699 (1956).

BITTNER, J. J.: Some possible effects of nursing on the mammary gland tumor incidence in mice. Science **84**, 162—163 (1936).

— Breast cancer and mother's milk. J. Hered. **28**, 363—365 (1937).

— Relation of nursing to the extrachromosomal theory of breast cancer in mice. Amer. J. Cancer **35**, 90—97 (1939a).

— The influence of transplanted normal tissue on breast cancer ratios in mice. Publ. Hlth Rep. (Wash.) **54**, 1827—1831 (1939b).

— Breast and lung carcinoma in "A" stock mice. Publ. Hlth Rep. (Wash.) **54**, 380—392 (1939c).

— Further studies on active milk influence in breast cancer production in mice. Proc. Soc. exp. Biol. (N. Y.) **45**, 804—810 (1940).

BITTNER, J. J.: The preservation by freezing and drying in vacuo of the milk influence for the development of breast cancer in mice. Science **93**, 527—528 (1941a).
— Changes in the incidence of mammary carcinoma in mice of the A stock. Cancer Res. **1**, 113—114 (1941b).
— The influence of foster nursing on experimental breast cancer. Trans. Coll. Phycns Philad. **9**, 129—143 (1941c).
— The milk influence of breast tumors in mice. Science **95**, 462—463 (1942a).
— Observations on the genetics of susceptibility for the development of mammary cancer in mice. Cancer Res. **2**, 540—545 (1942b).
— Possible relationship of the estrogenic hormones, genetic susceptibility, and milk influence in the production of mammary cancer in mice. Cancer Res. **2**, 710—721 (1942c).
— Inciting influences in the etiology of mammary cancer in mice. In: Research Conference on Cancer, pp. 63—96, American Association for the Advancement of Science, Washington 1945a.
— Characteristics of the mammary tumor milk agent in serial dilution and blood studies. Proc. Soc. exp. Biol. (N. Y.) **59**, 43—44 (1945b).
— Causes and control of mammary cancer in mice. Harvey Lect. **42**, 221—246 (1946).
— Transplantability of mammary cancer in mice associated with source of mammary tumor milk agent. Cancer Res. **7**, 741—745 (1947).
— Some enigmas associated with the genesis of mammary cancer in mice. Cancer Res. **8**, 625—639 (1948a).
— Propagation of the mammary tumor milk agent in tumors from C57 black mice. Proc. Soc. exp. Biol. (N. Y.) **67**, 219—221 (1948b).
— Recovery of the mammary tumor milk agent following transfer by the male parent. Cancer Res. **10**, 204 (1950).
— Inherited hormonal mechanisms and mammary cancer in virgin female mice. Cancer Res. **11**, 237 (1951).
— Transfer of the agent for mammary cancer in mice by the male. Cancer Res. **12**, 387—398 (1952a).
— Studies on the inherited susceptibility and inherited hormonal influence in the genesis of mammary cancer in mice. Cancer Res. **12**, 594—601 (1952b).
— Influence of the mammary-tumor agent on the genesis of mammary cancer in agent-free mice after male transmission. J. nat. Cancer Inst. **25**, 177—199 (1960).
— Biological assay and serial passage of the mouse mammary tumour agent in mammary tumours from mothers and their hybrid progeny. In: A Ciba Foundation Symposium on Tumour Viruses of Murine Origin, pp. 56—81, G. E. W. WOLSTENHOLME and M. O'CONNOR eds. London: J. & A. Churchill Ltd. 1962.
— C. A. EVANS, and R. G. GREEN: Survival of the mammary tumor milk agent of mice. Science **101**, 95—97 (1945).
—, and M. J. FRANTZ: Sensitivity of females of C stock to male infection with mammary tumor agent. Proc. Soc. exp. Biol. (N. Y.) **86**, 698—701 (1954).
— R. A. HUSEBY, M. B. VISSCHER, Z. B. BALL, and F. W. SMITH: Mammary cancer and mammary structure in inbred stocks of mice and their hybrids. Science **99**, 83—85 (1944).
BLAIR, P. B.: A new strain of the mouse mammary tumor virus. Science **127**, 518 (1958).
— A mutation in the mouse mammary tumor virus. Cancer Res. **20**, 635—642 (1960).
— S. M. BLAIR, W. R. LYONS, H. A. BERN, and C. H. LI: Effect of hormones and of parity on the occurrence of hyperplastic alveolar nodules and tumors in the mammary glands of female A/Crgl mice. Cancer Res. **20**, 1640—1645 (1960).
—, and K. B. DEOME: Mammary tumor development in transplanted hyperplastic alveolar nodules of the mouse. Proc. Soc. exp. Biol. (N. Y.) **108**, 289—291 (1961).
— —, and S. NANDI: The characteristics of the preneoplastic state in mouse mammary carcinogenesis. In: A Henry Ford Hospital International Symposium on Biological Interactions in Normal and Neoplastic Growth, pp. 371—389, M. J. BRENNAN and W. L. SIMPSON eds. Boston: Little, Brown & Company 1962.
BONSER, G. M.: The effect of oestrone administration on the mammary glands of male mice of two strains differing greatly in their susceptibility to spontaneous mammary carcinoma. J. Path. Bact. **42**, 169—176 (1936).
— A microscopical study of the evolution of mouse mammary cancer: the effect of the milk factor and a comparison with the human disease. J. Path. Bact. **57**, 413—422 (1946).
— The evolution of mammary cancer induced in virgin female IF mice with minimal doses of locally-acting methylcholanthrene. J. Path. Bact. **68**, 531—546 (1954).
BOOT, L. M., O. MÜHLBOCK, G. RÖPCKE, and W. VAN EGGENHORST TENGBERGEN: Further investigations on induction of mammary cancer in mice by isografts of hypophyseal tissue. Cancer Res. **22**, 713—727 (1962).

Brunschwig, A., and A. D. Bissel: Estrus cycles in mice of cancerous and non-cancerous strains. Arch. Surg. **33**, 515—520 (1936).

Bryan, W. R., H. Kahler, and V. T. Riley: Attempts to demonstrate a viruslike principle in mammalian tumors by the yolk injection technique. In: Research Conference on Cancer, pp. 40—53, American Association for the Advancement of Science, Washington 1945.

— — M. B. Shimkin, and H. B. Andervont: Extraction and ultracentrifugation of mammary tumor inciter of mice. J. nat. Cancer Inst. **2**, 451—455 (1942).

Burrows, H.: Biological actions of sex hormones, 2nd edition. London: Cambridge University Press 1949.

—, and C. Hoch-Ligeti: Effect of progesterone on the development of mammary cancer in C3H mice. Cancer Res. **6**, 608—609 (1946).

Caschera, F.: La «menopausa» nei topi femmine vergini (RIII/Dm/Se, C3Hb/Se, A/He/Se substrains). Lav. Ist. Anat. Univ. Perugia **19**, 13—20 (1959).

— La «pseudogravidanza spontanea» in topi femmine vergini, isolate e coabitanti, del BALB/c_f substrain. Lav. Ist. Anat. Univ. Perugia **20**, 17—30 (1960a).

— Le variazioni cicliche estrali e le relative modificazioni degli organi sessuali, in relazione all'età ed alla coabitazione, in topi femmine vergini del BALB/cf substrain (sull'esame di 580 cicli). Lav. Ist. Anat. Univ. Perugia **20**, 63—74 (1960b).

— e N. Maltzeff: Modificazioni nel topo in rapporto con l'attenuazione della funzione ovarica (in vergini del BALB/c_f/Cb/Se substrain). Lav. Ist. Anat. Univ. Perugia **20**, 253—262 (1960).

Cloudman, A. D.: Spontaneous neoplasms in mice. In: Biology of the Laboratory Mouse, pp. 168—233, G. D. Snell ed., New York: Dover Publications Inc. 1956.

Cole, H. A.: The mammary gland of the mouse during oestrous cycle, pregnancy and lactation. Proc. Roy. Soc. B **114**, 136—161 (1933).

Consolandi, G., e U. Veronesi: La diffusione metastatica del cancro della mammella. IV. Parallelo sull'andamento del fenomeno nell'uomo e negli "inbred strains" del topo. Lav. Ist. Anat. Univ. Perugia **17**, 213—240 (1957).

— — La diffusione metastatica del cancro mammario negli "inbred strains" del topo. Atti Soc. ital. Cancer. **1**, 159—216 (1958).

Cori, C. F.: The influence of ovariectomy on the spontaneous occurrence of mammary carcinoma in mice. J. Cancer Res. **10**, 265—266 (1926).

— The influence of ovariectomy on the spontaneous occurrence of mammary carcinoma in mice. J. exp. Med. **45**, 983—991 (1927).

Cowie, A. T., and S. J. Folley: Endocrine aspects of mammary growth and function, particularly in relation to pituitary hormones. In: Endocrine Aspects of Breast Cancer, pp. 266—275, A. R. Currie ed., London: E. & S. Livingstone Ltd. 1958.

DeBruyn, W. M., and E. L. Benedetti: Ultrastructure of virus-like particles found in long-term cultures of mouse. In: Proceedings of the European Regional Conference on Electron Microscopy, Vol. 2, pp. 999—1003, A. L. Houwink and B. J. Spit eds., Delft: De Nederlandse Vereniging voor Electronenmicroscopie 1960.

DeOme, K. B.: The role of the mammary tumor virus in mouse mammary noduligenesis and tumorigenesis. In: Viruses, Nucleic Acids and Cancer, 17th Annual Symposium on Fundamental Cancer Research at the University of Texas M. D. Anderson Hospital and Tumor Institute, pp. 498—507. Baltimore: The Williams and Wilkins Company 1963.

— H. A. Bern, W. E. Berg, and L. E. Pissott: Radiophosphorus uptake by normal, hyperplastic and tumorous mammary tissues of mice. Proc. Soc. exp. Biol. (N. Y.) **92**, 55—58 (1956).

— — S. Nandi, D. R. Pitelka, and L. J. Faulkin jr.: The precancerous nature of the hyperplastic alveolar nodules found in the mammary glands of old female C3H/Crgl mice. In: Genetics and Cancer, pp. 327—348. Austin: Univ. Texas Press 1959a.

— P. B. Blair, and L. J. Faulkin jr.: Some characteristics of the preneoplastic hyperplastic alveolar nodules of the C3H/Crgl mice. Acta Un. int. Cancr. **17**, 973—982 (1961).

— L. J. Faulkin jr., H. A. Bern, and P. B. Blair: Development of mammary tumors from hyperplastic alveolar nodules transplanted into gland-free mammary fat pads of female C3H mice. Cancer Res. **19**, 515—520 (1959b).

— S. Nandi, H. A. Bern, P. Blair, and D. Pitelka: The preneoplastic hyperplastic alveolar nodule as the morphological precursor of mammary cancer in mice. In: The Morphological Precursors of Cancer, pp. 349—368, L. Severi ed., Division of Cancer Research, Perugia 1962.

Deringer, M. K.: Occurrence of tumors, particularly mammary tumors, in agent-free strain C3HeB mice. J. nat. Cancer Inst. **22**, 995—1002 (1959).

— W. E. Heston, and H. B. Andervont: Estrus in virgin strain C3H (high-tumor) and virgin strain A (low-tumor) mice and in the reciprocal $(A \times C3H)F_1$ hybrids. J. nat. Cancer Inst. **5**, 403—405 (1945).

DMOCHOWSKI, L.: Comparative potency of the mammary tumour agent of mice of different genetic constitutions. Brit. J. exp. Path. **26**, 267—269 (1945).
— Preservation of mammary tumour agent by desiccation of breast tumour tissue of mice. Brit. J. exp. Path. **27**, 391—393 (1946).
— Mammary tumour inducing factor and genetic constitution. Brit. J. Cancer **2**, 94—102 (1948).
— Some data on the distribution of the milk factor. Brit. J. Cancer **3**, 525—533 (1949).
— A study of the development of mammary tumours in hybrid mice. Brit. J. Cancer **7**, 73—119 (1953a).
— The milk agent in the origin of mammary tumors in mice. Advanc. Cancer Res. **1**, 103—172 (1953b).
— Progress in mammalian genetics and cancer. Discussion. J. nat. Cancer Inst. **15**, 785—787 (1954).
— A biological and biophysical approach to the study of the development of mammary cancer in mice. Acta Un. int. Cancr. **12**, 582—618 (1956).
— Viruses and tumors in the light of electron microscope studies: A review. Cancer Res. **20**, 977—1015 (1960).
— Some recent studies on mouse tumor viruses: the Bittner mammary tumor virus and the Gross leukemia virus. Ann. Med. (Perugia) **54**, 753—771 (1963a).
— The electron microscopic view of virus-host relationship in neoplasia. In: Progress in Tumor Research, Vol. 3, pp. 35—147, F. HOMBURGER ed., New York: S. Karger 1963b.
—, and C. E. GREY: Subcellular structures of possible viral origin in some mammalian tumors. Ann. N. Y. Acad. Sci. **68**, 559—615 (1957).
— — F. PADGETT, and J. A. SYKES: Studies on the structure of the mammary tumor-inducing virus (BITTNER) and of leukemia virus (GROSS). In: Viruses, Nucleic Acids and Cancer, 17th Annual Symposium on Fundamental Cancer Research at the University of Texas M. D. Anderson Hospital and Tumor Institute, pp. 85—121. Baltimore: The Williams and Wilkins Company 1963a.
—, and C. D. HAAGENSEN: The distribution of the mammary-tumor inducing agent in the various constituents of the cytoplasm of mammary tumor cells in mice. Acta Un. int. Cancr. **11**, 646—653 (1955).
— —, and D. H. MOORE: Studies of sections of normal and malignant cells of high and low-cancer-strain mice by means of electron microscope. Acta Un. int. Cancr. **11**, 640—645 (1955).
—, and R. D. PASSEY: Unpublished data 1951. Quoted by L. DMOCHOWSKI, 1953a.
— — Attempts at tumor virus isolation. Ann. N. Y. Acad. Sci. **54**, 1035—1066 (1952).
— L. O. PEARSON, C. E. GREY, and J. A. SYKES: Studies on the behavior of the Bittner virus in mice of some apparently virus-free strains. Acta Un. int. Cancr. **19**, 276—279 (1963b).
DUNN, T. B.: Morphology of mammary tumours in mice. In: The Physiopathology of Cancer, pp. 123—148, F. HOMBURGER and W. H. FISHMAN eds., London: Cassell & Co. 1953.
DURAN-REYNALS, F.: Virus-induced tumors and the virus theory of cancer. In: The Physiopathology of Cancer, 2nd edition, pp. 238—292, F. HOMBURGER ed., London: Cassell & Co. 1958.
EVERSOLE, W. J.: Inhibition of azo dye carcinogenesis by adrenalectomy and treatment with desoxicorticosterone trimethylacetate. Proc. Soc. exp. Biol. (N. Y.) **96**, 643—646 (1957).
— The rôle of the adrenal cortex in azo dye carcinogenesis. Lav. Ist. Anat. Univ. Perugia **18**, 25—36 (1958).
FEKETE, E.: A comparative morphological study of the mammary gland in a high and a low tumor strain of mice. Amer. J. Path. **14**, 557—578 (1938).
— Observations on three functional tests in a high tumor and a low tumor strain of mice. Amer. J. Cancer **38**, 234—238 (1940).
— A comparative study of the ovaries of virgin mice of the dba and C57 black strains. Cancer Res. **6**, 263—269 (1946).
—, and C. C. LITTLE: Observations on mammary tumor incidence of mice born from transferred ova. Cancer Res. **2**, 525—530 (1942).
—, and H. K. OTIS: Observations on leukemia in AKR mice born from transferred ova and nursed by low leukemic mothers. Cancer Res. **14**, 445—447 (1954).
FIORE-DONATI, L., and L. CHIECO-BIANCHI: Influence of host factors on development and type of leukemia induced in mice by Graffi virus. J. nat. Cancer Inst. **32**, 1083—1107 (1964).
FOULDS, L.: Mammary tumours in hybrid mice: A sex-factor in transplantation. Brit. J. Cancer **1**, 362—370 (1947).
— Mammary tumours in hybrid mice: The presence and transmission of the mammary tumour agent. Brit. J. Cancer **3**, 230—239 (1949a).
— Mammary tumours in hybrid mice: Growth and progression of spontaneous tumours. Brit. J. Cancer **3**, 345—375 (1949b).

FOULDS, L.: Mammary tumours in hybrid mice: Hormone responses of transplanted tumours. Brit. J. Cancer **3**, 240—246 (1949c).
— The experimental study of tumor progression: A review. Cancer Res. **14**, 327—339 (1954).
— The histologic analysis of mammary tumors of mice. I. Scope of investigation and general principles of analysis. J. nat. Cancer Inst. **17**, 701—711 (1956a).
— The histologic analysis of mammary tumors of mice. II. The histology of responsiveness and progression. The origins of tumors. J. nat. Cancer Inst. **17**, 713—753 (1956b).
— The histologic analysis of mammary tumors of mice. III. Organoid tumors. J. nat. Cancer Inst. **17**, 755—781 (1956c).
— The histologic analysis of mammary tumors of mice. IV. Secretion. J. nat. Cancer Inst. **17**, 783—801 (1956d).
— The development of mammary tumours. In: Proceedings of the II International Symposium on Mammary Cancer, pp. 501—503, L. SEVERI ed., Division of Cancer Research, Perugia 1958.
FRIEND, C.: Cell-free transmission in adult Swiss mice of a disease having the characters of a leukemia. J. exp. Med. **105**, 307—318 (1957).
FULLER, R. H., E. BROWN, and C. A. MILLS: Environmental temperatures and spontaneous tumors in mice. Cancer Res. **1**, 130—133 (1941).
FURTADO-DIAS, M. T.: Spontaneous testicural tumours in mice of the H strain. In: Proceedings of the II International Symposium on Mammary Cancer, pp. 505—512, L. SEVERI ed., Division of Cancer Research, Perugia, 1958.
GARDNER, W. U.: Estrogens in carcinogenesis. Arch. Path. **27**, 138—170 (1939).
— Growth of the mammary glands in hypophysectomized mice. Proc. Soc. exp. Biol. (N. Y.) **45**, 835—838 (1940).
— The effect of estrogen on the incidence of mammary and pituitary tumors in hybrid mice. Cancer Res. **1**, 345—358 (1941).
— Persistence and growth of spontaneous mammary tumors and hyperplastic nodules in hypophysectomized mice. Cancer Res. **2**, 476—488 (1942).
— Hormonal aspects of experimental tumorigenesis. Adv. Cancer Res. **1**, 173—232 (1953).
—, and E. ALLEN: Malignant and non-malignant uterine and vaginal lesions in mice receiving estrogens and estrogens and androgens simultaneously. Yale J. Biol. Med. **12**, 213—234 (1939).
— C. A. PFEIFFER, J. J. TRENTIN, and J. T. WOLSTENHOLME: Hormonal factors in experimental carcinogenesis. In: The Physiopathology of Cancer, pp. 225—297, F. HOMBURGER and W. H. FISHMAN eds., Cassell & Co., London 1953.
— G. M. SMITH, and L. C. STRONG: Stimulation of abnormal mammary growth by large amounts of estrogenic hormone. Proc. Soc. exp. Biol. (N. Y.) **33**, 148—150 (1935).
— L. C. STRONG, and G. M. SMITH: The mammary glands of mature female mice of strains varying in susceptibility to spontaneous tumor development. Amer. J. Cancer **37**, 510—517 (1939).
GILLMAN, J., C. GILBERT, and I. SPENCE: Phaeochromocytoma in the rat. Cancer **6**, 494—511 (1953).
GOMEZ, E. T., and C. W. TURNER: Effects of thyroxine and galactin on lactation in hypophysectomized guinea pig. Proc. Soc. exp. Biol. (N. Y.) **36**, 80—81 (1937).
GORER, P. A., and L. W. LAW: Attempt to demonstrate neutralizing antibodies to the mammary tumour "milk agent" in mice. Brit. J. Cancer **3**, 90—93 (1949).
GRAD, B.: The influence of hyper- and hypothyroidism on the incidence of lymphatic leukemia in AKR mice. Cancer Res. **17**, 266—271 (1957).
GRAFF, S., D. H. MOORE, W. M. STANLEY, H. T. RANDALL, and C. D. HAAGENSEN: The milk agent. Acta Un. int. Cancr. **6**, 191—196 (1948).
— — — — — Isolation of mouse mammary carcinoma virus. Cancer **2**, 755—762 (1949).
— H. T. RANDALL, G. E. CARPENTER, and C. D. HAAGENSEN: The milk factor in blood. Science **104**, 289 (1946).
GRAFFI, A.: Chloroleukemia of mice. Ann. N. Y. Acad. Sci. **68**, 540—558 (1957).
GREEN, R. G.: Cytotoxic property of mouse cancer antiserum. Proc. Soc. exp. Biol. (N. Y.) **1**, 113—114 (1946).
—, and J. J. BITTNER: Neutralization of mouse mammary cancer virus with antiserum. Cancer Res. **6**, 499 (1946).
— M. M. MOSEY, and J. J. BITTNER: Antigenic character of cancer milk agent in mice. Cancer Res. **5**, 588 (1945).
— — — Antigenic character of the cancer milk agent in mice. Proc. Soc. exp. Biol. (N. Y.) **61**, 115—117 (1946).
GREENE, H. S. N.: Toxemia of pregnancy in the rabbit: Clinical manifestations and pathology. J. exp. Med. **65**, 809—832 (1937).

GREENE, H. S. N.: Toxemia of pregnancy in the rabbit: II. Etiological considerations with special reference to hereditary factors. J. exp. Med. **67**, 369—388 (1938).
— Uterine adenomata in the rabbit: III. Susceptibility as a function of constitutional factors. J. exp. Med. **73**, 273—292 (1941).
—, and B. L. NEWTON: Evolution of cancer of the uterine fundus in the rabbit. Cancer **1**, 82—99 (1948).
—, and J. A. SAXTON JR.: Uterine adenomata in the rabbit: I. Clinical history, pathology and preliminary transplantation experiments. J. exp. Med. **67**, 691—708 (1938).
GROSS, L.: "Spontaneous" leukemia developing in C3H mice following inoculation, in infancy, with AK leukemic extracts, or AK embryos. Proc. Soc. exp. Biol. (N. Y.) **76**, 27—32 (1951a).
— Pathogenic properties and "vertical" transmission of the mouse leukemia agent. Proc. Soc. exp. Biol. (N. Y.) **8**, 342—348 (1951b).
— Development and serial cell-free passage of a highly potent strain of mouse leukemia virus. Proc. Soc. exp. Biol. (N. Y.) **94**, 761—771 (1957).
— Viral etiology of mouse leukemia. Advanc. Cancer Res. **6**, 149—180 (1961a).
— Oncogenic viruses. New York: Pergamon Press 1961b.
— Studies on pathogenic properties and natural transmission of a mouse leukaemia virus. In: A Ciba Foundation Symposium on Tumour Viruses of Murine Origin, pp. 159—175, G. E. W. WOLSTENHOLME and M. O'CONNOR eds., London: J. & A. Churchill Ltd. 1962.
GUÉRIN, M.: Coprs d'inclusion dans les adénocarcinomes mammaires de la souris. Bull. Cancer **42**, 14—28 (1955).
GULIK, P. J. VAN, and R. KORTEWEG: Susceptibility to follicular hormone and disposition to mammary cancer in female mice. Amer. J. Cancer **38**, 506—515 (1940a).
— — The anatomy of the mammary gland in mice with regard to the degree of its disposition for cancer. Ned. Akad. Wettenschappen **43**, 891—900 (1940b).
HAALAND, M.: Spontaneous tumours in mice. A. R. imp. Cancer Res. Fd. **4**, 1—113 (1911).
HADDOW, A.: The breast as the fountain of cancer lore. In: Proceedings of the II International Symposium on Mammary Cancer, Opening Lecture, pp. XXXVII—XLVIII, L. SEVERI ed., Division of Cancer Research, Perugia, 1958.
HAMILTON, J. B., M. HOLLANDER, and H. B. ANDERVONT: Note on the increased rate of nail growth in mice carrying the milk agent for mammary cancer. J. nat. Cancer Inst. **20**, 409—415 (1958).
HARKNESS, M. N., H. A. BERN, M. ALFERT, and N. O. GOLDSTEIN: Cytochemical studies of hyperplastic alveolar nodules in the mammary gland of the C3H/HeCRGL mouse. J. nat. Cancer Inst. **19**, 1023—1033 (1957).
HARVEN, E. DE: Etudes au microscope électronique de la leucémie de Friend et d'autres cancers de la souris également associés à la présence de particules virusales. Rev. belge Path. **28**, 7—136 (1961).
—, and C. FRIEND: Electron microscopy of Swiss mouse leukemia virus. In: Symposium on Phenomena of the Tumor Viruses, J. W. BEARD ed., National Cancer Institute Monograph No. 4, 291—297, 1960.
HEILMAN, F. R.: On yolk sac cultivation and virus induction of malignant tumors. In: Research Conference on Cancer, pp. 54—55, Americal Association for the Advancement of Science, Washington, 1945.
HEIMAN, J.: The effect of progesterone and testosterone propionate on the incidence of mammary cancer in mice. Cancer Res. **5**, 426—430 (1945).
HESTON, W. E.: Genetic analysis of susceptibility to induced pulmonary tumors in mice. J. nat. Cancer Inst. **3**, 69—78 (1942a).
— Inheritance of susceptibility to spontaneous pulmonary tumors in mice. J. nat. Cancer Inst. **3**, 79—82 (1942b).
— Genetics of mammary tumors in mice. In: A Symposium on Mammary Tumors in Mice, pp. 55—84, F. R. MOULTON ed., American Association for the Advancement of Science, Washington, 1945.
— Paths of gene action in mammary-tumor development in mice. J. nat. Cancer Inst. **7**, 79—85 (1946).
— Rôle of genes and their relationship to extrachromosomal factors in the development of mammary gland tumours in mice. Brit. J. Cancer **2**, 87—90 (1948).
— Localization of gene action in the causation of lung and mammary gland tumors in mice. J. nat. Cancer Inst. **15**, 775—783 (1954).
— Mammary tumors in agent-free mice. Ann. N. Y. Acad. Sci. **71**, 931—942 (1958).
— Complete inhibition of occurrence of spontaneous hepatomas in highly susceptible (C3H × YBR)F_1 male mice by hypophysectomy. J. nat. Cancer Inst. **31**, 467—474 (1963).
— Induction of mammary gland tumors in strain C57BL/He mice by isografts of hypophyses. J. nat. Cancer Inst. **32**, 947—955 (1964).

HESTON, W. E., and H. B. ANDERVONT: Importance of genetic influence on the occurrence of mammary tumors in virgin female mice. J. nat. Cancer Inst. **4**, 403—407 (1944).
— M. K. DERINGER, and H. B. ANDERVONT: Gene-milk agent relationship in mammary tumor development. J. nat. Cancer Inst. **5**, 289—307 (1945).
—, and T. B. DUNN: Tumor development of susceptible strain A and resistant strain L lung transplants in LAF_1 hosts. J. nat. Cancer Inst. **11**, 1057—1071 (1951).
— G. VLAHAKIS, and M. K. DERINGER: High incidence of spontaneous hepatomas and the increase of this incidence with urethan in C3H, C3Hf, and C3He male mice. J. nat. Cancer Inst. **24**, 425—435 (1960).
— —, and Y. TSUBURA: Strain DD, a new high mammary tumor strain, and comparison of DD with strain C3H. J. nat. Cancer Inst. **32**, 237—251 (1964).
HUMMEL, K. P., and C. C. LITTLE: Studies on the mouse mammary tumor agent. I. The agent in blood and other tissues in relation to physiologic or endocrine state of the donor. Cancer Res. **9**, 129—134 (1949).
— — Comparison of the virulence of the mammary-tumor agent from four strains of mice. J. nat. Cancer Inst. **23**, 813—821 (1959).
— —, and S. B. HEDDY: Studies on the mouse mammary tumor agent. II. The neutralization of the agent by placenta. Cancer Res. **9**, 135—136 (1949).
HUSEBY, R. A., Z. B. BALL, and M. B. VISSCHER: Further observations on the influence of simple caloric restriction on mammary cancer incidence and related phenomena in C3H mice. Cancer Res. **5**, 40—46 (1945).
— C. P. BARNUM, and J. J. BITTNER: Titration of the milk agent virus in milk and lactating mammary gland cells. Cancer Res. **10**, 516—520 (1950).
—, and J. J. BITTNER: A comparative morphological study of the mammary glands with reference to the known factors influencing the development of mammary carcinoma in mice. Cancer Res. **6**, 240—255 (1946).
— — Comparative studies of estrous cycles in relation to mammary tumor milk agent. Cancer Res. **7**, 722 (1947).
— — Studies on the inherited hormonal influence. Acta Un. int. Cancr. **6**, 197—205 (1948).
ICHIKAWA, Y., and S. AMANO: A new type of virus found in a spontaneous mammary tumor of SL mice and its proliferating modus observed in ultra-thin sections under the electron microscope. Gann **49**, 57—64 (1958).
IGLESIAS, R., W. H. STERNBERG, and A. SEGALOFF: A functional ovarian tumor occurring spontaneously in a rat. Cancer Res. **10**, 226 (1950).
IMAGAWA, D., J. J. BITTNER, and J. T. SYVERTON: Cytotoxic studies on mouse mammary cancer cells. Cancer Res. **10**, 226—227 (1950).
— R. G. GREEN, and H. O. HALVORSON: A precipitin test for antigens present in mouse tissue containing the milk agent. Proc. Soc. exp. Biol. (N. Y.) **68**, 162—166 (1948).
— J. T. SYVERTON, and J. J. BITTNER: The cytotoxic effect *in vitro* of antiserum upon heterologous mouse mammary cancer cells. Cancer Res. **11**, 259 (1951).
— — — The cytotoxicity of serum for mouse mammary cancer cells. I. The effects of admixture *in vitro* upon homoiotransplantability. Cancer Res. **14**, 1—7 (1954).
JESSE, M. J., and C. D. HAAGENSEN: Unpublished data, 1963. Quoted by D. H. MOORE and M. J. LYONS, 1963b.
JONES, E. E.: A comparative study of hyperplastic nodules in mammary glands of mice with and without the mammary tumor inciter. Acta Un. int. Cancr. **7**, 263—265 (1951).
KAPLAN, H. S., C. S. NAGAREDA, and M. B. BROWN: Endocrine factors and radiation-induced lymphoid tumors of mice. In: Recent Progress in Hormone Research, Vol. X, pp. 293—338, G. PINCUS ed., New York: Academic Press 1954.
KINOSITA, R., J. O. ERICKSEN, D. M. ARMEN, M. E. DOLCH, and J. P. WARD: Electron microscope study of mouse mammary carcinoma tissue. Exp. Cell Res. **4**, 353—361 (1953).
KIRSCHBAUM, A., J. R. SAPHIRO, and H. W. MIXER: Synergistic action of leukemogenic agents. Cancer Res. **13**, 262—268 (1953).
KLEIN, E., and G. KLEIN: A system for the detection of single gene mutations in mouse tumors. In: Proceedings of the II International Symposium on Mammary Cancer, pp. 709—712, L. SEVERI ed., Division of Cancer Research, Perugia, 1958a.
KLEIN, G., and E. KLEIN: Some experiments on the mechanism of progression in mouse mammary carcinomas. In: Proceedings of the II International Symposium on Mammary Cancer, pp. 713—717, L. SEVERI ed., Division of Cancer Research, Perugia, 1958b.
KORTEWEG, R.: Genetically determined differences in hormone production possible factor influencing susceptibility to mammary cancer in mice. Brit. J. Cancer **2**, 91—94(1948).
LACASSAGNE, A.: Tentatives pour modifier, par la progéstérone ou par la testostérone, l'apparition des adénocarcinomes mammaires provoqués par l'oestrone chez la souris. C. R. Soc. Biol. (Paris) **126**, 385—387 (1937).

LASFARGUES, E. Y.: Concerning the rôle of insulin in the differentiation and functional activity of mouse mammary tissues. Exp. Cell. Res. (1963) (in press).
—, and D. G. FELDMAN: Hormonal and physiological background in the production of B particles by the mouse mammary epithelium in organ cultures. Cancer Res. **23**, 191—196 (1963).
— D. H. MOORE, and M. R. MURRAY: Maintenance of the milk factor in cultures of mouse mammary epithelium. Cancer Res. **18**, 1281—1285 (1958).
— — —, and C. D. HAAGENSEN: Production of the milk agent in cultures of mouse mammary carcinoma. J. Biophys. Biochem. Cytol. **5**, 93—96 (1959).
—, and M. R. MURRAY Hormonal influences on the differentiation and growth of embryonic mouse mammary glands in organ cultures. Develop. Biol. **1**, 413—435 (1959).
— —, and D. H. MOORE: Cultivation of the mouse mammary carcinoma virus. In: Symposium on Phenomena of the Tumor Viruses, J. W. BEARD ed., National Cancer Institute Monograph, No. 4, 151—166, 1960.
LATHROP, A. E. C., and L. LOEB: The influence of pregnancies on the incidence of cancer in mice. Proc. Soc. exp. Biol. (N. Y.) **11**, 38—41 (1913).
LAW, L. W.: Effect of pseudopregnancy on mammary carcinoma incidence in mice of the A stock. Proc. Soc. exp. Biol. (N. Y.) **48**, 486—487 (1941).
— The effect of gonadectomy and adrenalectomy on the appearance and incidence of spontaneous lymphoid leukemia in C58 mice. J. nat. Cancer Inst. **8**, 157—159 (1947).
— Genetic studies in experimental cancer. Advanc. Cancer Res. **2**, 281—352 (1954).
— Present status of nonviral factors in the etiology of reticular neoplasms of the mouse. Ann. N. Y. Acad. Sci. **68**, 616—635 (1957).
LEONARD, S. L., and R. P. REECE: Failure of steroid hormones to induce mammary growth in hypophysectomized rats. Endocrinology **30**, 32—36 (1942).
LIEBERMAN, M., and H. S. KAPLAN: Leukemogenic activity of filtrates from radiation-induced lymphoid tumors of mice. Science **130**, 387—388 (1959).
LIPPINCOTT, S. W., J. E. EDWARDS, H. G. GRADY, and H. L. STEWART: A review of some spontaneous neoplasms in mice. J. nat. Cancer Inst. **3**, 199—210 (1942).
LITTLE, C. C.: Evidence that cancer is not a simple mendelian recessive. J. Cancer Res. **12**, 30—46 (1928).
—, and J. PEARSON: The results of a "functional test" in a strain of mice (C57 Black) with a low breast tumor incidence. Amer. J. Cancer **38**, 224—233 (1940).
LOEB, L.: Further investigations on the origin of tumors in mice. Internal secretion as a factor in the origin of tumors. J. Med. Res. **40**, 477—496 (1919).
—, and M. M. KIRTZ: The effects of transplants of anterior lobes of the hypophysis on the growth of the mammary gland and on the development of mammary gland carcinoma in various strains of mice. Amer. J. Cancer **36**, 56—82 (1939).
LYONS, M. J., and D. H. MOORE: Purification of the mouse mammary tumour virus. Nature (Lond.) **194**, 1141—1142 (1962).
MACDOWELL, E. C., J. S. POTTER, and M. J. TAYLOR: Mouse leukemia. XII. The rôle of genes in spontaneous cases. Cancer Res. **5**, 65—83 (1945).
MAN, J. C. H. DE, and T. G. VAN RIJSSEL: Electron microscopy of tissue of the mammary glands and tumors in old mice with special reference to mitochondrial size. J. nat. Cancer Inst. **26**, 919—947 (1961).
MARTINEZ, C.: Factors affecting the tranplantability and metastatic growth of tumors in mice. Ann. Med. (Perugia) **48**, 315—328 (1957).
MCENDY, D. P., M. C. BOON, and J. FURTH: On the role of thymus, spleen and gonads in the development of leukemia in a high-leukemia stock of mice. Cancer Res. **4**, 377—383 (1944).
METCALF, D.: The thymic origin of the plasma lymphocytosis stimulating factor. Brit. J. Cancer **10**, 442—457 (1956).
— Thymus lymphocytosis stimulating activity in high and low leukemia strains of mice. Proc. Amer. Ass. Cancer Res. **2**, 231—232 (1957).
— Adrenal cortical function in high- and low-leukemia strains of mice. Cancer Res. **20**, 1347—1353 (1960).
MILLER, E. W., J. W. ORR, and F. O. PYBUS: The effect of oestrone on the mouse skeleton, with particular reference to the Newcastle bone tumor (NBT) strain. J. Path. Bact. **55**, 137—150 (1943).
—, and F. C. PYBUS: Effect of foster nursing on incidence of spontaneous mammary carcinoma in two inbred strains of mice. Cancer Res. **5**, 94—101 (1945).
MILLER, J. F. A. P.: Etiology and pathogenesis of mouse leukemia. Advanc. Cancer Res. **6**, 291—368 (1961).
— Rôle of the tymus in virus-induced leukaemia. In: A Ciba Foundation Symposium on Tumour Viruses of Murine Origin, pp. 262—283, G. E. W. WOLSTENHOLME and M. O'CONNOR eds., London: J. & A. Churchill Ltd. 1962.

Miroff, G., and D. G. Feldman: Production and release of virus-like particles by cultures of agent-free ascites cells. J. nat. Cancer Inst. **31**, 807—825 (1963).

Mixner, J. P., and C. W. Turner: Role of estrogen in the stimulation of mammary lobule-alveolar growth by progesterone and by the mammogenic lobule-alveolar growth factor of the anterior pituitary. Endocrinology **30**, 591—597 (1942).

Moloney, J. B.: Biological studies on a lymphoid-leukemia virus extracted from sarcoma 37. I. Origin and introductory investigations. J. nat. Cancer Inst. **24**, 933—951 (1960).

— Discussion of the Gross's paper. In: A Ciba Foundation Symposium on tumour Viruses of Murine Origin, pp. 171—172, G. E. W. Wolstenholme and M. O'Connor eds., London: J. & A. Churchill Ltd. 1962.

Moore, D. H.: Some preparations of the mouse mammary carcinoma agent. In: Proc. nat. Cancer Conf. **1**, 299—303 (1952).

— On the identification and characterization of the milk agent. In: A Ciba Foundation Symposium on Tumour Viruses of Murine Origin, pp. 107—137, G. E. W. Wolstenholme and M. O'Connor eds., London: J. & A. Churchill Ltd. 1962.

— Mouse mammary tumour agent and mouse mammary tumours. Nature (Lond.) **198**, 429—433 (1963).

— H. C. Chopra, P. D. Lunger, and M. J. Lyons: Unpublished data. Quoted by D. H. Moore, 1963.

— E. Y. Lasfargues, M. R. Murray, C. D. Haagensen, and E. C. Pollard: Correlation of physical and biological properties of mouse mammary tumor agent. J. biophys. biochem. Cytol. **5**, 85—92 (1959).

—, and M. J. Lyons: Purification and subsequent studies of the mouse mammary tumor virus. In: Electron Microscopy, Fifth International Congress for Electron Microscopy, Vol. 2, pp. MM-6, Sidney S. Breese jr. ed., New York: Academic Press Inc. 1962.

— — Electrophoretic separation of the mouse mammary tumor virus. J. nat. Cancer Inst. **31**, 1255—1273 (1963a).

— — Studies of replication and properties of the Bittner virus. In: Viruses, Nucleic Acids and Cancer (17th Annual Symposium on Fundamental Cancer Research at the University of Texas M. D. Anderson Hospital and Tumor Institute), pp. 224—242. Baltimore: Williams and Wilkins Company, 1963b.

— E. C. Pollard, and C. D. Haagensen: Further correlations of physical and biological properties of mouse mammary tumor agent. Fed. Proc. **21**, 942—946 (1962).

Morris, H. P.: Diet and some other environmental influences in the genesis and growth of mammary tumours in mice. In: A Symposium on Mammary Tumors in Mice, pp. 140—161, F. R. Moulton ed., American association for the Advancement of Science, Washington, 1945a.

— Some nutritional factors influencing the origin and development of cancer. J. nat. Cancer Inst. **6**, 1—17 (1945b).

Mühlbock, O.: On the susceptibility of different inbred strains of mice for oestrone. Acta brev. neerl. Physiol. **15**, 18—20 (1947).

— The oestrone sensitivity of the mammary gland in female mice of various strains. Acta brev. neerl. Physiol. **16**, 22—27 (1948).

— The sensitivity of the mammary gland to oestrone in different strains of mice with and without mammary tumor agent. Acta endocr. (Kbh.) **3**, 105—110 (1949).

— Mammary tumor-agent in the sperm of high-cancer-strain male mice. J. nat. Cancer Inst. **10**, 861—864 (1950a).

— Non occurrence of mammary-tumor agent in the excreta of high-cancer-strain mice. Acta physiol. pharmacol. neerl. **1**, 645—650 (1950b).

— Note on the influence of the number of litters upon the incidence of mammary tumors in mice. J. nat. Cancer Inst. **10**, 1259—1262 (1950c).

— Studies on the transmission of the mouse mammary tumor agent by the male parent. J. nat. Cancer Inst. **12**, 819—837 (1952).

— Experimentelle Untersuchungen über die Genese des Mammakarzinoms. Schweiz. Med. Wschr. **85**, 387—390 (1955a).

— Tumours of the hypophysis and thyroid in mice. Acta endocr. (Kbh.) **18**, 445—446 (1955b).

— The hormonal genesis of mammary cancer. Advanc. Cancer Res. **4**, 371—391 (1956).

— Hormones as carcinogenic factors. Ann. Med. (Perugia) **48**, 125—132 (1957).

— Studies on the hormone dependence of experimental breast tumours in mice. In: Endocrine Aspects of Breast Cancer, pp. 291—296, A. R. Currie ed., London: E. & S. Livingstone Ltd. 1958a.

— Mammary cancer in human beings and in animals. A comparison. In: Proceedings of the II International Symposium on Mammary Cancer, pp. 811—816, L. Severi ed., Division of Cancer Research, Perugia, 1958b.

MÜHLBOCK, O., and L. M. BOOT: Induction of mammary cancer in mice without the mammary tumor agent by isografts of hypophyses. Cancer Res. **19**, 402—412 (1959).

— — Natural factors influencing host responses. In: Symposium of Phenomena of the Tumor Viruses, J. W. BEARD ed., National Cancer Institute Monograph No. 4, 129—140, 1960.

— W. VAN EBBENHORST TENGBERGEN, and T. G. VAN RIJSSEL: Studies on the development of mammary tumors in dilute-brown DBAb mice without the agent. J. nat. Cancer Inst. **13**, 505—531 (1952).

MURPHY, J. B.: The effect of castration, theelin and testosterone on the incidence of leukemia in a Rockefeller Institute strain of mice. Cancer Res. **4**, 622—624 (1944).

—, and E. STURM: The effect of diethylstilbestrol on the incidence of leukemia in male mice of the Rockefeller Institute Leukemia strain (RIL). Cancer Res. **9**, 88—89 (1949).

MURRAY, W. S.: Ovarian secretion and tumor incidence. Science **66**, 600—601 (1927).

— Ovarian secretion and tumor incidence. J. Cancer Res. **12**, 18—25 (1928).

— Studies on inheritance of mammary carcinoma in mouse. Concentration of extrachromosomal factor. Physiological stability of individual. Cancer Res. **1**, 123—129 (1941a).

— Studies on effect of foster nursing and its relation to the development of mammary carcinoma in mouse. Cancer Res. **1**, 790—792 (1941b).

—, and C. C. LITTLE: Chromosomal and extrachromosomal influence in relation to the incidence of mammary tumors in mice. Amer. J. Cancer **37**, 536—552 (1939).

—, and S. G. WARNER: Segregation mammary cancer to no mammary cancer in the Marsh albino strain of mice. J. nat. Cancer Inst. **7**, 183—188 (1947).

NAGAREDA, C. S., and H. S. KAPLAN: The effect of hypophysectomy and X irradiation on lymphoid organs and on the induction of lymphoid tumors in C57 Bl mice. J. nat. Cancer Inst. **16**, 139—152 (1955).

NANDI, S.: Role of somatotropin in mammogenesis and lactogenesis in C3H/He Crgl Mice. Science **128**, 772—774 (1958).

— Hormonal control of mammogenesis and lactogenesis in the C3H/He Crgl mouse. Univ. Calif. Publ. Zool. **65**, 1—128 (1959).

— Effect of the mammary tumor agent (MTA) and of multiple pregnancies on the responsiveness of C3H mammary tissue to somatotropin-containing hormonal combinations. Proc. Amer. Ass. Cancer Res. **3**, 254 (1961a).

— Differential responsiveness of A and C3H mouse mammary tissues to somatotropin-containing hormonal combinations. Proc. Soc. exp. Biol. (N. Y.) **108**, 1—3 (1961b).

— Effect of hormones on the maintenance of hyperplastic alveolar nodules in the mammary glands of various strains of mice. J. nat. Cancer Inst. **27**, 187—201 (1961c).

—, and H. A. BERN: Relation between mammary gland responses to lactogenic hormone combinations and tumor susceptibility in various strains of mice. J. nat. Cancer Inst. **24**, 907—931 (1960).

— — Effect of hormones on mammary tumor development from transplanted hyperplastic alveolar nodules in hypophysectomized-ovariectomized-adrenalectomized C3H/Crgl mice. J. nat. Cancer Inst. **27**, 173—185 (1961).

— —, and K. B. DEOME: Hormonal induction and maintenance of precancerous hyperplastic alveolar nodules in the mammary glands of hypophysectomized female C3H/He Crgl mice. Acta Un. int. Cancr. **16**, 211—224 (1960c).

— — — Effect of hormones on growth and neoplastic development of transplanted hyperplastic alveolar nodules of the mammary glands of C3H/Crgl mice. J. nat. Cancer Inst. **24**, 883—905 (1960b).

NICOD, J. L.: Essai de classification des cancers spontanés de la glande mammaire chèz la souris blanche. Bull. Cancer **25**, 1—16 (1936).

OLIVI, M., C. BIANCIFIORI e G. BARBIERI: Il carcinoma spontaneo della mammella del topo ad alta incidenza. Introduzione nello schema classificativo del carcinoma tipo M (mucoso). Lav. Ist. Anat. Univ. Perugia **15**, 5—33 (1955).

—, e F. CASCHERA: Modificazioni mammarie nel topo sottoposto a pennellature di metilcolantrene (in vergini del BALB/c/Cb/Se substrain). Lav. Ist. Anat. Univ. Perugia **20**, 199—211 (1960).

— — e G. BARBIERI: La fase precancerosa biologica e la genesi dei noduli iperplastici alveolari nella mammella del topo (RIII/Dm/Se substrain). Lav. Ist. Anat. Univ. Perugia **18**, 5—24 (1958a).

— — — Mammary cancer development in the RIII/Dm/Se substrain of mice studied by the histological and "whole mount" methods. In: Proceedings of the II International Symposium on Mammary Cancer, pp. 617—626, L. SEVERI ed., Division of Cancer Research, Perugia, 1958b.

— — e E. BUCCIARELLI: Contributo alla conoscenza della patogenesi dei noduli di iperplasia alveolare nella mammella del topo (RIII/Dm/Se e BALB/cf/Cb/Se substrains). Lav. Ist. Anat. Univ. Perugia **21**, 107—117 (1961).

OLIVI, M., e G. CONSOLANDI: Rilievi sul cancro estrogenico della mammella nel topo "h.m.c.". Lav. Ist. Anat. Univ. Perugia **15**, 241—270 (1955).
ORR, J. W.: The chemical induction of mammary and ovarian tumours. Acta Un. int. Cancr. **12**, 682—689 (1956).
PASSARETTI, J. R., e F. CASCHERA: Il ciclo estrale nei topi femmina vergini del ceppo C+. Lav. Ist. Anat. Univ. Perugia **16**, 169—175 (1956).
PASSEY, R. D., L. DMOCHOWSKI, W. T. ASTBURY, and R. REED: Electron microscope studies of normal and malignant tissues of high- and low-breast-cancer strains of mice. Nature (Lond.) **160**, 565 (1947).
— — — —, and P. JOHNSON: Ultracentrifugation and electron microscope studies of tissues of inbred strains of mice. Nature (Lond.) **161**, 759 (1948).
— — — — — Electron microscope studies of normal and malignant tissues of high- and low-breast-cancer strains of mice. Nature (Lond.) **165**, 107 (1950a).
— — R. REED, and W. T. ASTBURY: Biophysical studies of extracts of tissues of high- and low-breast-cancer strain of mice. Biochim. Biophys. Acta **4**, 391—409 (1950b).
PEACOCK, A.: A possible mode of transmission of the mouse mammary tumor agent by the male parent. Brit. J. Cancer **7**, 352—357 (1953).
PIKOVSKI, M. A.: The survival of the mammary tumor agent in cultures of heterologous cells. J. nat. Cancer Inst. **13**, 1275—1282 (1953).
PITELKA, D. R., H. A. BERN, K. B. DEOME, C. N. SCHOOLEY, and S. R. WELLINGS: Virus-like particles in hyperplastic alveolar nodules of the mammary gland of the C3H/HeCRGL mouse. J. nat. Cancer Inst. **20**, 541—553 (1958).
— K. B. DEOME, and H. A. BERN: Viruslike particles in precancerous hyperplastic mammary tissues of C3H and C3Hf mice. J. nat. Cancer Inst. **25**, 753—777 (1960).
PORTER, K. R., and H. P. THOMPSON: A particulate body associated with epithelial cells cultured from mammary carcinomas of mice of a milk-factor strain. J. exp. Med. **88**, 15—24 (1948).
PREHN, R. T.: Transfer of the mammary tumor milk agent from implant to host. J. nat. Cancer Inst. **12**, 1127—1139 (1952).
PULLINGER, B. D.: Cystic disease of the breast human and experimental. Lancet **16**, 567—572 (1947).
— Tests for mammary tumour agent in C3Hf and RIIIf mouse strains. Brit. J. Cancer **14**, 279—284 (1960).
—, and S. IVERSEN: Mammary tumour incidence in relation to age and number of litters in C3Hf and RIIIf mice. Brit. J. Cancer **14**, 267—278 (1960).
PYBUS, F. C., and E. W. MILLER: A sex difference in the incidence of bone tumors in mice. Amer. J. Cancer **34**, 248—251 (1938).
— — The gross pathology of spontaneous bone tumors in mice. Amer. J. Cancer **40**, 47—53 (1940).
RANADIVE, J. K.: The influence of "milk borne tumor agent" on some endocrine glands in intact and castrated mice. Acta Un. int. Cancr. **12**, 701—710 (1956).
RAUSCHER, F. J.: A virus-induced disease of mice characterized by erythrocytopoiesis and lymphoid leukemia. J. nat. Cancer Inst. **29**, 515—543 (1962).
RICHARDSON, F. L., and G. HALL: Mammary tumors and mammary-gland development in hybrid mice treated with diethylstilbestrol for varying periods. J. nat. Cancer Inst. **25**, 1023—1033 (1960).
—, and K. P. HUMMEL: Mammary tumors and mammary-gland development in virgin mice of strains C3H, RIII and their F_1 hybrids. J. nat. Cancer Inst. **23**, 91—100 (1959).
SAMUELS, L. T., J. J. BITTNER, and B. K. SAMUELS: Excretion of steroids in the feces of mice of various strains with and without the mammary tumor milk agent. Cancer Res. **7**, 722 (1947).
SEVERI, L., C. BIANICFIORI, M. OLIVI, and F. SQUARTINI: On hormone dependence in the transmission of mammary tumour agent from males. In: Endocrine Aspects of Breast Cancer, pp. 283—290, A. R. CURRIE ed., London: E. & S. Livingstone Ltd. 1958.
— — — — A microscopical study of mammary cancer in hybrid mice, with particular reference to histogenesis. Acta Un. int. Cancr. **15**, 227—231 (1959).
— M. OLIVI e C. BIANCIFIORI: Istopatologia del carcinoma mammario negli "inbred strains" del topo. Atti Soc. ital. Cancer. **1**, 85—158 (1958).
—, and F. SQUARTINI: A parallel study of human and experimental breast cancer. In: Proceedings of the II International Symposium on Mammary Cancer, pp. 835—845, L. SEVERI ed., Division of Cancer Research, Perugia, 1958.
— — Discussion of the Mühlbock's paper. In: A Ciba Foundation Symposium on Carcinogenesis, Mechanisms of Action, p. 94, G. E. W. WOLSTENHOLME and M. O'CONNOR eds., London: J. & A. Churchill Ltd. 1959.
— — Problems arising in the control of breast cancer. Acta Un. int. Cancr. **18**, 755—759 (1962).

Shimkin, M. B.: Unpublished data, 1943. Quoted by M. B. Shimkin, 1945.
— Hormones and mammary cancer in mice. In: A Symposium on Mammary Tumors in Mice, pp. 85—122, F. R. Moulton ed., American Association for the Advancement of Science, Washington, 1945.
—, and H. B. Andervont: Effect of foster nursing on the response of mice to estrogens. J. nat. Cancer Inst. **1**, 599—605 (1941).
— — Effect of foster nursing on the induction of mammary and testicular tumors in mice injected with stilbestrol. J. nat. Cancer. Inst. **2**, 611—622 (1942).
Silberberg, M., and R. Silberberg: Susceptibility to estrogen of breast, vagina, and endometrium of various strains of mice. Proc. Soc. exp. Biol. (N. Y.) **76**, 161—164 (1951).
— — Leukemogenic action of adrenocorticotrophic hormone (ACTH) in mice of various ages. Cancer Res. **15**, 291—293 (1955).
Silberberg, R., M. Silberberg, and J. J. Bittner: Relative rôle of milk agent and tissue sensitivity in estrogen induced mammary growth. Proc. Soc. exp. Biol. (N. Y.) **77**, 473—477 (1951).
Sinkovics, J. G., C. C. Shullenberger, and D. H. Clifton: Comparative studies on leukemogenesis in mice inoculated with murine and human leukemic materials. In: Atti di un Simposio Internazionale su I Virus nelle Leucemie dei Mammiferi, pp. 171—188, Accademia Nazionale dei Lincei, Roma, 1964.
Slye, M., H. F. Holmes, and H. G. Wells: Primary spontaneous tumors of the ovary in mice. J. Cancer Res. **5**, 205—226 (1920).
Smith, F. W.: Castration effects of inherited hormonal influence. Science **101**, 279—281 (1945).
— Castration effects on the inherited hormonal influence. Cancer Res. **6**, 494 (1946).
— Relationships of the inherited hormonal influence to the production of adrenal cortical tumors by castration. Cancer Res. 8, 641—651 (1948).
—, and J. J. Bittner: Castration effects in relation to inherited hormonal influence in mice. Cancer Res. **5**, 588 (1945).
Smoller, C. G., D. R. Pitelka, and H. A. Bern: Cytoplasmic inclusion bodies in cortisol-treated mammary tumors of C3H/Crgl mice. J. biophys. biochem. Cytol. **9**, 915—920 (1961).
Squartini, F.: Momenti di applicazione dei fattori eziologici del cancro mammario spontaneo del topo. Lav. Ist. Anat. Univ. Perugia **15**, 153—161 (1955).
— Il significato dell' "agente" nella risposta iperplastica della mammella del topo a stimoli ormonici. Lav. Ist. Anat. Univ. Perugia **16**, 143—167 (1956a).
— Il significato della suscettibilità ereditaria nella risposta iperplastica della mammella del topo a stimoli ormonici. Lav. Ist. Anat. Univ. Perugia **16**, 177—198 (1956b).
— La patogenesi del cancro spontaneo della mammella del topo. Lav. Ist. Anat. Univ. Perugia **16**, 211—269 (1956c).
— A new method for the study of the mammary gland of the mouse: Surface area of the glandular tree in section. Cancer **10**, 179—182 (1957).
— Eziopatogenesi del carcinoma mammario negli "inbred strains" del topo. Atti Soc. ital. Cancer. **1**, 7—84 (1958).
— Mammogenesis and breast carcinogenesis in virgin female mice of BALB/cf substrain with the milk agent. J. nat. Cancer Inst. **23**, 1227—1238 (1959).
— Mammary tumors in mice as a model in studies on carcinogenesis. In: Recent Contributions to Cancer Research in Italy, Vol. 1, pp. 289—335, P. Bucalossi and U. Veronesi eds., Casa Editrice Ambrosiana, Milano, 1960.
— Strain differences in growth of mouse mammary tumors. J. nat. Cancer Inst. **26**, 813—828 (1961).
— Responsiveness and progression of mammary tumors in high-cancer-strain mice. J. nat. Cancer Inst. **28**, 911—926 (1962a).
— Progress Report to USPHS Research Grant C-3844 Path: "A study of mammary cancer". Lav. Ist. Anat. Univ. Perugia **22**, 97—145 (1962b).
— E. Barola, I. Paoletti, e G. Rossi: Gravidico-dipendenza dei tumori mammari nei topi del C3H/Cb/Se substrain. Lav. Ist. Anat. Univ. Perugia **24**, 29—37 (1964).
—, e C. Biancifiori: Comportamento del "mammary tumor agent" dopo introduzione nell'ospite suscettibile. Lav. Ist. Anat. Univ. Perugia **18**, 119—123 (1958).
— C. Bolli, and G. Rossi: On the factors controlling breast susceptibility to estradiolbenzoate in mice. In: Proceedings of the II International Symposium on Mammary Cancer, pp. 523—538, L. Severi ed., Division of Cancer Research, Perugia, 1958.
—, e F. Caschera: Sviluppo mammario, noduli di iperplasia alveolare e tumori nei topi femmina vergini BALB/cf. Lav. Ist. Anat. Univ. Perugia **18**, 175—204 (1958).
—, e G. Lotti: Morfologia e funzione delle strutture mammarie del topo (con riferimenti alla mammella umana). Lav. Ist. Anat. Univ. Perugia **15**, 61—76 (1955).

SQUARTINI, F., e R. RIBACCHI: Irregolarità nella propagazione del "mammary tumor agent" attraverso i topi RIII. Lav. Ist. Anat. Univ. Perugia **20**, 5—16 (1960).

—, e G. ROSSI: Accrescimento e progressione dei tumori mammari nei topi femmina del substrain RIII/Dm/Se. Lav. Ist. Anat. Univ. Perugia **19**, 105—124 (1959a).

— — Analisi morfologica della "responsiveness" e della progressione nei tumori mammari del "substrain" RIII/Dm/Se. Lav. Ist. Anat. Univ. Perugia **19**, 165—214 (1959b).

— — Studio dei tumori mammari nel BALB/cf/Cb/Se substrain: accrescimento "responsiveness" e progressione, origine istologica, morfologia. Lav. Ist. Anat. Univ. Perugia **20**, 133—165 (1960).

— — Cancerogenesi e caratteri dei tumori mammari nei topi (RIII/Dm/Se substrain) sottoposti ad una singola gravidanza. Lav. Ist. Anat. Univ. Perugia **21**, 53—68 (1961a).

— — Comportamento dei tumori mammari nei topi (RIII/Dm/Se substrain) accoppiati con maschi vasectomizzati. Lav. Ist. Anat. Univ. Perugia **21**, 119—137 (1961b).

— — Responsiveness and progression of the morphological precursors of breast cancer in inbred mice: A review. In: The Morphological Precursors of Cancer, pp. 319—327, L. SEVERI ed., Division of Cancer Research, Perugia, 1962.

— — Alta incidenza di leucemia nei topi BALB/c allattati da RIII. In: Atti di un Simposio Internazionale su I Virus nelle Leucemie dei Mammiferi, pp. 129—148, Accademia Nazionale dei Lincei, Roma, 1964a.

— — Unpublished data, 1964b.

— — N. MALTZEFF e O. SACCO: Influenza del "forced breeding" sulla "responsiveness" dei tumori mammari (RIII/Dm/Se substrain). Lav. Ist. Anat. Univ. Perugia **20**, 237—251 (1960).

— — e I. PAOLETTI: Trasmissione extracromosomica dei caratteri tumorali: effetto del "foster-nursing" sul comportamento biologico e morfologico dei tumori mammari del topo. Lav. Ist. Anat. Univ. Perugia **22**, 203—211 (1962a). Tumori **48**, 273 (1962b).

— — — Characters of mammary tumours in BALB/c female mice foster-nursed by C3H and RIII mothers. Nature (Lond.) **197**, 505—506 (1963).

—, and L. SEVERI: Strain differences in the mammary tumour-inducing virus as detected by the characters and behaviour of neoplasms. In: A Ciba Foundation Symposium on Tumour Viruses of Murine Origin, pp. 82—106, G. E. W. WOLSTENHOLME and M. O'CONNOR eds., London: J. & A. Churchill Ltd. 1962.

— — Analisi statistica dei fattori che influenzano la trasmissione del "mammary tumour virus" da parte del maschio. In: La Statistica nelle Ricerche sui Tumori, Proceedings of a Symposium held in Rome, Oct. 27—28, 1963 (in press).

Staff of the Roscoe B. Jackson Memorial Laboratory: The existence of nonchromosomal influence in the incidence of mammary tumors in mice. Science **78**, 465—466 (1933).

STEWART, H. L.: Experimental cancer of the alimentary tract. In: The Physiopathology of Cancer, pp. 3—45, F. HOMBURGER and W. H. FISHMAN eds., London: Cassell and Company Ltd. 1953a.

— Endometrial cancer of the rabbit. In: The Physiopathology of Cancer, pp. 165—170, F. HOMBURGER and W. H. FISHMAN eds., London: Cassell and Company Ltd. 1953b.

— Pulmonary tumors in mice. In: The Physiopathology of Cancer, 2nd edition, pp. 18—37, F. HOMBURGER ed., London: Cassell and Company Ltd. 1958.

STONE, R., and D. H. MOORE: Purification of the mouse mammary carcinoma agent by means of a fluorocarbon. Nature (Lond.) **183**, 1275—1276 (1959).

STRONG, L. C.: Latent period in growth of spontaneous mammary carcinoma in female mice of the A strain. Arch. Path. **26**, 814—819 (1938).

SUZUKI, T.: Electron microscopic cyto-histopathology. III. Electron microscopic studies on spontaneous mammary carcinoma of mice. Gann **48**, 39—56 (1957).

TANNENBAUM, A.: The dependence of tumor formation on the degree of caloric restriction. Cancer Res. **5**, 609—615 (1945a).

— The dependence of tumor formation on the composition of the caloric-restricted diet as well as on the degree of restriction. Cancer Res. **5**, 616—625 (1945b).

—, and H. SILVERSTONE: The genesis and growth of tumors. IV. Effects of varying the proportion of protein (casein) in the diet. Cancer Res. **9**, 162—173 (1949a).

— — Dependence of formation of spontaneous mammary carcinoma in mice on the proportion of dietary fat. Cancer Res. **9**, 607—608 (1949b).

— — Nutrition in relation to cancer. Advanc. Cancer Res. **1**, 451—501 (1953).

TAYLOR, A., N. CARMICHAEL, and T. NORRIS: Further report on yolk sac cultivation of tumor tissue. Cancer Res. **8**, 264—269 (1948).

— R. E. HUNGATE, and D. R. TAYLOR: Yolk sac cultivation of tumors. Cancer Res. **3**, 537—541 (1943).

— J. THACKER, and D. PENNINGTON: The growth of cancer tissue in the yolk sac of the chick embryo. Science **96**, 342—343 (1942).

TAYLOR, H. C., and C. A. WALTMAN: Hyperplasias of the mammary gland in the human being and in the mouse. Arch. Surg. **40**, 733—820 (1940).
THUNG, P. J., L. M. BOOT, and O. MÜHLBOCK: Senile changes in the oestrous cycle and in ovarian structure in some inbred strains of mice. Acta Endocr. (Kbh.) **23**, 8—32 (1956).
TRENTIN, J. J.: Vaginal sensitivity to estrogens as related to mammary tumor incidence in mice. Cancer Res. **10**, 580—583 (1950).
— The effect of the presence or absence of the milk factor and of castration on mammary response to estrogen in male mice of strains of known mammary tumor incidence. Cancer Res. **11**, 286—287 (1951).
— Unpublished data, 1953. Quoted by W. U. GARDNER et al., 1953.
—, and C. W. TURNER: Quantitative study of the effect of inanition on responsiveness of the mammary gland to estrogens. Endocrinology **29**, 984—989 (1941).
TURNER, C. W. and E. T. GOMEZ: The normal development of the mammary gland of the male and female albino mouse. II. Extrauterine. Mo. Agr. exp. Sta. Res. Bull. **182**, 21—43 (1933).
TWOMBLY, G. H., and H. C. TAYLOR: Inactivation and conversion of estrogens *in vitro* by liver and other tissues from human cancer patients and from mice of strains susceptible to mammary carcinoma. Cancer Res. **2**, 811—817 (1942).
UPTON, A. C., and J. FURTH: The effects of cortisone on the development of spontaneous leukemia in mice and on its induction by irradiation. Blood **9**, 686—695 (1954).
VISSCHER, M. B., R. G. GREEN, J. J. BITTNER, Z. B. BALL, and H. A. SIEDENTOPF: Characterization of milk influence in spontaneous mammary carcinoma. Proc. Soc. exp. Biol. (N. Y.) **49**, 94—96 (1942).
VOGT, M., and R. DULBECCO: Studies on cells rendered neoplastic by polyoma virus: The problem of the presence of virus-related materials. Virology **16**, 41—51 (1962).
WALLACE, E. W., H. WALLACE, and C. A. MILLS: Influence of environmental temperature upon the incidence and course of spontaneous tumors in C3H mice. Cancer Res. **4**, 279—281 (1944).
— — — Influence of environmental temperature upon the incidence and course of spontaneous tumors in spayed C3H mice. Cancer Res. **5**, 47—48 (1945).
WHITE, F. R., and J. WHITE: Effect of a low-lysine diet on mammary-tumor formation in strain C3H mice. J. nat. Cancer Inst. **4**, 41—42 (1944).
— — G. B. MIDER, M. G. KELLY, and W. E. HESTON: Effect of caloric restriction on mammary-tumor formation in strain C3H mice and on the response of strain DBA to painting with methylcholanthrene. J. nat. Cancer Inst. **5**, 43—48 (1944).
WHITE, J., and G. B. MIDER: Effect of certain dietary constituents on the incidence of leukemia produced by methylcholanthrene in dilute brown mice. Cancer Res. **3**, 129—130 (1943).
WOOLLEY, G. W., E. FEKETE, and C. C. LITTLE: Mammary tumor development in mice ovariectomized at birth. Proc. nat. Acad. Sci. **25**, 277—279 (1939).
— — — Differences between high and low breast tumor strains of mice when ovariectomized at birth. Proc. Soc. exp. Biol. (N. Y.) **45**, 796—798 (1940).
— — — Gonadectomy and adrenal neoplasms. Science **97**, 291 (1941a).
— — — Effects of castration in the dilute brown strain of mice. Endocrinology **28**, 341—343 (1941b).
— L. W. LAW, and C. C. LITTLE: The occurrence on whole blood of material influencing the incidence of mammary carcinoma in mice. Cancer Res. **1**, 955—956 (1941).

Erzeugung von Tumoren durch endogenhormonelle Faktoren

Von

Walter Dontenwill

Mit 45 Abbildungen

Einleitung

Der Besprechung der endogen-hormonell bedingten Geschwülste soll zunächst ein formelles Einteilungsprinzip aller bösartigen Tumoren zugrunde gelegt werden. Ein solches Einteilungsprinzip kann nach histogenetischen oder kausalgenetischen Prinzipien erfolgen, es darf aber andererseits die Dignität der Geschwülste nicht vernachlässigen. Siegmund hatte schon 1941 die Ansicht vertreten, daß ein großer Teil von dem, was damals noch als „gutartige Geschwulst“ bezeichnet wurde, nichts anderes als eine resorptiv und reparativ bedingte Gewebsproliferation darstelle, wozu unter anderem die Riesenzellepuliden und braunen Tumoren des Knochens sowie die Xanthome zu rechnen sind, oder daß es sich um „regulativ-kompensatorisch bedingte organische Proliferationen handele, die meist durch hormonelle Impulse in einer durchaus funktionsmäßigen Weise die Form in Bewegung bringen, ohne sie aufzulösen oder der ganzheitlichen Ordnung zu entziehen“. Zu diesen Proliferationen, die die Bezeichnung „Tumor“ nicht verdienen, rechnete er die Strumen der verschiedenen endokrinen Organe, die sog. Adenome der Prostata, die Fibroadenome der Mamma und die Myome des Uterus. Für die Frage, woran sich diese Proliferationen „anpassen“ und wer sie „reguliert“, sind inzwischen in der in- und ausländischen Literatur so viele überzeugende Daten beigebracht worden, daß der Begriff der „Anpassungshyperplasie“ sich fest eingebürgert hat, auch wenn er von manchen Autoren, die sich von der Vorstellung des Tumorösen in diesen Hyperplasien nicht trennen können, in „hyperplasiogenes Gewächs“ abgewandelt wird (Büngeler). Das unserer Betrachtung zugrunde gelegte Einteilungsprinzip wurde 1951 von Büngeler formuliert und sollte ein heuristisches Arbeitsprinzip, d. h. ein Versuch sein, zu klaren Begriffsbestimmungen in der Geschwulstpathologie zu gelangen.

Büngeler (1951) trennt bei dieser Geschwulstdefinition die eigengesetzlichen Gewebsproliferationen als *autonome* Geschwülste von den nicht autonomen geschwulstähnlichen Gewebsproliferationen, die er als „Anpassungshyperplasien“ bzw. hyperplasiogene Geschwülste bezeichnet. Später wurde auch von Furth (1953) ein ähnliches Einteilungsprinzip vertreten. Er unterschied zwischen "conditioned and autonomous neoplasms". Außerdem prägte er den Begriff des hormonabhängigen Tumor oder "dependent tumor". Wenn wir nach der Definition von Büngeler hier die hormonell ausgelösten Geschwülste als nicht vollkommen autonome Gewächse behandeln, so glauben wir, damit insbesondere die Frage nach dem Einfluß der Hormone auf Wachstum und Proliferation von Geweben, insbesondere aber auf die Tumorentwicklung am ehesten beantworten zu können.

Zweifellos echte Geschwülste (Carcinome und Sarkome) sind nach BÜNGELER und der weitgehend übereinstimmenden Definition von Klinikern und Pathologen selbständige, von den Regulationseinrichtungen des Körpers nicht mehr beeinflußbare Zellproliferationen, deren völlige Autonomie vor allem in der Metastasenbildung, noch eindrucksvoller aber im Experiment bei der Überführung eines Organkrebses in die sog. Ascitesform und die damit gegebene Übertragbarkeit mittels einer einzelnen Tumorzelle in Erscheinung tritt, wie das YOSHIDA (1957) in seinen Untersuchungen am Buttergelb-Krebs der Leber zeigen konnte. Die völlige Entziehung von den das Wachstum regulierenden Einflüssen wird bei diesen frei in der Ascitesflüssigkeit schwimmenden Krebszellen dadurch deutlich, daß sie auch bei Übertragung auf ein gesundes und nicht vorbehandeltes Tier ihre Neigung zum schrankenlosen Wachstum beibehalten und sich ähnlich verhalten wie ein echter Parasit. Daß für diese vollkommene *Autonomie* entscheidende Änderungen in den Steuerungseinrichtungen der Zelle maßgebend sein müssen, liegt auf der Hand: Die Zelle selbst ist also offenbar nicht mehr regulierbar, während die Regulierungssysteme des Organismus noch intakt sein können. Das Wesentliche in der Begriffsbestimmung „maligner Tumor" liegt demnach in der vollkommenen Autonomie der mit Formverfall verknüpften Wachstumssteigerung, welche nicht mehr den ordnenden Einflüssen der Gefäßversorgung, des Nervensystems und der inneren Sekretion unterliegt.

Schwieriger ist die Definition bei denjenigen Wachstumsstörungen, welche in der Regel noch — und vor allem einem praktischen Bedürfnis Rechnung tragend — als gutartige Geschwülste bezeichnet werden, wobei zwischen ihnen und den „echten Krebsen" oft nur graduelle Unterscheidungen gemacht wurden, was besonders auch in den immer wieder behaupteten fließenden Übergängen zwischen beiden Geschwulstformen zum Ausdruck kommt („Stufen der Malignität", RÖSSLE). Bei den gutartigen Geschwülsten handelt es sich um lokal begrenzte, in der Regel expansiv wachsende und nicht metastasierende Wachstumssteigerungen, wobei Struktur und Leistung der Einzelzelle noch weitgehend denjenigen der normalen Körperzelle entsprechen, also offenbar noch den Wachstumsregulationen des Organismus unterworfen sind. Gerade in endokrinen Drüsen, die in ihrer Wachstumsregulation vom Bedarf des Organismus, d. h. von der übergeordneten Regulierung durch Hypophyse und ZNS abhängig sind, können bei Störungen der normalen Wachstumskorrelation Hyperplasien entstehen, die aber, ebenso wie die durch vermehrte hormonelle Stimulierung entstandenen Hyperplasien, in endokrin gesteuerten Geweben in der Regel als durchaus regulierte Wachstumsvorgänge zu betrachten sind. Bei der Entscheidung über Gut- oder Bösartigkeit dürfen bei diesen hyperplastischen Gewebsproliferationen weniger morphologische Kriterien, insbesondere Änderungen der Zellstrukturen, als vielmehr die biologischen Verhaltensweisen gewertet werden.

Wir sind uns darüber im klaren, daß das vorgenommene Einteilungsprinzip nicht widerspruchslos angenommen wird, möchten jedoch glauben, daß dem Leser die als Arbeitsprinzip gedachte, aus unseren Vorstellungen und Erfahrungen resultierende Einteilung verständlich erscheinen wird.

Literatur

BÜNGELER, W.: Die Definition des Geschwulstbegriffes und die Abgrenzung der Hyperplasien gegenüber den Geschwülsten. Verh. dtsch. Ges. Path. **35**, 10 (1951).

— Geschwülste und regulierte abhängige Wachstumsstörungen (Hyperplasien) im Rahmen der Cellular- und Relationspathologie. Z. Krebsforsch. **58**, 72 (1951).

—, u. W. DONTENWILL: Hormonell ausgelöste geschwulstartige Hyperplasien, hyperplasiogene Geschwülste und ihre Verhaltensweisen. Dtsch. med. Wschr. **1959**, 1885.

FURTH, J.: Conditioned and Autonomous Neoplasms. A Review. Cancer Res. **13**, 477—492 (1953).
YOSHIDA, T.: Studien über das Ascites Hepatom. Zugleich ein Beitrag zum Begriff der cellulären Autonomie im Wachstum der malignen Geschwulst einerseits und der Individualität der einzelnen Geschwulst andererseits. Virchows Arch. Path. Anat. **330**, 85 (1957).

I. Geschwulstartige Hyperplasien im Tierexperiment

A. In endokrinen Drüsen oder in endokrin gesteuerten Geweben nach Hormonbehandlung, bzw. nach Störung der hormonellen Korrelation, usw.

a) Hypophyse

Über Hypophysenadenome nach langdauernder Oestrogenbehandlung berichteten:

ZONDEK (1936, 1938), CRAMER und HORNING (1936), MCEUEN, SELYE und COLLIP (1936), LACASSAGNE und NYKA (1937), WOLFE und WRIGHT (1938), DEANESLEY (1939), WEIL und ZONDEK (1939), GARDNER und STRONG (1940), GARDNER (1941), NELSON (1941), NOBLE und COLLIP (1941), SEGALOFF und DUNNING (1945), DUX (1948), MEYER und CLIFTON (1956), CLIFTON und MEYER (1956).

Diese meist chromophoben Hypophysenadenome wurden oft als Nebenbefunde bei Versuchen zur experimentellen Erzeugung von Brustdrüsenkrebs durch Follikelhormon bei bestimmten Ratten- und Mäusestämmen beobachtet. SELYE (1944) sah in den Adenomen z. T. polymorphe Zellen und sog. polynucleäre Gigantzellen. DEANSLEY (1939), NELSON (1941), NOBLE und COLLIP (1941) beobachteten eine Abhängigkeit zwischen Behandlungsdauer und der Größe der Adenome, die nach langer Behandlung das höchste Gewicht erkennen ließen.

Ratten erhielten drei Monate lang dreimal wöchentlich 10 μg Oestradiol. Die Hypophyse vergrößerte sich von 2,5—4 mg auf 14—15 mg. Bei höheren Dosen Oestradiol (80 μg) per Injektion wurde eine Hypophysenvergrößerung bis 200 mg beobachtet.

Bei gleichartigen Versuchen sahen OBERLING und GUÉRIN und GUÉRIN (1936) Adenome der Hypophyse bei männlichen Ratten, denen nach Kastration (Technik s. KARG, Krankheiten der Genitalorgane) Ovarien von gleichaltrigen Weibchen eingepflanzt worden waren. Es handelte sich um adenomatöse Neubildungen von Kastrationszellen bzw. Hauptzellen oder sog. Schwangerschaftszellen.

SPAMPINATO (1950) sah nach einer Behandlung (266 Tage) mit täglich 0,5 mg Diäthylstilbendioxyd bei der weißen Ratte eine Zunahme des Hypophysengewichtes auf das 3—4fache, in 63% sah er chromophobe oder eosinophile Hyperplasien in Kombination mit gemischten Adenomen. EGAÑA, SZABO und LECANNELIER (1941) fanden Adenome nach täglichen Injektionen von 10 μg Oestrogen über 3 Monate, d. h. nach insgesamt 3000 μg.

Bei einem Mäusestamm, der nach Kastration zu hyperplastischen bzw. neoplastischen Nebennierenveränderungen neigt, beobachteten CHRISTY, DICKIE, ATKINSON und WOOLLEY (1951) neben den Zeichen der Oestrogenüberproduktion Adenome der Hypophyse. OBERLING, GUÉRIN, LAPLANE DE SÈZE und LACOUR (1950) behandelten weiße Ratten mit Oestrogen (Dihydro-Follikulin) allein (die Ratten erhielten, beginnend im Alter von 4—6 Wochen, jede Woche eine subcutane Injektion von "benzoat dihydrofolliculine" in Öl; 0,05—0,1 cm³ einer 1—5% Lösung Follikulin, daneben erhielten einzelne Tiere wöchentlich 0,2 cm³ einer 5—10% Lösung Testosteron, Progesteron oder Desoxycorticosteron) oder zusammen mit anderen Hormonen (Progesteron, Testosteron, Desoxycorticosteron). Es entstanden dabei Hypophysenadenome, die sich z. T. spontan wieder zurückbildeten. Testosteron hemmt nach OBERLING, GUÉRIN, LAPLANE DE SÈZE und LACOUR (1950) bei genügend hoher Dosis die Wirkung des Follikelhormons auf die Hypophyse, Progesteron und Desoxycorticosteron verstärken dagegen die Wirkung der Oestrogene auf die Hypophyse. Bei diesen Versuchen traten Mammacarcinome nur dann auf, wenn Oestrogene mit einem anderen Hormon zusammen, besonders mit Desoxycorticosteron, gegeben wurden.

GILLMAN und GILBERT (1955) beobachteten eine Förderung der Adenomentstehung des HVL nach Oestrogenbehandlung bei gleichzeitiger *Thyroxingabe* und eine hochgradige Hemmung bei Behandlung mit Thiouracil.

Hypophysenadenome konnten auch bei Parabiose eines kastrierten mit einem normalen Weibchen beobachtet werden, wobei die veränderte Gonadotropinsekretion des kastrierten Tieres beim nichtkastrierten eine Wucherung der Hypophyse auslöste [BIELSCHOWSKY und HALL (1951), HALL, HALL und CUNNINGHAM (1953), CUNNINGHAM, HALL und HALL (1954)]. LACOUR (1951) sah in der Hypophyse eine Hyperplasie der basophilen Zellen bei Tieren, deren Gonaden im Anschluß an die Autotransplantation in die Milz hyperplastisches Wachstum zeigten. CLIFTON und MEYER (1956) injizierten Ratten im Alter von 30 Tagen subcutan Pelotten von je 15 mg Diäthylstilboestrol und wiederholten dann diese Behandlung alle 4 Monate. Die ersten Hypophysenadenome fanden sie nach etwa 9 Monaten. In der Hypophyse waren die acidophilen und die nicht granulierten Zellen vermehrt. Es fanden sich viele Mitosen. Ähnliche Hypophysenadenome beobachtete auch RICHARDSON (1957) bei einem Stamm von hybriden Mäusen, die mit Stilboestrol behandelt wurden. MÜHLBOCK (1957) sah sogar nach kontinuierlicher Fütterung von Mäusen mit Trinkwasser, dem er pro Liter 1 mg Oestrogen zufügte, in 85% Hypophysenadenome. Wenn aber die Tiere in Intervallen von 5 Tagen mit der doppelten Menge Oestrogen gefüttert wurden, traten nur 5% Adenome auf, und nach Absetzen der Behandlung zeigten schon entwickelte Adenome keine Gewichtszunahme mehr.

VASQUEZ-LOPEZ berichtet 1944 über Adenome der *Pars intermedia* der Hypophyse des Goldhamsters nach langdauernder Behandlung mit normalen und synthetischen Oestrogenen und MCEUEN, SELYE und COLLIP (1939) über Adenome des Mittellappens der Ratte nach Oestrogenbehandlung.

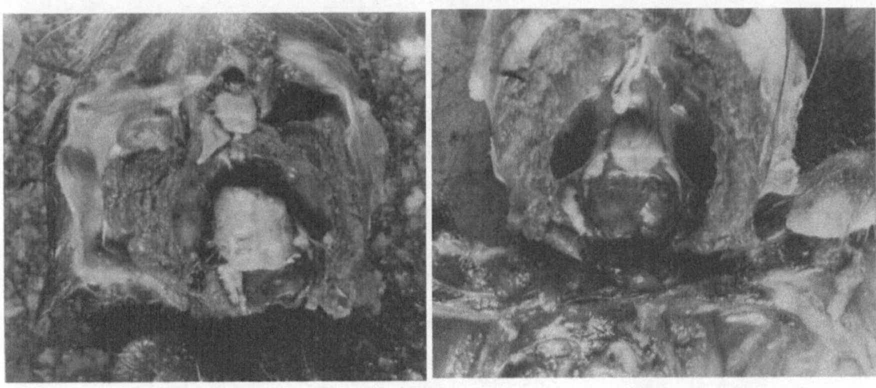

Abb. 1 Abb. 2

Abb. 1. Über erbsengroßes Hypophysenadenom beim Goldhamster. Behandlung 531 Tage Cyren A. (Jeden 2. Tag 0,6 mg)

Abb. 2. Linsengroßes Hypophysenadenom. Behandlung 531 Tage Cyren A. (Jeden 2. Tag 0,6 mg)

Daß zwischen den einzelnen Tierspecies und Tierstämmen starke Unterschiede hinsichtlich der Hypophysenveränderungen bestehen, zeigen die nachfolgenden Beispiele.

Beim *Meerschweinchen* beobachtete LIPSCHUTZ (1950) auch nach über ein Jahr dauernder Oestrogenbehandlung keine Hypophysenadenome, sondern lediglich eine Vergrößerung. Beim

Degu (Nager) beobachtete LIPSCHUTZ (1950) nur bei einem von 29 Tieren nach 8monatiger Behandlung eine Vergrößerung der Hypophyse.

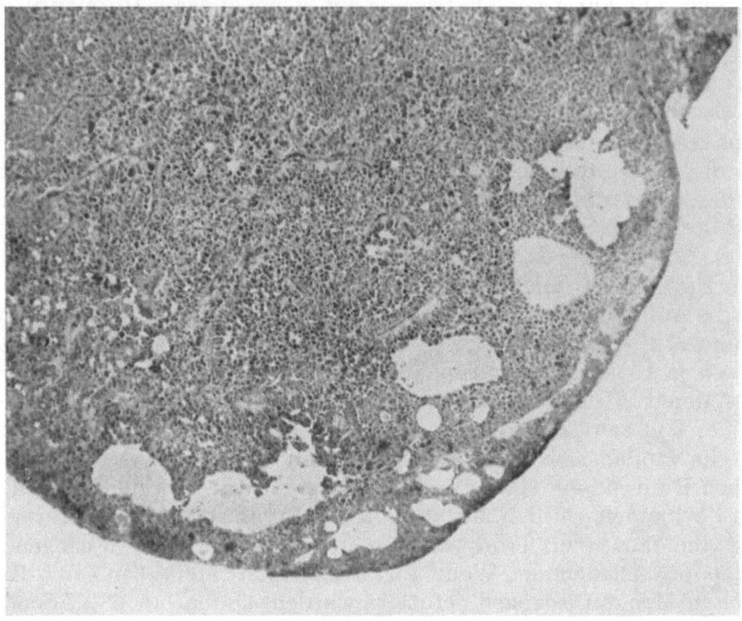

3a

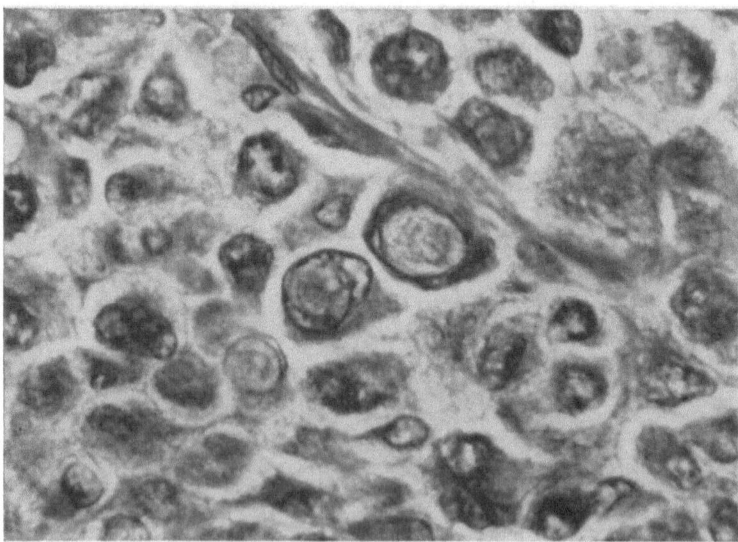

3b

Abb. 3a u. b. Hypophysenadenom beim Goldhamster mit polymorphen, meist basophilen Zellen mit Vacuolen. Behandlung 8 Monate, 9 Tage Cyren B. (Jeden 2. Tag 0,6 mg)

Besonders häufig traten auch z. T. außerordentlich große Hypophysenadenome (Abb. 1 u. 2) bei langdauernder Follikelhormonbehandlung (jeden 2. Tag 0,6 mg Cyren A oder B über etwa 12 Monate) des Goldhamsters auf [KIRKMAN und BACON

(1952), HORNING (1956), DONTENWILL und EDER (1959)]. Wir sahen dabei fast immer basophile Adenome mit z. T. hochgradiger Zellpolymorphie und typischen Crooke-Zellen mit Vacuolen (Abb. 3a u. b). Die Adenome führten häufig zu Deformierungen der Schädelbasis. Bei diesen Adenomen konnten keine Veränderungen an den endokrinen Drüsen oder endokrin gesteuerten Organen nachgewiesen werden, die auf eine Mehrsekretion der vergrößerten Hypophyse hindeuten.

1. Spezielle Hypophysenadenome

Während bei den bisher angeführten Adenomen oder Hyperplasien keine bestimmte Differenzierung nach ihrer Sekretion bzw. Leistung vorgenommen werden konnte, wurden in den letzten Jahren besonders von FURTH (1955, 1957, 1958), FURTH und CLIFTON (1957), CLIFTON (1959) eine Reihe von verschiedenartigen Hypophysenadenomen beschrieben [Übersicht über diese Hypophysenadenome, ihre Ursachen, ihre hormonelle Leistung bzw. Struktur zeigt ein Schema (Tab. 1) aus der Monographie von KWA HONG GIOG (1961)], die als mammatrope, adrenocorticotrope, thyreotrope, somatothyreotrope und amphophile Adenome bezeichnet wurden. Die Differenzierung dieser Adenome bezieht sich z. T. auf ihre spezifische Leistung, z. T. auf ihre typische Zellstruktur. RUSSFIELD, FRIEDLER

Tabelle 1. *Schematische Einteilung der Hypophysentumoren bei Maus und Ratte*

Proliferierender Zelltyp		anzunehmende Hormonbildung	Experimentelle Bedingungen	Art der Hypophysenstimulierung
ıeoretisch erwartet	tatsächlich beobachtet			
ısophiler β-Z	entgranulierter basophiler β-Z. chromophober	TSH („thyrotrophin" usw.)	Chirurgische Schilddrüsenentfernung; „Radiothyreoidektomie"; schilddrüsenblockierende Substanzen; Jodmangeldiät	Unterbrechung des Wechselmechanismus zwischen Schilddrüse und Hypophyse, durch chronischen Mangel an Schilddrüsenhormon
ɪidophil „Prolactin-produzierender Typ"	entgranulierter acidophiler; chromophober	Prolactin (Luteotrophin, mammotropes Hormon, lactogenes Hormon usw.)	Kontinuierliche Oestrogen behandlung, übermäßige Oestrogenwirkung, durch Dysfunktion der Gonaden und/oder Nebennieren, spontan, durch Bestrahlung, nach frühzeitiger Kastration	Oestrogenwirkung als spezifisches Stimulans der prolactinproduzierenden Zellen
ɪidophil „ACTH-produzierender Typ"	„vorwiegend chromophober einzelne Zellen mit groben acidophilen Granula"	ACTH	Durch Bestrahlung induziert	Durch Bestrahlung ausgelösteSchädigung der Nebennieren: Unterbrechung des Wechselmechanismus zwischen Nebenniere und Hypophyse
ɪidophil „wachstumshormonproduzierender Typ"	schmaler chromophober	Wachstumshormon (STH)	Durch Bestrahlung induziert	Unbekannt
ɪlta-basophil „FSH-produzierender Typ"	basophiler	FSH	Frühzeitige Kastration	Unterbrechung des Wechselmechanismus zwischen Gonaden und Hypophyse
ɪlta-basophil „LH-produzierender Typ"	basophiler	LH (ICSH usw.)	Frühzeitige Kastration	Unterbrechung der Wechselbeziehung zwischen Gonaden und Hypophyse

und FRENKEL berichteten 1963 über einen Hypophysentumor der 24 Monate nach Transplantation des Ovars in die Milz eines kastrierten Rattenweibchens entstanden war. Dieser Tumor war transplantabel.

2. *Mammotrope Adenome*

CLIFTON und MEYER (1956), FURTH, BUFFETT und GADSDEN (1957), FURTH, GADSDEN, CLIFTON und ANDERSON (1956), CLIFTON und FURTH (1957), FURTH und CLIFTON (1958), FURTH, CLIFTON, GADSDEN und BUFFET (1956), YOKORO, FURTH und HARAN-GHERA (1964) beschrieben in verschiedenen Arbeiten Hypophysenadenome nach langdauernder Behandlung mit Oestrogenen, aber auch nach Ganzkörperbestrahlung (s. Artikel WRBA). Sie sahen dabei Hyperplasien vorwiegend der acidophilen Zellen bei gleichzeitiger Hyperplasie aller Elemente der Brustdrüse und starker Milchsekretion. Eine gleichzeitig beobachtete Nebennierenrindenverbreiterung ging nicht mit einem Hypercorticoidismus einher, konnte also nicht als Zeichen einer Mehrsekretion von ACTH gedeutet werden. Die Veränderungen der Brustdrüse zeigten eindeutig, daß die mammotrope Hormonbildung die wesentliche Leistung der Adenome darstellt [BATES, CLIFTON und ANDERSON (1956)]. Bei diesen Adenomen trat auch ein somatotroper Effekt auf [FURTH, GADSDEN, CLIFTON und ANDERSON (1956), CLIFTON und FURTH (1957)], der sich in der Vergrößerung von Organen und Zellen nach Transplantation des Hypophysenadenoms beim Wirtstier zeigte. Prolactinproduktion in Hypophysenadenomen die nach Hypophysentransplantationen auftraten, wurde von BOOT, RÖPCKE und MÜHLBOCK (1964) festgestellt. Nach mehreren Passagen sah FURTH bei dem durch Diäthylstilbestrol induzierten Hypophysenadenomen autonomes Wachstum. Die Struktur des von FURTH (Furth MT F 4) beschriebenen Hypophysentumors wurde 1964 von SCHELIN, LUNDIN und BARTHOLDSON licht- und elektronenmikroskopisch untersucht. Der Tumor hat mammotrope, somatotrope und adrenocorticotrope Wirkung. Die Tumorzellen enthalten sehr schwach anfärbbare Granula. Elektronenmikroskopisch gibt es nur einen Typ sekretorischer Granula mit einem Durchmesser von ungefähr 350 μ. Er entspricht den acidophilen Granula des sog. STH-Typs. Es wird vermutet, daß sich funktionell pluripotente Zellen morphologisch ausdifferenzieren können und angenommen, daß sich der Furth-Tumor von einer pluripotenten Zelle ableitet und in dem Sinne pathologisch ist, daß er die Fähigkeit zur Bildung von drei verschiedenen Hormonen erworben hat.

3. *Thyreotrope Adenome*

Thyreotrope Adenome wurden nach chirurgischer Schilddrüsenentfernung [DENT, GADSDEN und FURTH (1955, 1956)] oder nach Zerstörung der Schilddrüse durch radioaktive Substanzen (bei Mäusen) sowie durch Hemmung der Thyroxinsynthese mit Thiouracil [MOORE, BRACKNEY und BOCK (1953)] [Versuchsanordnung siehe Schilddrüse] beobachtet. In allen 3 Versuchsanordnungen entsteht eine Mehrsekretion von thyreotropem Hormon, offenbar um die verminderte oder fehlende Schilddrüsenhormonproduktion wieder in Gang zu bringen. Die Hypophyse erfährt eine fortschreitende Aktivierung gerade derjenigen Zellart, die das thyreotrope Hormon bildet. Hier liegt also eine echte Anpassung der Hypophyse an eine veränderte hormonelle Korrelation vor. Die Hyperplasie stellt eine geschwulstähnliche Proliferation mit dem Ziel des Ausgleichs der Korrelationsstörung dar. Behandlung von C57Bl-Mäusen mit 0,5–2,4 g Dinitrophenol/kg als Nahrungszusatz reduziert die Häufigkeit von Hypophysenadenomen nach Behandlung mit 6-n-Propyl-2-Thiouracil [KING, BOCK, MOORE (1963)]. Die Ursachen der Entstehung thyreotroper Hypophysenadenome zeigt Abb. 4.

FURTH (1954), GADSDEN und FURTH (1953), FURTH, BURNETT und GADSDEN (1953), DENT, GADSDEN und FURTH (1956), FURTH, GADSDEN und BURNETT (1952), FURTH und BURNETT (1951), GORBMAN (1949, 1952, 1956), GORBMAN und EDELMAN (1952, 1955) haben in zahlreichen Experimenten bei Ratten die Wirkung der Bestrahlung mit J^{131} und der totalen sowie subtotalen chirurgischen Entfernung der Schilddrüse auf die Entstehung von Hypophysenadenomen untersucht. Sie konnten dabei zeigen, daß eine totale Entfernung bzw. Zerstörung der Schilddrüse nicht notwendig ist, sondern ein länger andauerndes Schilddrüsenhormondefizit zur Erzeugung eines thyreotropen Hypophysenadenoms genügt.

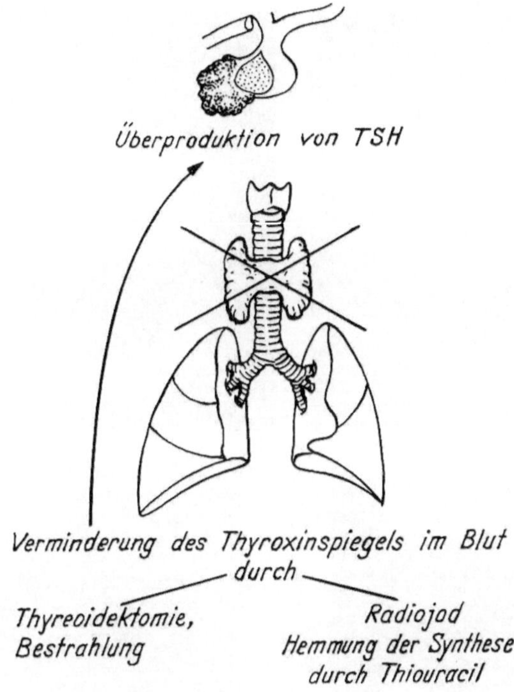

Abb. 4. Hormonelle Dysregulation bei der Entwicklung von thyreotropen Hypophysenadenomen

Der Mechanismus ist immer der gleiche, d. h. ausschlaggebend ist der Schilddrüsenhormonspiegel bzw. die Störung der Synthese durch Jodmangel oder Thiouracilbehandlung [BIELSCHOWSKY (1953)]. Welche Ausmaße ein Hypophysenadenom annehmen kann, zeigt Abb. 5.

Die erzeugten Hypophysenadenome zeigten in der ersten Passage nur Wachstum bei Abwesenheit der Schilddrüse, d. h. nur dann, wenn sie auf ein Tier transplantiert wurden, bei dem durch eine Hypothyreose eine vermehrte Thyreotropinsekretion erzeugt worden war. Nach einigen Passagen im hypothyreotischen Tier wurden die Adenome autonom [FURTH (1955), DENT, BURNETT und GADSDEN (1955)]. Die Adenome zeigten auf das Wirtstier eine gleiche Wirkung wie eine starke Thyreotropininjektion. Es fanden sich oft erhebliche adenomatöse Wucherungen des Schilddrüsengewebes mit Einbruch in Blutgefäße.

Neben diesen Adenomen wurde von FURTH (1954, 1955, 1957) ein besonderer Typ beschrieben, der als somatotrop-thyreotrop bezeichnet wird. Bei diesem Adenom traten neben der Wirkung des thyreotropen Hormons Wachstumssteigerungen der Brustdrüse und einzelner Organe auf, die als Folge der Mehrsekretion von Wachstumshormon gedeutet werden.

4. *Adenocorticotrope Adenome*

Adenocorticotrope Adenome wurden erstmals 1953 von FURTH, GADSDEN und UPTON beobachtet. Diese Adenome traten nach Ganzkörperbestrahlung (Dosis s. Abschnitt WRBA) auf. Die Mehrsekretion von ACTH wird erkennbar an der Nebenniere, die eine Hyperplasie der Zona fasciculata zeigt. Außerdem findet sich als

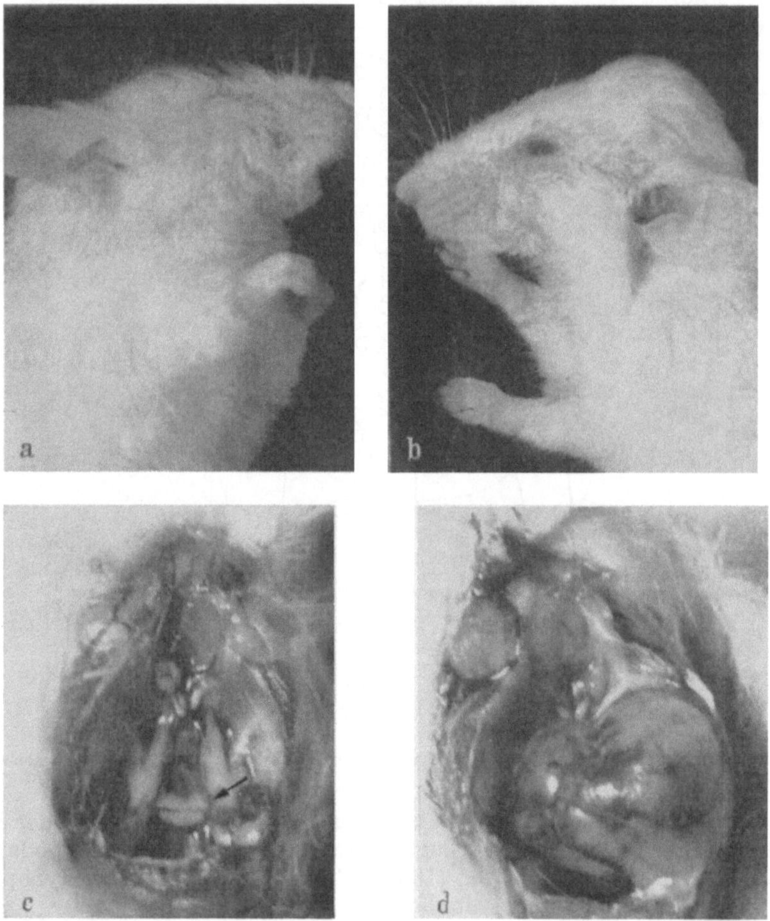

Abb. 5a—d. Großer, fast die ganze Schädelbasis ausfüllender Hypophysentumor nach Radiothyreoidektomie (Abb. nach FURTH). Erläuterung der Abbildung: 2a Normale Maus; 2b Normale Hypophyse der Maus; 3a Ausbuchtung der hinteren Schädelkalotte durch den Hypophysentumor; 3b Großer Hypophysentumor, der die Schädelhöhle halb ausfüllt

Zeichen des Hypercorticoidismus eine Leukopenie, eine Thymus- und Milzatrophie, eine Polyurie und Hyperglykämie. Die Genese der adrenocorticotropen Adenome ist noch keineswegs geklärt, kann aber nach GORBMAN (1956) durchaus als Folge einer Streßwirkung gedeutet werden. Durch die Ganzkörperbestrahlung kommt es wahrscheinlich zu einer langdauernden Überbelastung des Hypophysen-Nebennierenrindensystems, woraus eine Mehranforderung an die adrenocorticotrope Partialfunktion der Hypophyse resultiert. Die adenomatöse Wucherung ist auch hier wahrscheinlich als Anpassung der Hypophyse an eine gestörte hormonelle Korrelation aufzufassen [MAYER, ZOMZELY und FURTH (1956), FURTH und CLIFTON (1957), FURTH (1957), FURTH, GADSDEN und UPTON (1953), UPTON und FURTH

(1955), BAHN, FURTH, ANDERSEN und GADSDEN (1957)]. Ein Modell der Entwicklung der adrenocorticotropen Hypophysenadenome zeigt Abb. 6.

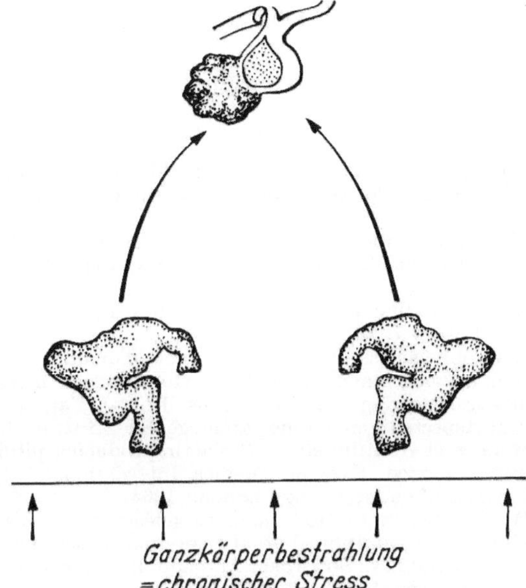

Abb. 6. Entwicklung des adrenocorticotropen Hypophysenadenoms

5. *Amphophile Hypophysenadenome*

Amphophile Hypophysenadenome sahen BURT, LANDING und SOMMERS (1954) nach Gabe von J^{131}. Auch hier ist eine Allgemeinwirkung auf die hormonelle Korrelation und nicht eine Direktwirkung auf die Hypophyse anzunehmen.

6. *Basophile Adenome*

Basophile Adenome der Hypophyse sahen, wie bereits kurz angeführt, verschiedene Untersucher bei Mäusen, die einige Tage post partum kastriert wurden. Für ihre Entstehung wird die verstärkte Follikelhormonsekretion der nach Kastration entstandenen Nebennierentumoren wesentlich verantwortlich gemacht [DICKIE und WOOLLEY (1949), DICKIE und LANE (1956), CHRISTY, DICKIE, ATKINSON und WOOLLEY (1951)].

7. *Wachstumshormon*

Bei Ratten, die bis zu 485 Tage in steigenden Dosen von 0,4—3,0 mg mit Wachstumshormon behandelt wurden, sahen die Untersucher Hyperplasien und Adenombildungen endokriner Organe oder endokrin gesteuerter Gewebe [MOON, SIMPSON, LI, EVANS (1950, 1951, 1952), KONEFF, MOON, SIMPSON, LI, EVANS (1951)], d. h. Adenome der Nebenniere, Hyperplasie des peribronchialen Lymphgewebes, Granulosazelltumoren, Fibroadenome und Myome bei gleichzeitiger Zunahme der basophilen Zellen und Abnahme der acidophilen Zellen der Hypophyse. Bei einem Tier trat auch ein kleines basophiles Adenom auf. Beim hypophysektomierten Tier konnten MOON, SIMPSON, LI und EVANS (1951, 1952) keine ähnlichen Veränderungen nachweisen.

Nach FURTH (1957) sind für die Entstehung der Hypophysenadenome drei Faktoren ausschlaggebend:

1. Eine verlängerte übermäßige Hormonapplikation.
2. Ein Mangel an spezifischen Einschränkungsvorrichtungen des HVL.
3. Ein Mangel an Beantwortungsvermögen der Zellen.

Immer handelt es sich bei den auslösenden Faktoren der Entstehung der Hypophysentumoren um Folgen einer hormonellen Korrelationsstörung zwischen HVL und gesteuertem Organ bzw. um eine Mehrbelastung einer bestimmten hormonellen Partialfunktion der Hypophyse.

Literatur

a) Hypophyse

BAHN, R., J. FURTH, E. ANDERSON and E. GADSDEN: Morphologic and Functional Changes Associated with Transplantable ACTH-producing Tumors of Mice. Amer. J. Path. **33**, 1075 (1957).

BATES, R. W., K. H. CLIFTON and E. ANDERSON: Prolactin and thyrotrophin content of functional transplantable pituitary tumors. Proc. Soc. exp. Biol. (N. Y.) **93**, 525—527 (1956).

BIELSCHOWSKY, F.: Chronic iodine deficiency as cause of neoplasia in thyroid and pituitary of aged rats. Brit. J. Cancer **7**, 203 (1953).

—, and W. H. HALL: Carcinogenesis in parabiotic rats. Tumours of the ovary induced by acetaminofluorene in intact females joined to gonadectomized litter-mates and the reaction of their pituitaries to endogenous oestrogens. Brit. J. Cancer **5**, 331 (1951).

—, and E. S. HORNING: Aspects of endocrine carcinogenesis. Brit. med. Bull. **14**, 106 (1958).

BOOT, L. M., G. RÖPCKE, and O. MÜHLBOCK: Prolactin-producing pituitary tumours arising in pituitary isografts in mice. Excerpta Medica International Congress Series No. 83. Proc. 2. intern. Congress of endocrinology London 1964.

BÜNGELER, W., u. W. DONTENWILL: Hormonell ausgelöste geschwulstartige Hyperplasien, hyperplasiogene Geschwülste und ihre Verhaltensweisen. Dtsch. med. Wschr. **1959**, 1885.

BURT, A. S., B. H. LANDING and S. C. SOMMERS: Amphophil tumors of the hypophysis induced in mice by I 131. Cancer Res. **14**, No. 7, 497 (1954).

CHRISTY, N. P., M. M. DICKIE, W. B. ATKINSON and G. W. WOOLLEY: The pathogenesis of uterine lesions in virgin mice and in gonadectomized mice bearing adrenal cortical and pituitary tumors. Cancer Res. **11**, 413 (1951).

CLIFTON, K. H.: Problems in experimental tumorigenesis of the pituitary gland, gonads, adrenal cortices, and mammary glands: a review. Cancer Res. **19**, 2 (1959).

—, and J. FURTH: Hormonal influences on growth and somatotropic actions of autonomous mammotropes. Proc. Soc. exp. Biol. (N. Y.) **94**, 809—814 (1957).

—, and R. K. MEYER: Mechanism of anterior pituitary tumor induction by estrogen. Anat. Rec. **125**, 65—81 (1956).

COHEN, A., and J. FURTH: Corticotropin assay with transplantable adrenal tumors slices. Application to the assay of adrenotropic pituitary tumors. Cancer Res. **19**, 72 (1959).

CRAMER, W., and E. S. HORNING: Experimental production by oestrin of pituitary tumors with hypo-pituitarism. Lancet **1936 I**, 247—249.

— — The effect of oestrin on the pituitary gland. Lancet **1936 I**, 1056.

CUNNINGHAM, A. W. B., C. E. HALL and O. HALL: Neoplasia in parabiotics. J. Path. Bact. **68**, 309 (1954).

DEANESLY, R.: Depression of hypophyseal activity by the implantation of tablets of oestrone and oestradiol. J. Endocr. **1**, 36 (1939).

—, and A. S. PARKES: Further experiments of the administration of hormones by the subcutaneous implantation of tablets. Lancet **1938 II**, 606.

DENT, J. N., E. L. GADSDEN and J. FURTH: On the relation between thyroid depression and pituitary tumor induction in mice. Cancer Res. **15**, 72—75 (1955).

— — — Further studies on induction and growth of thyrotropic pituitary tumors in mice. Cancer Res, **16**, 171—174 (1956).

DICKIE, M. M., and P. W. LANE: Adrenal tumors, pituitary tumors, and other pathological changes in F_1 hybrids of strain DE X strain Dba. Cancer Res. **16**, 48—52 (1956).

—, and G. W. WOOLLEY: Spontaneous basophilic tumors of the pituitary glands in gonadectomized mice. Cancer Res. **9**, 372—384 (1949).

DONTENWILL, W., u. M. EDER: Histogenese und biologische Verhaltensweise hormonell ausgelöster Geschwülste. Beitrag path. Anat. **120**, 270 (1959).

DUNNING, W. F., and M. R. CURTIS: The incidence of diethylstilbestrol-induced cancer in reciprocal F_1 hybrids obtained from crosses between rats of inbred lines that are susceptible and resistant to the induction of mammary cancers by this agent. Cancer Res. **12**, 702 (1952).

DUX, C.: Recherches microscopiques sur les adénomes hypophysaires du rat. Bull. Cancer (Paris) **35**, 201 (1948).

EDELMAN, A., and A. GORBMAN: Endocrine factors influencing the development of hypophyseal tumors in mice. Proc. Amer. Ass. Cancer Res. 2, 13—14 (1955).

EGAÑA, E., J. SZABO y S. LECANNELIER: Acciones tóxicas y tumorígenas del caprilato de estradiol en rata. Rev. chil. Hig. 3, 39 (1941).

FURTH, J.: Morphologic changes associated with thyrotrophin-secreting pituitary tumors. Amer. J. Path. 30, 421—463 (1954).

— Thyroid-pituitary tumorigenesis. J. nat. Cancer Inst. 15, 687 (1954).

— Experimental pituitary tumors. Recent Progr. Hormone Res. 11, 221 (1955).

— Experimental pituitary tumors. In: G. PINCUS (ed.), Recent Progr. Hormone Res. 11, 221—249 (1955).

— Hormonal factors and tumor growth. Cancer Res. 17, 454 (1957).

— R. F. BUFFETT and E. L. GADSDEN: On the pathogenesis of pituitary tumor induction by ionizing radiation. Proc. Amer. Ass. Cancer Res. 2, 204 (1957).

—, and W. T. BURNETT: Hormone-secreting transplantable neoplasms of the pituitary induced by I^{131}. Proc. Soc. exp. Biol. (N. Y.) 78, 222 (1951).

— —, and E. L. GADSDEN: Quantitative relationship between thyroid function and growth of pituitary tumors secreting TSH. Cancer Res. 13, 298—307 (1953).

—, and K. H. CLIFTON: Experimental pituitary tumors and the role of pituitary hormones in tumorigenesis of the breast and thyroid. Cancer 10, 842—853 (1957).

— — Experimental pituitary tumors. In: G. E. W. WOLSTENHOLME and M. O'CONNOR (eds.), Ciba Foundation Colloquia on Endocrinology, 12, 3—17. London: J. & A. Churchill, Ltd. 1958.

— — Experimental observations on mammotropes and the mammary gland. In: A. R. CURRIE and C. F. W. ILLINGWORTH (eds.), Endocrine Aspects of Breast Cancer, 276—282. Edinburgh: E. & S. Livingstone, Ltd. 1958.

— — E. L. GADSDEN and R. F. BUFFETT: Dependent and autonomous mammotropic pituitary tumors in rats; their somatotropic features. Cancer Res. 16, 608—616 (1956).

— J. N. DENT, W. T. BURNETT and E. L. GADSDEN: The mechanism of induction and the characteristics of pituitary tumors induced by thyroidectomy. J. clin. Endocr. 15, 81 (1955).

— E. L. GADSDEN and W. T. BURNETT jr.: Autonomous transplantable pituitary tumors arising in growths dependent on absence of the thyroid gland. Proc. Soc. exp. Biol. (N. Y.) 80, 4—7 (1952).

— — K. H. CLIFTON and E. ANDERSON: Autonomous mammotropic pituitary tumors in mice; their somatotropic features and responsiveness to estrogens. Cancer Res. 16, 600—607 (1956).

—, and A. C. UPTON: ACTH-secreting transplantable pituitary tumors. Proc. Soc. exp. Biol. (N. Y.) 84, 253—254 (1953).

GADSDEN, E. L., and J. FURTH: Effect of thyroid hormone on growth of thyrotrophin-secreting pituitary tumors. Proc. Soc. exp. Biol. (N. Y.) 83, 511—514 (1953).

GARDNER, W. U., and L. C. STRONG: Strain-limited development of tumors of the pituitary gland in mice receiving estrogen. Yale J. Biol. Med. 12, 543—548 (1940).

— The effect of estrogen on the incidence of mammary and pituitary tumors in hybrid mice. Cancer Res. 1, 345 (1941).

— The effect of steroid hormones on experimental pituitary and gonadal tumorigenesis. Ciba Found. Coll. Endocr. 1, 52 (1952).

GILMAN, J., and C. GILBERT: Modulating action of the thyroid on oestrogen-induced pituitary tumors in rats. Nature (Lond.) 175, 724 (1955).

GORBMAN, A.: Tumorous growths in the pituitary and tracheae following radiotoxic dosages of I^{131}. Proc. Soc. exp. Biol. (N. Y.) 71, 237—240 (1949).

— Factors influencing development of hypophyseal tumors in mice after treatment with radioactive iodine. Proc. Soc. exp. Biol. (N. Y.) 80, 538—540 (1952).

— Pituitary tumors in rodents following changes in thyroid function: a review. Cancer Res. 16, 99—105 (1956).

—, and A. EDELMAN: The role of ionizing radiation in eliciting tumors of the pituitary gland in mice. Proc. Soc. exp. Biol. (N. Y.) 81, 348—350 (1952).

GRIFFIN, A. C., H. L. RICHARDSON, C. H. ROBERTSON, M. A. O'NEAL and J. D. SPAIN: The role of hormones in liver carcinogenesis. J. nat. Cancer Inst. (Suppl.). 15, 1623 (1955).

HALL, C. E., O. HALL and A. W. B. CUNNINGHAM: Spontaneous neoplasia in female parabiotic rats. Tex. Rep. Biol. Med. 11, 448 (1953).

HORNING, E. S.: Endocrine factors involved in the induction, prevention and transplantation of kidney tumors in the male golden hamster. Z. Krebsforsch. 61, 1 (1956).

KING, D. W., F. G. BOCK, and G. E. MOORE: Dinitrophenol inhibition of pituitary adenoma formation in mice fed propylthiouracil. Proc. Soc. exp. Biol. (N. Y.) 112, 365—366 (1963.)

KIRKMAN, H.: Steroid tumorigenesis. Cancer Chicago **10**, 757 (1957).
—, and R. L. BACON: Estrogen-induced tumors of the kidney. I. Incidence of renal tumors in intact and gonadectomized male golden hamsters treated with diethylstilbestrol. J. nat. Cancer Inst. **13**, 745 (1952).
KIRSCHBAUM, A.: The role of hormones in cancer: Laboratory animals. Cancer Res. **17**, 432 (1957).
KONEFF, A. A., H. D. MOON, M. E. SIMPSON, CH. H. LI and H. M. EVANS: Neoplasms in rats treated with pituitary growth hormone. IV. Pituitary gland. Cancer Res. **11**, 113 (1951).
KWA HONG GIOG: An experimental study of Pituitary Tumours. Berlin-Göttingen-Heidelberg: Springer-Verlag 1961.
LACASSAGNE, A.: Les cancers produits par des substances chimiques endogènes. Paris: Hermann & Cie. 1950.
— et W. NYKA: Différence de réaction de l'hypophyse à l'administration de substances oestrogènes dans diverses lignées sélectionnées de souris. C. R. Soc. Biol. (Paris) **136**, 1112 (1937).
LACOUR, F.: Studie über die Hypophyse von Ratten, bei denen nach BISKIND Tumoren der Sexualdrüsen erzeugt worden waren. Bull. Ass. franç. Cancer **42**, 421 (1951).
LIPSCHUTZ, A.: Steroid hormones and tumors. Baltimore: Williams & Wilkins Comp. 1950.
— Steroid homeostasis hypophysis and tumorigenesis. Cambridge: W. Heffer & Sons, Ltd. 1957.
MAYER, J., C. ZOMZELY and J. FURTH: Body composition and energetics in obesity induced in mice by adrenotropic tumors. Science **123**, 184—185 (1956).
MCEUEN, C. S., H. SELYE and J. B. COLLIP: Some effects of prolonged administration of oestrin in Rats. Lancet **1936 I**, 775—776.
— — — A pigmented adenoma of the intermediate lobe in a rat chronically treated with oestrin. Proc. Soc. exp. Biol. (N. Y.) **40**, 241 (1939).
MEYER, R. K., and K. H. CLIFTON: Effect of diethylstilbestrol-induced tumorigenesis on the secretory activity of the rat anterior pituitary gland. Endocrinology **58**, 686—693 (1956).
MOON, H. D., M. E. SIMPSON and H. M. EVANS: Inhibition of methylcholanthrene carcinogenesis by hypophysectomy. Science **16**, 331 (1952).
— — CH. H. LI and H. M. EVANS: Neoplasms in rats treated with pituitary growth hormone. III. Reproductive organs. Cancer Res. **10**, 549 (1950).
— — — — Neoplasms in rats treated with pituitary growth hormone. V. Absence of neoplasms in hypophysectomized rats. Cancer Res. **11**, 535 (1951).
— — — — Effect of pituitary growth hormone in mice. Cancer Res. **12**, 448 (1952).
MOORE, G. E., E. L. BRACKNEY and F. G. BOCK: Production of pituitary tumors in mice by chronic administration of a thiouracil derivative. Proc. Soc. exp. Biol. (N. Y.) **82**, 643 (1953).
MÜHLBOCK, O.: Karzinogenese, Endogenese und Exogenese. Krebsforschung und Krebsbekämpfung. Band II. München-Berlin: Urban & Schwarzenberg 1957.
NELSON, W. O.: The occurrence of hypophyseal tumors in rats under treatment with diethylstilbestrol. Proc. Amer. Physiol. Soc. 20, 210 (1941).
NOBLE, R. L., and J. B. COLLIP: Regression of oestrogen-induced mammary tumors in female rats following removal of the stimulus. Canad. med. Ass. J. **44**, 1—5 (1941).
NORMAN, J.: On the relation between thyroid depression and pituitary tumor induction in mice. Rep. Cancer Res. **15**, 70—75 (1955).
OBERLING, CH., M. GUÉRIN et P. GUÉRIN: La production expérimentale de tumeurs hypophysaires chez le rat. C. R. Soc. Biol. (Paris) **123**, 1152 (1936).
— — M. LAPLANE DE SEZE et M. LACOUR: Production de tumeurs hypophysaires et mammaires chez le rat par injections de fulliculine seule ou associée à d'autres hormones. Extr. Bull. Cancer **3**, 176—192 (1950).
RICHARDSON, F. L.: Incidence of mammary and pituitary tumors in hybrid mice treated with stilbestrol for varying periods. J. nat. Cancer Inst. 18, 813—830 (1957).
RUSSFIELD, A. B., G. FRIEDLER, and J. K. FRENKEL: Biological Characteristics of two transplantable pituitary tumors of syrian hamsters. Cancer Res. **23**, 720—724 (1963).
SCHELIN, U., P. M. LUNDIN, and L. BARTHOLDSON: Light and electron microscopic studies on an autonomous stilbestrol-induced pituitary tumor in rats. Endocrinology **75**, 893—900 (1964).
SEGALOFF, A., and W. F. DUNNING: The effect of strain, estrogen, and dosage on the reaction of the rat's pituitary and adrenal to estrogenic stimulation. Endocrinology **36**, 238 (1945).
SELYE, H.: Atypical cell proliferation in the anterior lobe adenomas of estradiol-treated rats. Cancer Res. **4**, 349 (1944).
SPAMPINATO, V.: Hypophysenadenome nach Oestrogenzufuhr bei der weißen Ratte. Endocrinologie **19**, 367 (1950).
UPTON, A. C., and J. FURTH: Induction of pituitary tumors by means of ionizing irradiation. Proc. Soc. exp. Biol. (N. Y.) **84**, 255 (1953).
— — Spontaneous and radiation-induced pituitary adenomas of mice. J. nat. Cancer Inst. **15**, 1001 (1955).

VASQUEZ-LOPEZ, E.: The relation of the pituitary gland and related hypotalamic centres in the hamster to prolonged treatment with oestrogens. J. Path. Bact. **56**, 1 (1944).
WEIL, A., and B. ZONDEK: The histopathology of the pituitary of the white rat injected with follicular hormone. Endocrinology **25**, 114 (1939).
WOLFE, J. M., and A. W. WRIGHT: Histologic effects induced in the anterior pituitary of the rat by prolonged injection of estrin with particular reference to the production of pituitary adenomata. Endocrinology **23**, 200 (1938).
YOKORO, K., J. FURTH, and N. HARAN-GHERA: Induction of mammotropic pituitary tumors by X-rays in rats and mice. The role of mammotropes in development of mammary tumors. Cancer Res. **21**, 178—186 (1961).
ZONDEK, B.: Tumour of the pituitary induced with follicular hormone. Lancet **1936 I**, 776.
— Hypophyseal tumours induced by estrogenic hormone. Amer. J. Cancer **33**, 555 (1938).

b) Schilddrüse

Ein experimentelles Modell für Hyperplasien endokriner Organe bei erhöhter Leistungsanforderung bzw. bei Störung der Korrelation stellt die Schilddrüsenveränderung nach Anwendung schwefelhaltiger, kropferzeugender Substanzen dar.

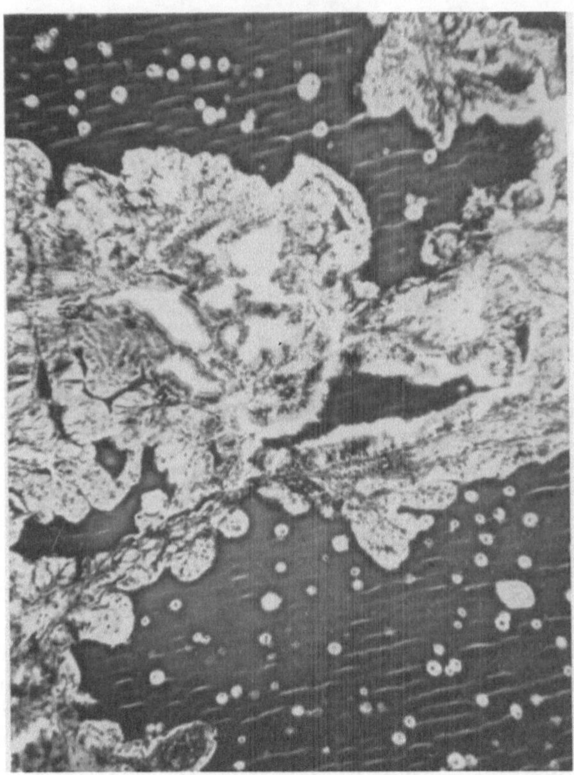

Abb. 7

Abb. 7 u. 8. Makro- und mikrofollikuläres, z. T. cystisches Adenom der Ratten-Schilddrüse. 12 Monate Behandlung mit Methylthiouracil tgl. 0,05 g oral (nach KRACHT)

Nach langdauernder Behandlung (über 15 Monate) von Ratten mit Methylthiouracil (tgl. 0,05 g) sahen u. a. BIELSCHOWSKY, GRIESBACH, HALL, KENNEDY und PURVES (1949) knotige Hyperplasien bzw. Adenome der Schilddrüse.

PURVES und GRIESBACH (1946, 1947) beobachteten bis zu 31% (später 50%) maligne Schilddrüsenadenome mit Einbruch in Blutgefäße und in die Kapsel. Über weitere ähnliche

Untersuchungen berichteten BIELSCHOWSKY (1945), BIELSCHOWSKY, GRIESBACH, HALL, KENNEDY und PURVES (1949), HALL (1948), HALL und BIELSCHOWSKY (1949), PURVES, GRIESBACH und KENNEDY (1951), BIELSCHOWSKY und HALL (1953). Gleiche Beobachtungen machten auch MONEY, RAWSON (1950) und MORRIS, DALTON, GREEN (1951), die aber bei der Beurteilung der Malignität zurückhaltender waren. Adenome der Schilddrüse sahen bei gleichen Versuchen auch DALTON, MORRIS und DUBNIK (1949), MORRIS und GREEN (1951), SELLERS, HILL und LEE (1953), VAN DYKE (1953), MOORE und BRACKNEY und BOCK (1953), FURTH (1954), MORRIS (1955) bei Mäusen. Während bei C-Mäusen nur ein metastasierendes Carcinom unter 30 Tieren beobachtet wurde, sahen DALTON, MORRIS, STRIEBICH und DUBNIK (1950) und GORBMAN (1947) bei C3H-Mäusen bis zu 50% bösartige Schilddrüsengeschwülste.

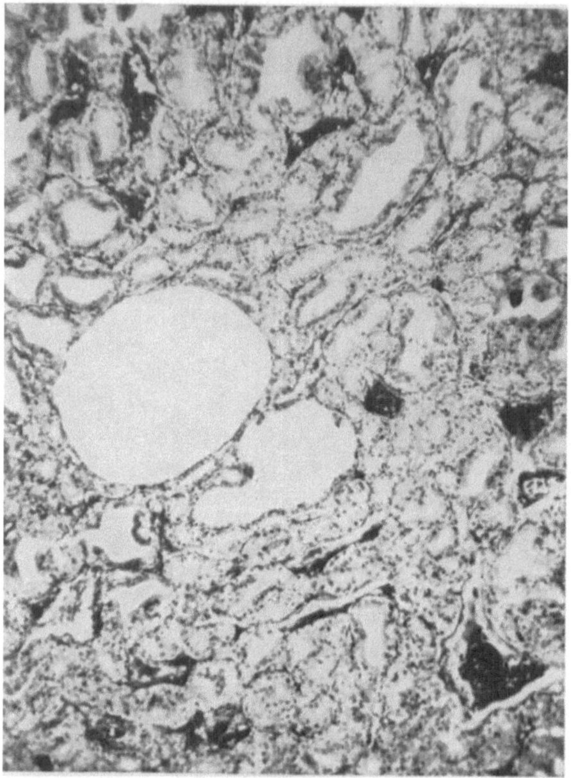

Abb. 8

Die knotigen Hyperplasien der Schilddrüse zeigen, wie später auch KRACHT (1954) (Abb. 7, 8, 9) nachweisen konnte, eine erhebliche Polymorphie der Kerne. Bei der Beurteilung der Malignität muß aber gerade bei der Schilddrüse, einem Organ, in dem normalerweise schon Gewebsverschleppungen auf dem Blutwege vorkommen, Zurückhaltung gewahrt werden. KRACHT (1954) sah an seinen eigenen Versuchen bei alleiniger Behandlung mit Methylthiouracil keinerlei echte Schilddrüsencarcinome. Die Entstehung der Schilddrüsenadenome ist Folge der Störung der Thyroxinsynthese. Es kommt durch den Jodmangelzustand bzw. die verminderte Hormonproduktion in der Schilddrüse zu einer Mehrsekretion thyreotropen Hormons [KRACHT (1954)], das wiederum zu einer Proliferation des Schilddrüsenepithels führt (Abb. 10). Die Hyperplasien sind transplantabel [BIELSCHOWSKY (1949)], aber nur auf Tiere, die eine gleichzeitige Thyreotropinübersekretion z. B. bei Thiouracilbehandlung [MORRIS, DALTON und GREEN (1951)] zeigen. Nach Behandlung von Ratten mit Thiuramen [GRIEPENTROG (1962)] (Diät mit Pomarsol 0,01%, Lutiram 0,013%, Polyram 0,01%) fand GRIEPENTROG (1961)

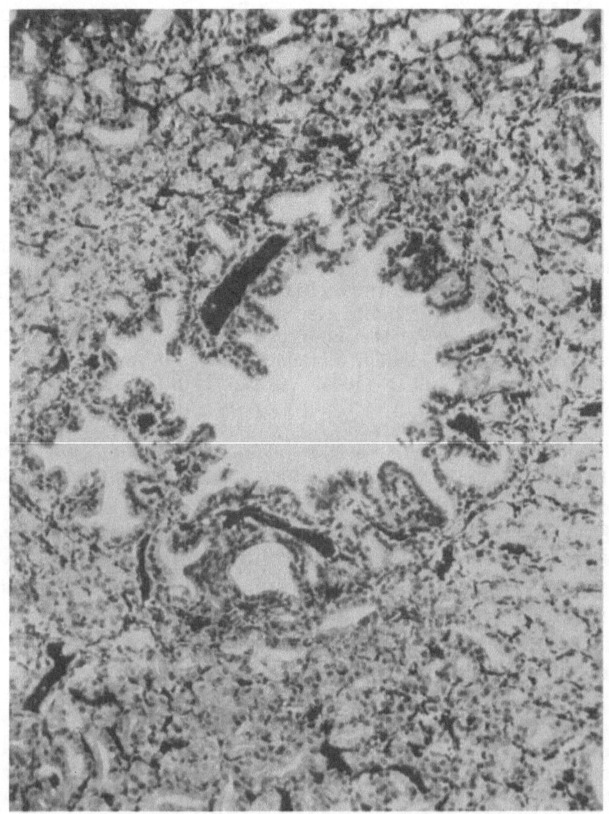

Abb. 9. Makrofollikulares hypochromatisches Adenom in zentralen Schilddrüsenanteilen. Methylthiouracil 7 Monate tgl. 0,05 g oral bei Ratten (nach KRACHT)

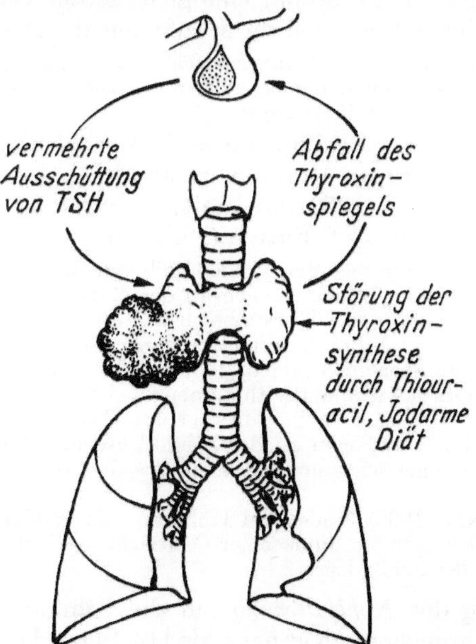

Abb. 10. Ursachen der Schilddrüsenadenomentwicklung

bei 20 von 65 Schilddrüsen Hyperplasien und Tumoren (1 malignes trabeculäres Adenom – 10 wuchernde Struma Langhans).

Bei kombinierter Behandlung von Methylthiouracil und dem Carcinogen Acetaminofluoren(0,05 g Methylthiouracil oral zusammen mit 12 mg Acetylaminofluoren) trat nicht nur eine Beschleunigung der Adenombildung, sondern auch eine Zunahme der Häufigkeit auf [DONIACH (1950), HALL und BIELSCHOWSKY (1949), PASCHKIS, CANTAROW und STASNEY (1948, 1951)]; es wurden vielfach maligne Tumoren beobachtet.

Durch den starken proliferativen Reiz des Thiouracils, durch Erzeugung einer Mehrsekretion des thyreotropen Hormons, kommt es zur Wirkung des Carcinogens (Acetaminofluoren) an der Schilddrüse [BIELSCHOWSKY (1947), HALL (1948), KRACHT (1954)]. Bei der kombinierten Behandlung mit Acetaminofluoren und Thiouracil bezeichneten BIELSCHOWSKY (1945, 1947) und HALL (1948) das Acetaminofluoren als carcinogenen Initialfaktor und das Thiouracil als "promoting" Faktor. Alleinige Behandlung mit Acetaminofluoren zeigt keine Wirkung an der Schilddrüse [GORBMAN (1947), AXELRAD und LEBLOND (1953, 1955)], und nach COX, WILSON und DE EDS (1947) treten nur einzelne Adenome auf. MONEY und RAWSON (1950) behandelten Ratten mit Thiouracil (0,1% wäßrige Lösung) und Dibenzanthracen (subcutan). Die Schilddrüsentumoren, die durch Thiouracil allein erzeugt wurden, waren histologisch nicht von den Tumoren zu unterscheiden, die bei Kombination beider Substanzen auftraten.

Knotige Hyperplasien nach Thiouracilbehandlung fand auch LAQUEUR (1949) bei Ratten. Er sah tubuläre, intraacinöse Proliferationen wie auch Knotenbildungen. TRAUTMANN und HILL (1950) beobachteten auch bei Meerschweinchen, Hund und Schwein nach Methylthiouracilbehandlung eine Gewichtszunahme der Schilddrüse (die Hypophyse zeigte gleichzeitig eine Gewichtszunahme). Maligne Entartungen konnten nicht nachgewiesen werden.

STUDER (1948) sah nach gleichzeitiger Behandlung von Thiouracil und Vitamin A eine Hemmung der Kropfentstehung.

MONEY berichtete 1950 über histologische Untersuchungen an durch Methylthiouracilbehandlung hervorgerufenen Adenomen der Schilddrüse. Nach seiner Ansicht scheinen sich die Adenome jeweils von einem Follikel aus zu entwickeln und sind nur zum Teil innersekretorisch wirksam. Dabei ist der Einbruch des proliferierenden Schilddrüsengewebes in Gefäße kein sicheres Kriterium der Malignität; MONEY konnte keine bösartigen Neubildungen nachweisen.

Nach DONIACH (1950, 1953) erhöht eine gleichzeitige Gabe von radioaktivem Jod zusammen mit Methylthiouracil die Häufigkeit der Adenomentstehung.

DALTON, MORRIS, STRIEBICH und DUBNIK (1950) sahen nach Behandlung mit Methylthiouracil neben den Schilddrüsenadenomen auch noch Veränderungen an der Nebenniere, am Respirationsepithel und an der Hypophyse.

Daß die Proliferation der Schilddrüse nach Methylthiouracilgaben über eine Mehrsekretion des thyreotropen Hormons zustande kommt, zeigen die Versuche von TRAUTMANN und HILL (1950) an hypophysektomierten Hunden und von KRACHT an hypophysektomierten Ratten (1952/53).

KRACHT konnte die Wirkung des Methylthiouracils auf die Schilddrüse, die Hypophyse und Nebenniere in zahlreichen Untersuchungen an der Ratte weitgehend abklären und beweisen, daß durch eine Hemmung der Thyroxinsynthese die Mehrsekretion des thyreotropen Hormons entsteht, das dann durch Proliferationsanregung zu den adenomatösen Wucherungen Anlaß gibt. KRACHT konnte aber auch zeigen (1954), daß die früher vielfach vertretene Ansicht der cancerogenen Wirkung des Methylthiouracils nicht zu Recht besteht. Der Grad der Thyroxinsynthesestörung ist nach FURTH, BURNETT und GADSDEN (1953) und FURTH (1953, 1954) entscheidend für die Reaktionen an der Schilddrüse und Hypophyse; diese Störung kann ebenso durch Jodmangel wie durch radioaktives Jod oder Thiouracil hervorgerufen werden.

OBERLING und GUÉRIN (1936) fanden bei Hühnern, die in Käfigen ohne Kies gehalten wurden, Knochenveränderungen im Sinne einer Ostitis fibrosa und gleichzeitig eine Hyperplasie und Überfunktion der Schilddrüse.

Über die Wirkung der *Kohlfütterung* auf die Schilddrüse berichtete bereits 1932 ZECKWER. Bei Kaninchen sah er nach bis 114 Tagen dauernder Kohlfütterung

Hyperplasien der Schilddrüse. Auch BIANCHI (1933) konnte diese Veränderungen nachweisen und spricht von einer beschleunigten saisonmäßigen Umwandlung der Sommerschilddrüse in eine Winterschilddrüse bzw. umgekehrt.

Die Wirkung konnte durch stärkere Belichtung der Tiere oder durch Jodgaben beeinflußt werden. AXHAUSEN (1937) sah nach Kohlfütterung Kropferzeugung auch bei Ziegen und Meerschweinchen.

Auch eine *Radiumemanation* kann, wie PIGHINI (1936) zeigen konnte, zu kropfartigen Veränderungen der Schilddrüse führen (bei Kaninchen, Tauben und Meerschweinchen), die durch Jodbehandlung verhindert werden. Maligne Schilddrüsentumoren bei Ratten wurden von GOLDBERG und CHAIKOFF (1951, 1952), GOLDBERG, LINDSAY, NICHOLS und CHAIKOFF (1964), MARKS und BUSTAD (1963) nach Behandlung mit radioaktivem Jod festgestellt. MONEY (1953) berichtete über einen fördernden Effekt des Thiouracils bei dieser Behandlung.

Über die Erzeugung von Hypophysenadenomen bei der Methylthiouracilbehandlung haben wir bereits berichtet [s. Hypophyse MOORE, BRACKNEY und BOCK (1953)]. Kleine Schilddrüsenadenome sahen BERG, GORDON und GORBMAN (1954) beim Schwertfisch nach Thiouracilgaben.

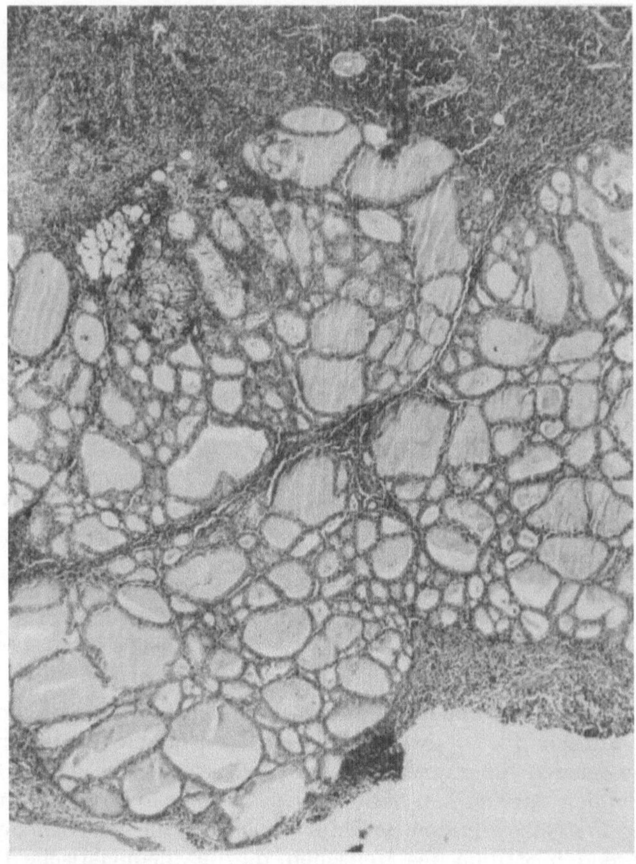

Abb. 11. Kleines Schilddrüsenregenerat mit trachea-ähnlichem Gewebe in der Milz, 10 Monate, 7 Tage nach Transplantation von embryonalem Schilddrüsengewebe

Schilddrüsenadenome bei chronischem *Jodmangel* (Diät s. Abschnitt Erkrankungen der Schilddrüse) alter Ratten sah BIELSCHOWSKY (1953), und von AXELRAD und LEBLOND (1953) wurden sogar solide Zellwucherungen der Schilddrüse mit den Zeichen der Malignität beobachtet. FORTNER, GEORGE und STERNBERG (1960) konnten durch Behandlung von Goldhamstern mit jodarmer Reis- und Karottendiät Schilddrüsencarcinome mit Metastasen in den Lymphknoten und Lungen erzeugen. Während bei ihren Untersuchungen von 620 Kontrolltieren, die länger als 181 Tage lebten, nur 1,5% bösartige Geschwülste der Schilddrüse erkennen ließen (von acht Carcinomen waren zwei papilläre und follikuläre Adenocarcinome und sechs Spindelzellcarcinome), nahm die Häufigkeit der Schilddrüsentumoren nach Behandlung mit jodarmer Diät stark zu. 12% der behandelten Tiere

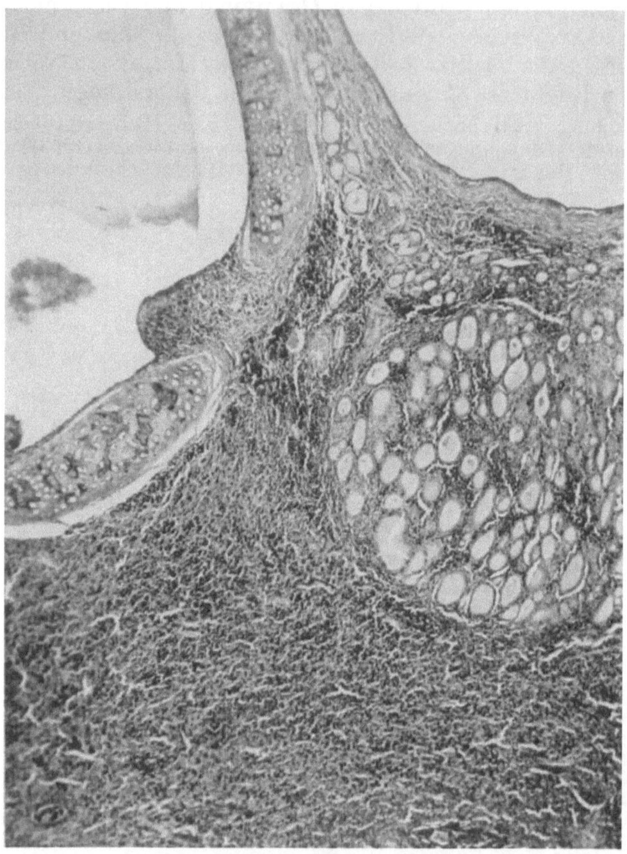

Abb. 12. Schilddrüsenregenerat in der Milz, 4 Monate, 21 Tage nach Transplantation von Schilddrüsengewebe einer erwachsenen Ratte

zeigten Schilddrüsencarcinome mit Metastasen in den Lymphknoten oder Lungen. 28% ließen in der Schilddrüse „wahrscheinlich" („probable", s. unten) Carcinome erkennen (ohne Zeichen von Metastasen) und 59% zeigten eine starke Schilddrüsenhyperplasie. Bei den Carcinomen handelte es sich um papilläre follikuläre Adenocarcinome. Die metastasierenden Schilddrüsencarcinome verglich der Autor mit der metastasierenden Struma des Menschen, da die „neoplastische Umwandlung der Schilddrüse diffus war". Die starke Aktivierung des Schilddrüsengewebes führten FORTNER u. Mitarb. (1960) auf eine Überproduktion von thyreotropem Hormon zurück, sie beobachteten bei einer größeren Zahl von Tieren eine Vergrößerung der Hypophyse. Bei 31 Goldhamstern, die 12 Monate mit hohen Dosen Tabakrauchkondensat behandelt worden waren, sahen wir [DONTENWILL und

Mohr (1962)] zum Teil außerordentlich große adenopapilläre Schilddrüsenhyperplasien. 13 der 31 Tiere zeigten Absiedlungen in den Lungen. Die Schilddrüsenhyperplasien wurden als „metastasierende Strumen" aufgefaßt und mit der metastasierenden Struma (v. Gierke) des Menschen verglichen. Der hohe Nicotingehalt der Tabakkondensate wird als Ursache der Aktivierung der Schilddrüsentätigkeit angesehen.

Nach *Implantation* von Schilddrüsengewebe in die Milz sahen Lacour, Oberling und Guérin (1953), Dosne de Pasqualini und Mancini (1951), Brachetto-Brian und Grinberg (1951) Adenome, nachdem die Schilddrüse entfernt worden war. Dempster und Doniach (1955) dagegen sprechen nicht von Adenomen und nehmen an, daß für das Angehen und Überleben der Implantate eine Unterfunktion der Schilddrüse nicht zwingende Notwendigkeit ist. Wir, Dontenwill und Ranz (1960), beobachteten nach Implantation der total entfernten Schilddrüse bei der Ratte nur eine bis zur Größe des ursprünglichen Organs reichende Regeneration, sprechen aber nicht von Adenomen (Abb. 11 u. 12). Das embryonale Schilddrüsengewebe zeigt eine wesentlich geringere Regeneration als die Schilddrüsentransplantate erwachsener Ratten. Für das Angehen der Transplantate ist die vollständige Schilddrüsenentfernung keine Vorbedingung.

Über maligne Hauttumoren der Ratte nach Thiouracilinjektion (intraperitoneal 6 Monate 3mal wöchentlich 3—4 cm^3 einer 10%igen Lösung) berichten Rosin und Rachmilewitz (1954).

Mit Absicht haben wir die z. T. umstrittenen *Schilddrüsencarcinome* nach Thiouracilbehandlung und jodarmer Diät mit den Adenomen zusammen abgehandelt, da dies sicher dem allgemeinen Verständnis dient und die Problematik der morphologischen Malignität der Schilddrüsenveränderungen besser hervorhebt.

Literatur

b) Schilddrüse

Axelrad, A., and C. P. Leblond: Thyroid tumor induction in rats by a low iodine diet with and without 2-acetylaminofluorene. Ass. Cancer Res. **1**, 2 (1953).

— — Induction of thyroid tumors in rats by low iodine diet. Cancer **8**, 339—367 (1955).

Axhausen, H.: Zur Frage der Kropferzeugung bei Ziegen, Kaninchen, Meerschweinchen durch Fütterung verschiedener Kohlarten. Diss. Freiburg 1937.

Berg, O., M. Gordon and A. Gorbman: Comparative effects of thyroidal stimulants and inhibitors of normal and tumorous thyroids in Xiphophorin fishes. Cancer Res. **14**, 527 (1954).

Bianchi, G. C.: Verhalten der Schilddrüse bei mit gekochtem Kohl gefütterten Kaninchen. Ein Beitrag zu den Saisonveränderungen der Schilddrüse. Beitr. path. Anat. **90**, 539 (1933); Zbl. Path. **58**, 247 (1933).

Bielschowsky, F.: Tumors of the thyroid produced by 2-acetylaminofluorene and allylthiourea. Brit. J. exp. Path. **25**, 90—95 (1944).

— Experimental nodular goitre. Brit. J. exp. Path. **26**, 270 (1945).

— The carcinogenic action of 2-acetylaminofluorene and related compounds. Brit. med. Bull. **4**, 406 (1947).

— The role of thyroxine deficiency in the formation of experimental tumours of the thyroid. Brit. J. Cancer **3**, 547 (1949).

— Chronic iodine deficiency as cause of neoplasia in thyroid and pituitary of aged rats. Brit. J. Cancer **7**, 203—213 (1953).

— W. E. Griesbach, W. H. Hall, T. H. Kennedy and H. D. Purves: Studies on experimental goitre: the transplantability of experimental thyroid tumours in the rat. Brit. J. Cancer **3**, 541 (1949).

—, and W. H. Hall: Carcinogenesis in the thyroid-ectomized rat. Brit. J. Cancer **7**, 358 (1953).

—, and E. S. Horning: Aspects of endocrine carcinogenesis. Brit. med. Bull. **14**, 106 (1958).

Brachetto-Brian, D., y R. Grinberg: Proceso histológico de los autoinjertos intra splenicos de tiroides en ratas tiroidectomizades. Rev. Soc. Biol. **27**, 199 (1951).

Cox, A. J., R. H. Wilson and F. de Eds: The carcinogenetic activity of 2-acetylaminofluorene: characteristics of the lesions in albino rats. Cancer Res. **7**, 647 (1947).

Dalton, A. J., H. P. Morris and C. S. Dubnik: Morphologic changes in the organs of female C3H mice after long-term ingestion of thiourea and thiouracil. J. nat. Cancer Inst. **9**, 201 (1949).

DALTON, A. J., H. P. MORRIS, M. J. STRIEBICH, and C. S. DUBNIK: Histologische Veränderungen bei Strain C-Mäusen nach langdauernder Fütterung mit Methylthiouracil. J. nat. Cancer Inst. **11**, 391 (1950).

DEMPSTER, W. J., and I. DONIACH: The survival of thyroid implants in relation to thyroid defiency. Arch. int. Pharmacodyn. **101**, 398 (1955).

DONIACH, I.: The effects of radioactive iodine alone and in combination with methylthiouracil and acetylaminofluorene upon tumour production in the rat's thyroid gland. Brit. J. Cancer **4**, 223 (1950).

— The effect of radioactive iodine alone and in combination with methylthiouracil upon tumor production in the rat thyroid gland. Brit. J. Cancer **7**, 181—202 (1953).

DONTENWILL, W.: Vergleichende Untersuchungen an in die Milz implantierten endokrinen Drüsen. Verh. dtsch. Ges. Path. **43**, 243 (1959).

—, u. H. RANZ: Vergleichende Untersuchungen an Transplantaten endokriner Drüsen. Im Druck.

DOSNE DE PASQUALINI, C., y R. E. MANCINI: Injerto del tiroides en el bazo. Rev. Soc. argent. Biol. **27**, 102 (1951).

DYKE, J. H. VAN: Influence of age on experimental thyroid tumorigenesis in female rats. Anat. Rec. **115**, 377 (1953).

FORTNER, J. G., PH. GEORGE, and ST. S. STERNBERG: Induced and spontaneous thyroid cancer in the syrian (golden) hamster. Endocrinology **66**, 364—376 (1960).

FURTH, J. Conditioned and autonomous neoplasms. A review. Cancer Res. **13**, 477 (1953).

— Thyroid-pituitary tumorigenesis. J. nat. Cancer Inst. **15**, 687—691 (1954).

— W. T. BURNETT and E. L. GADSDEN: Quantitative relationship between thyroid function and growth of pituitary tumors secreting TSH. Cancer Res. **13**, 298 (1953).

GOLDBERG, R. C., and I. L. CHAIKOFF: Development of thyroid neoplasms in the rat following a single injection of radioactive iodine. Proc. Soc. exp. Biol. (N. Y.) **76**, 563—566 (1951).

— — Induction of thyroid cancer in the rat by radioactive iodine. Arch. Path. (Chicago) **53**, 22 (1952).

— S. LINDSAY, C. W. NICHOLS, and I. L. CHAIKOFF: Induction of neoplasms in thyroid glands of rats by subtotal thyroidectomy and by the injection of one microcurie of I^{131}. Cancer Res. **24**, 35—43 (1964).

GORBMAN, A.: Thyroidal and vascular changes in mice following chronic treatment with goitrogens and carcinogens. Cancer Res. **7**, 746 (1947).

GRIEPENTROG, F.: Tumorartige Schilddrüsenveränderungen in chronisch-toxikologischen Tierversuchen mit Thiuramen. Beih. path. Anat. **126**, 243—255 (1962).

HALL, W. H.: The role of initiating and promoting factors in the pathogenesis of tumours of the thyroid. Brit. J. Cancer **2**, 273 (1948).

—, and F. BIELSCHOWSKY: The development of malignancy in experimentally-induced adenomata of the thyroid. Brit. J. Cancer **3**, 534 (1949).

KRACHT, J.: Die Schilddrüse und ihre Beziehungen zum Hypophysenvorderlappen und zur Nebennierenrinde. Jahresbericht 1952/53 Tuberkulose-Forschungsinstitut Borstel S. 367.

— Über Wechselbeziehungen zwischen Nebennierenrinde und Schilddrüse im Tierexperiment. Verh. dtsch. Ges. Path. **36**, 202 (1952).

— Geschwulstartige Anpassungshyperplasien der Schilddrüse im Tierexperiment. Verh. dtsch. Ges. Path. **38**, 372 (1954).

—, u. U. KRACHT: Zur Histopathologie und Therapie der Schreckthyreotoxikose des Wildkaninchens. Virchows Arch. path. Anat. **321**, 238 (1952).

—, u. H. SPAETHE: Über Wechselbeziehungen zwischen Schilddrüse und Nebennierenrinde. I. Mitt. Virchows Arch. path. Anat. **323**, 174 (1953).

— — Über Wechselbeziehungen zwischen Schilddrüse und Nebennierenrinde. II. u. III. Mitt. Virchows Arch. path. Anat. **323**, 83, u. **323**, 629 (1953).

LACOUR, F., C. OBERLING et M. GUÉRIN: Tumeurs par greffe intrasplénique de thyroïde chez des rats thyroidectomisés. Bull. Ass. franç. Cancer **39**, 390—396 (1953).

LAQUEUR, G. L.: Knotige Hyperplasie der Schilddrüsen durch Thiouracil. Cancer Res. **9**, 247 (1949).

MARKS, S., and L. K. BUSTAD: Thyroid neoplasms in sheep fed radioiodine. J. nat. Cancer Inst. **30**, 661—673 (1963).

MONEY, W. L.: The effect of thiouracil on the collection of radioactive iodine in exper. induced thyroid tumors. Cancer **6**, Nr. 1 (1953).

—, and R. W. RAWSON: The experimental production of thyroid tumors in the rat exposed to prolonged treatment with thiouracil. Cancer **3**, 321-335 (1950).

MOORE, G. E., E. L. BRACKNEY and F. G. BOCK: Production of pituitary tumors in mice by chronic administration of a thiouracil derivative. Proc. Soc. exp. Biol. (N. Y.) **82**, 643—645 (1953).

MORRIS, H. P.: Experimental thyroid tumors. In: The Thyroid. Brookhaven Symposia in Biology 7, 192 (1955); Upton, N. Y. Brookhaven National Laboratory.
— A. DALTON and C. GREEN: Malignant thyroid tumors occurring in the mouse after prolonged hormonal imbalance during the ingestion of thiouracil. J. clin. Endocr. 11, 1281—1295 (1951).
—, and C. D. GREEN: Role of thiouracil in the induction, growth and transplantability of mouse thyroid tumors. Science 114, 44—46 (1951).
OBERLING, CH., u. M. GUÉRIN: Schilddrüsenhyperplasie und Struma bei Hühnern, die in Käfigen ohne Kies gehalten wurden. C. R. Soc. Biol. 121, Nr. 10, 947 (1936); Zbl. Path. 65, 328 (1936).
PASCHKIS, K. E., A. CANTAROW and J. STASNEY: Influence of thiouracil on carcinoma induced, by 2-acetaminofluorene. Cancer Res. 8, 257 (1948).
— — — Competitive action of 2-thiouracil and uracil in AAF-induced cancer. Science 114, 264 (1951).
PIGHINI, G.: Schilddrüsenkröpfe, hervorgerufen durch Radiumemanation in Meerschweinchen Kaninchen und Tauben — mit und ohne Jodbehandlung. Riv. sper. Freniat. 60, 563 (1936); Zbl. Path. 68, 215 (1937).
PURVES, H. D., and W. E. GRIESBACH: Studies on experimental goitre. — VII: Thyroid carcinomata in rats treated with thiourea. Brit. J. exp. Path. 27, 294 (1946); 28, 46 (1947).
— —, and T. H. KENNEDY: Studies in experimental goitre: malignant change in a transplantable rat thyroid tumour. Brit. J. Cancer 5, 301 (1951).
ROSIN, A., and M. RACHMILEWITZ: The development of malignant tumors of the face in rats after prolonged treatment with thiourea. Cancer Res. 14, 494 (1954).
SELLERS, E. A., J. M. HILL and R. B. LEE: Effect of iodine and thyroid on the production of tumors of the thyroid and pituitary by propylthiouracil. Endocrinology 52, 188 (1953).
STUDER, A.: Hemmung des Thiouratkropfes der Ratte durch synthetischen Vitamin A-Methyläther. Experientia (Basel) 4, 232—233 (1948).
TRAUTMANN, D. A., u. H. HILL: Die Beeinflussung von endokrinen Drüsen durch Methylthiouracil. Endokrinologie 27, 267 (1950).
ZECKWER, I.: Wirkung der Kohlfütterung auf die Morphologie der Kaninchenschilddrüse. Amer. J. Path. 8, Nr. 2 (1932); Zbl. Path. 56, 119 (1932/33).

c) Epithelkörperchen und Pankreas

Bei einer Reihe von Störungen des Mineralhaushaltes durch Änderung der Zufuhr von Calcium und Phosphat in der Nahrung, durch Nierenschädigung oder

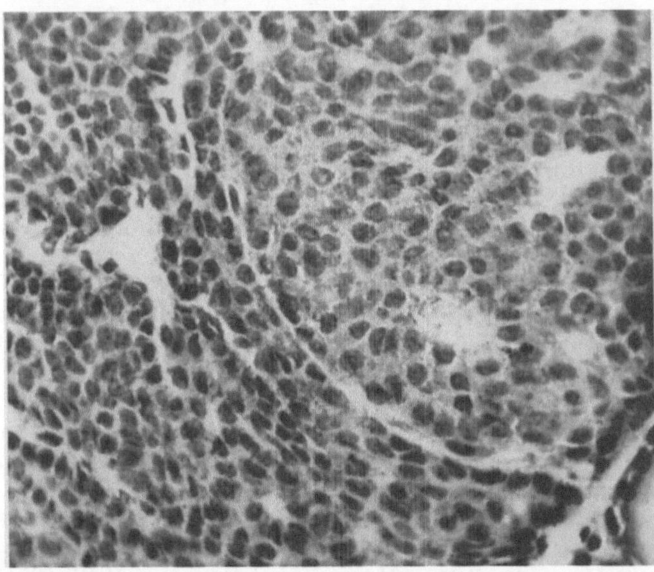

Abb. 13. Adenomatöse Hyperplasie des Epithelkörperchens (re. obere Bildhälfte) nach Behandlung mit Ammonphosphatlösung 2—4% Lösung 0,5 cm³ pro Tag bei Ratten (20 Monate in Intervallen) (nach EDER)

durch Störung des Säure-Basen-Gleichgewichtes im Blut, sowie durch Änderung der Vitaminzufuhr, konnten Veränderungen an den Epithelkörperchen beobachtet werden, die recht verschieden gedeutet werden. Die meisten Untersucher sahen eine Vergrößerung der Zellkerne und eine Gewichtszunahme der Epithelkörperchen und bezeichnen diese Veränderungen als Hyperplasie. Dabei handelt es sich meist um diffuse Hyperplasien der hormonell wirksamen Zellen oder um herdförmige und diffuse Hyperplasien [EDER (1960, 1961)] Abb. 13. EGER (1956) spricht bei seinen Untersuchungen von adenomatöser Wucherung und knotiger Hyperplasie der Epithelkörperchens, die EGER vorwiegend nach Nierenschädigung mit Uranylnitrat und Bleiacetat sah. Bei diesen Experimenten kommt es über eine Störung der Ausscheidungsfunktion der Tubuli offenbar zu einer Phosphatretention und zu einer Acidose, die durch eine Mobilisierung des Calciums ausgeglichen werden muß. Die Mobilisierung des Calciums ist nur durch eine Mehrleistung der Epithelkörperchens möglich, die dann die von vielen Untersuchern beschriebene Hyperplasie oder Hyperaktivität zeigt.

In zahlreichen experimentellen Untersuchungen gelang es nicht, Adenome der Inselzellen des *Pankreas* zu erzeugen, es wurden lediglich Zellvergrößerungen oder eine Vermehrung einzelner Zellarten der Inseln beobachtet [Lit. KRACHT (1956), FASSBENDER (1956), TONUTTI (1956), SEIFERT (1956)].

Literatur

c) Epithelkörperchen usw.

EDER, M.: Morphologische Untersuchungen über herdförmige Epithelkörperchenhyperplasien. Virchows Arch. path. Anat. **334**, 301 (1961).

— Experimentelle und histochemische Untersuchungen über herdförmige Hyperplasien im Epithelkörperchen. Virchows Arch. path. Anat. **334**, 324 (1961).

EGER, W.: Der experimentelle Hyperparathyroidismus. Verh. dtsch. Ges. inn. Med. **62**, 403 (1956).

FASSBENDER, H. G.: In KAUFMANN: Lehrbuch der speziellen pathologischen Anatomie. Berlin: Walter de Gruyter 1956.

KRACHT, J.: Das Inselzellsystem bei Über- und Unterfunktion der Nebennierenrinde. Verh. dtsch. Ges. Path. **40**, 272 (1956).

SEIFERT, G.: Die Pathologie des kindlichen Pankreas. Leipzig: Thieme 1956.

TONUTTI, E.: In KAUFMANN: Lehrbuch der speziellen pathologischen Anatomie. Berlin: Walter de Gruyter 1956.

d) Nebenniere

Eine große Zahl Untersucher konnte zeigen, daß bei einer Belastung des Hypophysen-Nebennieren-Systems eine Aktivierung der Nebenniere erfolgt, die meist in Form einer diffusen Hyperplasie der Nebennierenrinde sichtbar wird. Nur selten treten bei allgemeiner Belastung durch Beanspruchung der Herz- und Skeletmuskulatur oder anderer Versuchsanordnungen herdförmige knotige Hyperplasien der Nebenniere auf [Lit. bei TONUTTI (1956) und FASSBENDER (1956) und bei LIEBEGOTT (1952, 1958)].

Neben dieser als Anpassung an eine gesteigerte Stoffwechselsituation aufzufassenden Aktivierung der Nebenniere im Sinne einer Hyperplasie finden wir bei bestimmten Versuchsanordnungen knotige Hyperplasien in Mark und Rinde, die meist als „Adenome" bezeichnet werden.

In einer Reihe von Versuchen haben vor allem WOOLLEY, DICKIE und LITTLE (1953), WOOLLEY, FEKETE und LITTLE (1940, 1943), FEKETE, WOOLLEY und LITTLE (1941), FEKETE und LITTLE (1945), WOOLLEY und LITTLE (1945, 1946, 1950), WOOLLEY (1945, 1949, 1950, 1953, 1954, 1958), FRANTZ und KIRSCHBAUM (1948, 1949), SMITH (1948), FLAKS (1949), HOUSSAY, HIGGINS, BENNET (1951), KING, CASAS und VISSCHER (1949), HUSEBY und BITTNER (1948, 1951), CHRISTY (1951), MARTINEZ und BITTNER (1955, 1956), DICKIE und LANE (1956) zeigen können, daß bei bestimmten *Mäuse*stämmen nach frühzeitig — meist in den ersten fünf Lebenstagen — erfolgter Kastration sowie nach partieller Ovarektomie [HUMMEL (1954)] und einseitiger Adrenalektomie [MARTINEZ-BITTNER (1955)] (Abb. 14 zeigt schematisch den Entstehungsmechanismus der Nebennierentumoren nach Kastration) bei einzelnen Tierstämmen z. B. nach etwa 6—9 Monaten eine knotige Hyperplasie der Nebenniere gefunden wird. Bei Tieren des CE-Stammes und des Donor-Stammes sahen die Untersucher Carcinome mit deutlicher Zellpolymorphie [WOOLLEY und LITTLE (1945, 1946), WOOLLEY (1958)].

Die Ansprechbarkeit der Nebenniere im Hinblick auf adenomatöse und carcinomatöse Veränderungen ist weitgehend an Mäusestämme gebunden, die eine bestimmte Anfälligkeit des endokrinen Systems zeigen [HUSEBY und BITTNER (1951), WOOLLEY und LITTLE (1945, 1946), WOOLLEY (1958)]. WOOLEY, DICKIE und LITTLE untersuchten 1953 bei Kreuzungsversuchen verschiedener Mäusestämme den Zeitpunkt und die Häufigkeit des Auftretens von Nebennieren-Hyperplasien und Nebennieren-Carcinomen. Nebennieren-Tumoren wurden nach 9 Monaten bei einer Kreuzung von DBA- und CE-Mäusen und nach 6 Monaten bei einer Kreuzung von CE- und kastrierten weiblichen DBA-Mäusen festgestellt. Nach 12 Monaten wurden sie gefunden bei Kreuzungen von DBA × CE-Mäusen und CE-Mäusen × kastrierten männlichen DBA-Mäusen. Eine andere Kreuzung erfolgte zwischen dem Stamm CE × C57BL und C57BL und CE-Mäusen. Hierbei fanden sich Nebennieren-Tumoren sowohl bei der Kreuzung CE × C57BL als auch bei der Kreuzung C57BL mit kastrierten weiblichen CE-Mäusen nach 10 Monaten. Bei der Kreuzung CE mit kastrierten C57BL-Männchen fand sich vor 16 Monaten kein Nebennieren-Tumorenauftreten. Außerdem war ihr Auftreten nur sporadisch. Bei Kreuzungen zwischen C57BL und kastrierten männlichen CE-Mäusen traten nach 10 Monaten erstmals Nebennierentumoren auf, nach 16 Monaten fanden sich bei allen Tieren der Kreuzung C57BL × kastrierten weiblichen CE-Mäusen Tumoren. Die Kreuzungen CE × C57BL-Mäuse hatten Mütter aus dem CE-Stamm. FLAKS (1949) sah nach Ovarektomie metastasierende Carcinome der Nebenniere.

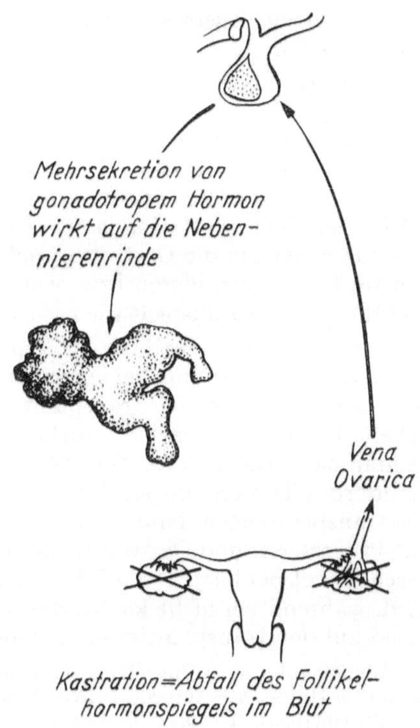

Abb. 14. Entstehungsmechanismus des Nebennierenadenoms nach Kastration

Die adenomartigen Wucherungen der Nebennierenrinde, die bei Ratten, Hamstern und Mäusen auch spontan vorkommen, entstehen nicht, wenn man z. B. nach der Exstirpation der Gonaden laufend Oestrogene und Androgene [WOOLLEY und LITTLE (1946), WOOLLEY (1950), MONSEN (1952)] zuführt. Die Nebenniere übernimmt bei den kastrierten Tieren die Funktion der Gonaden, d. h. die weiter vorhandene trope Steuerung der Sexualhormonproduktion wirkt sich nun an der Nebenniere aus und führt hier zu einer adenomatösen Wucherung der Rinde.

Die oestrogene Hormonsekretion der Nebennierenadenome bei gonadektomierten Tieren ist auch am Uterus [GARDNER (1941), CHRISTY (1951), MONSEN (1952), MONSEN und KIRSCHBAUM (1954)] und der Mamma [SILBERBERG, SILBERBERG und OPDYKE (1953)] sichtbar in Form von hormonell bedingten Gewebswucherungen wie Adenomyosis und adenomatöser Hyperplasie. Oestrogenausscheidung bei Tieren mit Nebennierenrindenadenomen konnten DORFMAN und GARDNER (1944) nachweisen.

Eine Androgensekretion der Nebennieren-Tumoren wiesen FRANTZ und KIRSCHBAUM (1948) nach. Daß die Tumoren Oestrogene produzieren, zeigt sich auch am gehäuften Auftreten von Mammacarcinomen bei einzelnen Mäuse-Stämmen [Christy (1951), Fekete, Woolley und Little (1941), Dickie und Lane (1956), Frantz und Kirschbaum (1948, 1949)] und von Hypophysenadenomen [Dickie und Woolley (1949)].

Die Entstehung adenomatöser Wucherungen der Nebennierenrinde konnte durch Behandlung mit Desoxycorticosteron gehemmt, aber nicht verhindert werden [Houssay, Higgins, und Bennet (1951)]. Nebennierenrindenadenome treten häufig bei alten Weibchen des NH-Stammes auf, bei denen früh eine Alterung der Ovarien auftritt. Die Ovarien werden dann refraktär für Gonadotropine, und so entsteht ein Zustand der physiologischen Kastration [Frantz und Kirschbaum (1949)].

Nach Hypophysektomie und Kastration traten keine Nebennierentumoren bzw. Hyperplasien auf [Ferguson und Visscher (1953)]. Die Injektion von Hypophysenvorderlappengewebe förderte die Entstehung der Nebennieren-Adenome nach Kastration [Silberberg, Silberberg und Opdyke (1953)]. Die Beeinflussung der Nebenniere erfolgt nach Houssay u. a. (1953, 1954) über den HVL, der genaue Mechanismus ist noch unklar; nicht verständlich ist insbesondere, warum die Oestrogenproduktion der Nebenniere nicht in der Lage ist, den HVL zu kontrollieren bzw. warum sich die Korrelation zwischen Nebenniere und HVL nicht so einspielt wie zwischen Nebenniere und Ovar [Lipschutz (1950)].

Browning (1958) sah bei der *Transplantation der nach Kastration entstandenen Nebennierentumoren* nur bei einzelnen eine hormonelle Abhängigkeit. Die Latenzzeit bis zum Angehen der transplantierten Tumoren war bei weiblichen und männlichen, bei kastrierten und nicht kastrierten Tieren verschieden. Testosteron hemmt nach Browning, White und Sadler (1959) das Wachstum des transplantierten Tumors am stärksten. Eine geringere Hemmung auf das Wachstum des transplantierten Tumors findet sich nach Behandlung kastrierter Männchen mit Progesteron und Oestrogen oder mit Oestrogen allein. Progesteronbehandlung beschleunigt bei kastrierten Männchen das Wachstum, wenn es allein verabreicht wird, während bei nicht kastrierten Männchen eine Progesteronbehandlung hemmend auf den transplantierten Tumor wirkt.

Adenomatöse oder diffuse Hyperplasien der Nebenniere nach früher Kastration beschrieben bei *Ratten* Houssay, Cardeza, Pinto, Burgos (1951), Houssay, Cardeza, Foglia, Houssay und Pinto (1953), Houssay, Houssay, Cardeza, Pinto und Foglia (1953), Houssay, Houssay, Cardeza, Pinto und Foglia (1954), Cardeza (1954); beim *Hamster* Woolley (1953); beim *Meerschweinchen* mit vermännlichender Wirkung Spiegel (1939) und Lipschutz (1935); beim *Hund* Lubimow und Feodossiev [s. Lipschutz (1957)]. Nebennierenadenome traten häufiger bei oestrogenbehandelten Ratten des August-Stammes auf (36% bei männlichen, 17% bei weiblichen), bei Kontrollen nur 1% [Dunning, Curtis und Segaloff (1947)]. Nebennierenhyperplasie bzw. Hypertrophie wurde von Morris (1953) nach Thyreoidektomie und Thiouracilbehandlung beim *Leghorn* Cockeral gefunden, nie aber ausgesprochene Adenome.

Nach Behandlung männlicher *Hamster* (Abb. 15) mit weiblichem Sexualhormon sahen wir vereinzelt Nebennierenadenome, z. T. mit reticularisähnlichen Strukturen. Die gleichen Beobachtungen machten Franks und Chesterman (1956) und Kirkman (1957), die bei Hamstern nach Behandlung mit männlichem Geschlechtshormon bei 46 von 64 Tieren Nebennierenadenome feststellten. Franks und Chesterman (1956) fanden auch nach Follikelhormonbehandlung des Hamsters Hyperplasie und Adenome der Nebennierenrinde in Verbindung mit Herz- und Nierenveränderungen bei starkem Kaliumdefizit; sie bewerten diese Adenome wie diejenigen des Menschen beim sog. Hyperaldosteronismus.

Kirkman und Robbins (1956) sahen bei 64% mit Testosteronpelotten behandelten Goldhamstern Adenome und Carcinome der Nebennierenrinde.

Interessant sind besonders die Beobachtungen geschwulstartiger Bildungen im *Nebennierenmark* der Ratte nach langdauernder Nicotinbehandlung, wie sie erstmals von STAEMMLER (1935, 1936) beschrieben wurden. STAEMMLER behandelte die Ratten bis zu 20 Monaten mit Nicotininjektionen (0,05—0,2 mg Nicotin puriss. [Merck] täglich in einer Lösung von 1 : 1000—1 : 10000), die nach seiner Ansicht eine kontinuierliche Mehrausschüttung von Adrenalin bedingen. Im Verlaufe mehrerer Monate kommt es dann zur Hyperplasie des Marks und in zwei Fällen zu Adenomen, die bis an die Oberfläche durchgebrochen waren. LUPULESCU (1965) fand bei Meerschweinchen nach Behandlung mit α-Oestradiol (tgl. 1 mg bei einem Durchschnittsgewicht der Tiere von 350 g) und Somatotropin – SPOFA (2mal wöchentlich 10 Evanseinheiten) Phäochromocytome der Nebenniere. Die Adrenalin und Noradrenalinausscheidung der Tiere war erheblich erhöht.

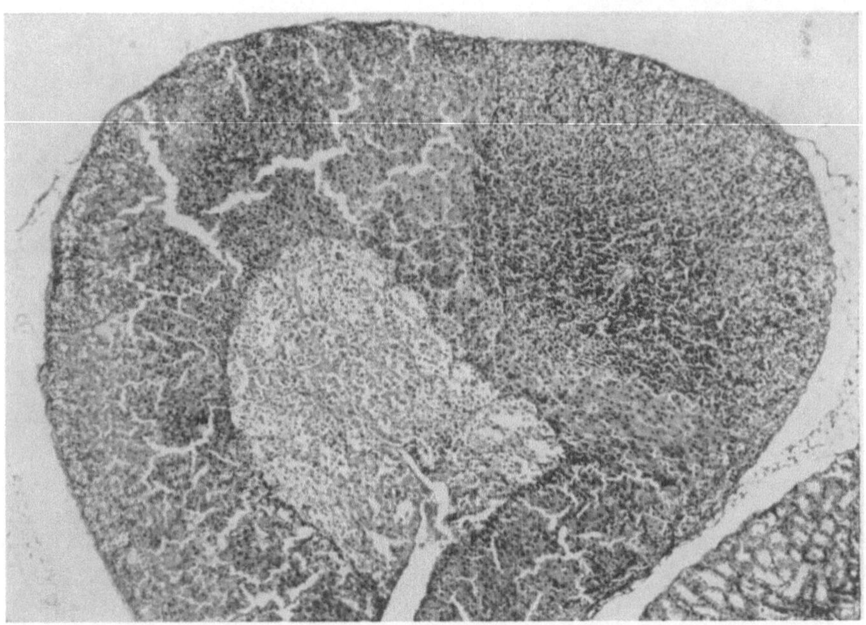

Abb. 15. Nebennierenrindenadenom beim Goldhamster. Behandlung Cyren B, 0,6 mg, jeden 2. Tag, 13 Mon. 20 Tg.

Daß durch eine Mehranforderung an das Nebennierenmark Hyperplasien entstehen können, ist nach den Beobachtungen beim Menschen und Tier wahrscheinlich, ob aber allein durch eine solche Regulationsstörung echte Phäochromocytome hervorgerufen werden, ist umstritten. Auch ERÄNKÖ (1955) beschrieb knotige Hyperplasien im Nebennierenmark der Ratte nach Nicotinbehandlung. Wir (DONTENWILL) haben in fast zwei Jahre dauernden Versuchen, die nach der Methodik von STAEMMLER (1935, 1936) durchgeführt wurden, keine Hyperplasien beobachtet, weder bei der Ratte noch beim Goldhamster.

Nach SMITH, GARDNER, LI und KAPLAN (1949) und YEAKEL (1947) treten Markadenome auch spontan auf und werden nach verschiedenen Versuchsanordnungen in einer geringen Zahl bei Mäusen und Ratten sowie Hamstern gefunden. Die Untersuchungen von GILMAN, GILBERT und SPENCE (1953) haben inzwischen gezeigt, daß Phäochromocytome bei Ratten im Alter häufiger werden. Im Alter von 13—18 Monaten traten bei weiblichen Ratten in 50% und bei männlichen Ratten in 82% Marktumoren auf. Spontane Nebennieren-Marktumoren bei Mäusen wurden auch von JONES und WOODWARD (1954) mitgeteilt.

Phäochromocytome wurden auch nach langdauernder Behandlung von Ratten mit Wachstumshormon beschrieben. Da auch hier die Behandlung bis zu 480 Tagen dauerte, ist fraglich, ob es sich nicht zum Teil um spontane Adenome handelt [MOON, SIMPSON, LI und EVANS (1950)].

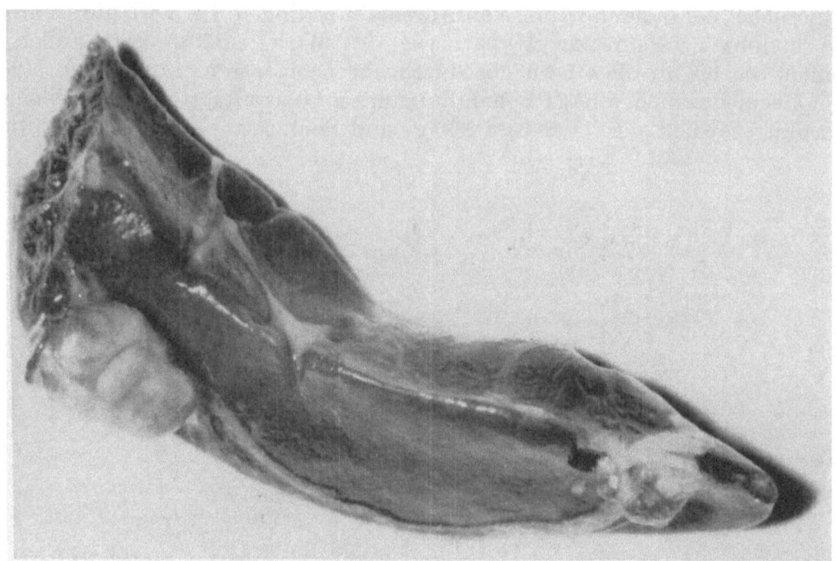

Abb. 16a. Knotige Regeneration von Nebennierenrindengewebe in der Milz, 4 Monate, 14 Tage nach Transplantation

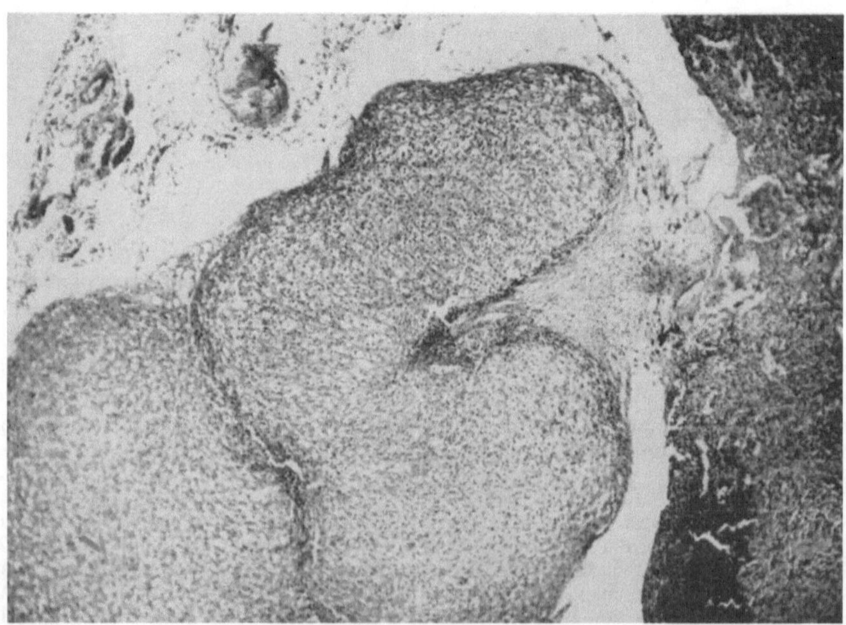

Abb. 16b. Das unter der Milzkapsel liegende knotige Nebennierenregenerat zeigt eine stielartige Verbindung mit der Milz (linker Bildrand)

Nach *Transplantation von Nebennierengewebe* in die Milz oder subcutan bei gleichzeitiger Entfernung beider Nebennieren sahen wir (Abb. 16a u. b), ebenso wie GREEP und DEANE (1949), INGLE und HIGGINS (1938), WILLIAMS (1947), EVERETT (1949), BERNSTEIN und ENOCH (1951), READ (1951) und DOSNE DE PASQUALINI und MANCINI (1951), WOODRUFF und BOSWELL (1953), DEMPSTER (1955), keine Adenombildung. Die Nebennieren-Regeneratgröße überstieg in unseren Versuchen [DONTENWILL und RANZ (1960)] nur bei Transplantation in die Milz in geringem Maße die Größe der entfernten Nebenniere, das Angehen des Transplantates war aber immer von einem absoluten Hormondefizit, d. h. von der Entfernung beider Nebennieren abhängig.

Literatur

d) Nebenniere

BERNSTEIN, D., and J. ENOCH: Effect of hypoglycemia on rats with intrasplenic adrenal transplants. Proc. Soc. exp. Biol. (N. Y.) **78**, 285 (1951).

BROWNING, H. C.: Hormonal dependence of adrenal cortical Tumors of CE and BALB/c mice in serial intraocular transfer. Cancer Res. **18**, 781 (1958).

BROWNING, H., W. WHITE and W. SADLER: Inhibition of growth of a transplanted adrenal cortical tumor by sex steroids. Cancer Res. **19**, 819 (1959).

CARDEZA, A. F.: Histologia de los tumores de la suprarenal en ratas castradas. Rev. Soc. argent. Biol. **30**, 200 (1954).

CHRISTY, N. P.: The pathogenesis of uterine lesions in virgin mice and in gonadectomized mice bearing adrenal cortical and pituitary tumors. Cancer Res. **11**, No. 6 (1951).

DEMPSTER, W. J.: The transplanted adrenal gland. Brit. J. Surg. **42**, 540 (1955).

DICKIE, M. M., and P. W. LANE: Adrenal tumors, and other pathological changes in F_1 hybrids of strain DE X strain DBA. Cancer Res. **16**, 48 (1956).

—, and G. W. WOOLLEY: Spontaneous basophilic tumors of the pituitary glands in gonadectomized mice. Cancer Res. **9**, 372 (1949).

DONTENWILL, W., u. H. RANZ: Vergleichende Untersuchungen an Transplantaten endokriner Drüsen.

DORFMAN, R. I., and W. U. GARDNER: Metabolism of the steroid hormones. The excretion of estrogenic material by ovariectomized mice bearing adrenal tumors. Endocrinology **34**, 421—423 (1944).

DOSNE DE PASQUALINI, CH., y R. E. MANCINI: Injerto de suprarrenal en el bazo. Rev. Soc. argent. Biol. **27**, 8 (1951); **27**, 67 u. 72 (1951).

DUNNING, W. F., M. R. CURTIS and A. SEGALOFF: Strain differences in response to diethylstilbestrol and the induction of mammary gland and bladder cancer in the rat. Cancer Res. **7**, 511—521 (1947).

ERÄNKÖ, O.: Nodular hyperplasia and increase of noradrenaline content in the adrenal medulla of nicotine-treated rats. Effect of insulin on chromaffin reaction, fluorescing islets and catechol amines in the adrenal medulla of the rat. Acta path. microbiol. scand. **36**, 3 (1955).

EVERETT, N. B.: Autoplastic and homoplastic transplants of the rat adrenal cortex and medulla to the kidney. Anat. Rec. **103**, 335 (1949).

FASSBENDER, H.: Pathologische Anatomie der endokrinen Drüsen. In: KAUFMANN: Lehrbuch der speziellen pathologischen Anatomie. Berlin: Walter de Gruyter & Co. 1956.

FEKETE, E., and C. C. LITTLE: Histological study of adrenal cortical tumors in gonadectomized mice of the Ce strain. Cancer Res. **5**, 220 (1945).

— G. W. WOOLEY and C. C. LITTLE: Histologic changes following ovarectomy in mice. J. exp. Med. **74**, 1 (1941).

FERGUSON, D. J., and M. B. VISSCHER: The effect of hypophysectomy on the development of adrenal tumors in C3H mice. Cancer Res. **13**, 405 (1953).

FLAKS, J.: Adrenal cortical carcinoma with metastases in an ovariectomized strong A mouse. J. Path. Bact. **61**, 266 (1949).

FRANKS, L., and F. C. CHESTERMAN: Experimental production of morphological changes resembling CONN's Syndrome. Lancet **1956 II**, 1193—1194.

— — Adrenal degeneration and tumour formation in the golden hamster following treatment with stilboestrol and methylcholanthrene. Brit. J. Cancer **11**, 105 (1957).

FRANTZ, M., and J. A. KIRSCHBAUM: Androgenic secretion by tumors of the mouse adrenal cortex. Proc. Soc. exp. Biol. (N. Y.) **69**, 357 (1948).

— — Development of adrenal cortical adenomas in ovariectomized mice injected with "physiologic" doses of sex hormone. Proc. Soc. exp. Biol. (N. Y.) **72**, 282 (1949).

— — Sex hormone secretion by tumors of the adrenal cortex of mice. Cancer Res. **9**, 257—266 (1949).

— —, and C. CASAS: Endocrine interrelationship and spontaneous tumors of the adrenal cortex in NH mice. Proc. Soc. exp. Biol. (N. Y.) **66**, 645—646 (1948).

GARDNER, W. U.: Estrogenic effects of adrenal tumors of ovariectomized mice. Cancer Res. **1**, 633 (1941).
GILMAN, J., CH. GILBERT and I. SPENCE: Phaeochromocytoma in the rats. Pathogenesis and collateral reactions and its relation to comparable tumours in man. Cancer (Chicago) **6**, 494 (1953).
GREEP, R. O., and H. W. DEANE: Histological, cytochemical and physiological observations on the regeneration of the rat's adrenal gland following enucleation. Endocrinology **45**, 42 (1949).
HOUSSAY, A., G. M. HIGGINS and W. A. BENNET: The influence exerted by desoxycorticosterone acetate upon the production of adrenal tumors in gonadectomized mice. Cancer Res. **11**, 297 (1951).
HOUSSAY, A. B., B. A. HOUSSAY, A. F. CARDEZA, R. M. PINTO and V. G. FOGLIA: Estrogenic adrenal tumors and gonadotrophic pituitary tumors in gonadectomized rats. 3rd Panamer. Congr. Endocrinol. (Santiago de Chile) 1954, p. 19.
— — V. G. FOGLIA, A. B. HOUSSAY y R. M. PINTO: Evolución anatómica y funcional de los tumores suprarenales de las ratas castradas. Rev. Soc. argent. Biol. **29**, 170—179 (1953).
— — — — — Evolution anatomique et fonctionelle des tumeurs surrénales chez les rats castrés. C. R. Soc. Biol. (Paris) **148**, 918—919 (1954).
HOUSSAY, B. A., A. F. CARDEZA, R. M. PINTO y M. H. BURGOS: Tumores suprarenales y acciones estrogénicas en ratas castradas. Rev. Soc. argent. Biol. **27**, 56 (1951).
— A. B. HOUSSAY, A. F. CARDEZA, V. G. FOGLIA and R. M. PINTO: Adrenal tumors in gonadectomized rats. Acta physiol. lat.-amer. **3**, 125 (1953).
HUMMEL, K. P.: Induced ovarian and adrenal tumours. J. nat. Cancer Inst. **15**, 711 (1954).
HUSEBY, R. A., and J. J. BITTNER: The relationship of the inherited hormonal influence to the production of adrenal cortical tumors by castration. Cancer Res. **8**, 641—651 (1948).
— — Postcastration adrenal changes and the subsequent development of mammary cancer in several inbred stocks of mice and their hybrids. Cancer Res. **10**, 226 (1950).
— — Differences in adrenal responsiveness to post-castrational alteration as evidenced by transplanted adrenal tissue. Cancer Res. **11**, No. 12, 954 (1951).
INGLE, D. J., and G. M. HIGGINS: Autotransplantation and regeneration of the adrenal gland. Endocrinology **22**, 458 (1938).
JONES, E. E., and L. J. WOODWARD: Spontaneous adrenal medullary tumors in hybrid mice. J. nat. Cancer Inst. **15**, 449—461 (1954).
KING, J. T., C. B. CASAS and M. B. VISSCHER: The influence of estrogen on cancer incidence and adrenal changes in ovariectomized mice on caloric restriction. Cancer Res. **9**, 436—437 (1949).
KIRKMAN, H.: Steroid Tumorigenesis. Cancer Res. **10**, 754 (1957).
—, and M. ROBBINS: The carcinogenicity of testosterone propionate in Syrian hamster. Proc. Amer. Ass. Cancer Res. **2**, 125 (1956).
LASNITZKI, I.: The effect of estrogen alone and combined with 20-methylcholanthren of mouse prostate glands grown in vitro. Cancer Res. **14**, 632 (1954).
LIEBEGOTT, G.: Die Pathologie der Nebennieren. Verh. dtsch. Ges. Path. **36**, 21 (1952).
— In: Pathologie der Laboratoriumstiere. Herausgegeben von D. COHRS, R. JAFFÉ u. H. MEESSEN. Berlin-Göttingen-Heidelberg: Springer 1958.
LIPSCHUTZ, A.: Steroid Hormons and Tumors. Baltimore: Williams & Wilkins Comp. 1950.
— Steroid Homeostasis Hypophysis and Tumorigenesis. Cambridge: W. Heffer & Sons, Ltd. 1957.
LUPULESCU, A.: Phäochromozytome nach gleichzeitiger Verabreichung von Oestradiol und somatotropem Hormon bei Meerschweinchen. Endokrinologie **48**, 164—170 (1965).
MARTINEZ, C., and J. J. BITTNER: Postcastrational adrenal tumors in unilaterally adrenalectomized C3H mice. Cancer Res. **15**, 612 (1955).
— — Función estrogénica de los tumores suprarenales producidos por la castración en ratones. Rev. argent. Endocr. **2**, 40 (1956).
MONSEN, H.: Effect of cortisone and sex steroids on the induction and maintenance of castration induced adrenal cortical adenomas of mice. Cancer Res. **12**, 284—285 (1952).
— and A. KIRSCHBAUM: Pituitary-adrenal gonadal interrelationship in the maintenance of adrenal cortical tumors of mice as determined by parabiosis. Proc. Amer. Ass. Cancer Res. **1**, 33—34 (1954).
MOON, H. D., A. A. KONEFF, CH. H. LI and M. E. SIMPSON: Pheochromocytomas of adrenals in male rats chronically injected with pituitary growth hormone (22667). Proc. Soc. exp. Biol. **93**, 74—77 (1956).
— M. E. SIMPSON, CH. H. LI and H. M. EVANS: Neoplasms in rats treated with pituitary growth hormone. II. Adrenal glands. Cancer Res. **10**, 364 (1950).
MORRIS, D. M.: Adrenal hypertrophy in the white leghorn cockerel after treatment with thiouracil and thyroidectomy. Science 16, **117**, 61 (1953).

READ, G.: Adrenal transplants into spleen and the inaktivation of adrenal cortical hormones. Aust. J. exp. Biol. med. Sci. **23**, 161 (1951).
SILBERBERG, R., M. SILBERBERG and M. OPDYKE: Effects of anterior hypophysis on mammary glands and adrenals. A. M. A. Arch. Path. **55**, 506—515 (1953).
SMITH, F. W.: The relationship of the inherites hormonal influence to the production of adrenal cortical tumors by castration. Cancer Res. **8**, 641 (1948).
— W. U. GARDNER, M. H. LI and H. KAPLAN: Adrenal medullary tumors (Pheochromocytomas) in mice. Cancer Res. **9**, 193—198 (1949).
SPIEGEL, A.: Auftreten von Adenomen der Nebennierenrinde mit vermännlichender Wirkung bei frühkastrierten Meerschweinchenmännchen. Klin. Wschr. **1939**, 1068; Zbl. allg. Path. path. Anat. **74**, 328 (1940).
— Über das Auftreten von Geschwülsten der Nebennierenrinde mit vermännlichender Wirkung bei frühkastrierten Meerschweinchenmännchen. Virchows Arch. path. Anat. **305**, 2, 367 (1939); Zbl. allg. Path. path. Anat. **77**, 249 (1941).
STAEMMLER, M.: Die chronische Vergiftung mit Nicotin. Ergebnisse experimenteller Untersuchungen an Ratten. Virchows Arch. path. Anat. **295**, 366 (1935).
— Über geschwulstartige Bildungen im Nebennierenmark als Folge exper. Nikotinvergiftung. Klin. Wschr. **12**, 404 (1936).
TONUTTI, E.: Normale Anatomie der endokrinen Drüsen und endokrine Regulation. In: KAUFMANN: Lehrbuch der speziellen pathologischen Anatomie. Berlin: Walter de Gruyter & Co. 1956.
WILLIAMS, R. G.: Studies of adrenal cortex: regeneration of the transplanted gland and the vital quality of autogenous grafts. Amer. J. Anat. **81**, 199 (1947).
WOODRUFF, M. F., and TH. BOSWELL: The effect of cortisone and ACTH on adrenal transplantats in the rat. J. Endocr. **10**, 86 (1953).
WOOLLEY, G. W.: The incidence of adrenal cortical carcinoma in gonadectomized male mice of the extreme dilution strain. Cancer Res. **5**, 211 (1945).
— The incidence of adrenal cortical carcinoma in male mice of the extreme dilution strain over one year of age. Cancer Res. **5**, 506 (1945).
— The adrenal cortex and its tumors. Ann. N. Y. Acad. Sci. **50**, 616—626 (1949).
— Effect of hormonal substances on adrenal cortical tumors formation in mice. Cancer Res. **10**, 250 (1950).
— Experimental endocrine tumors with special reference to the adrenal cortex. Recent Progr. Hormone Res. **5**, 383 (1950).
— Evidence that adrenal cortical tumors in aged, gonadectomized hamsters produce sexlike hormones. Anat. Rec. **115**, 381 (1953).
— Carcinogenesis in the adrenal. J. nat. Cancer Inst. **15**, 717 (1954).
— Tumors of the adrenal cortex. In: G. E. W. WOLSTENHOLME and M. O'CONNOR (eds.), Ciba Found. Coll. Endocrinol. **12**, 122—133 (1958). (London: J. & A. Churchill, Ltd.)
— M. M. DICKIE and C. C. LITTLE: Adrenal tumors and other pathological changes in reciprocal crosses in mice. I. Strain DBA x Strain CE and the reciprocal. Cancer Res. **12**, 142—152 (1953).
— — — Adrenal tumors and other pathological changes in reciprocal crosses in mice. II. An introduction to results of four reciprocal crosses. Cancer Res. **13**, 231—245 (1953).
— E. FEKETE and C. C. LITTLE: Differences between high and low breast tumor strains of mice when ovariectomized at birth. Proc. Soc. exp. Biol. (N. Y.) **45**, 796 (1940).
— — — Gonadectomy and adrenal tumors. Science **97**, 291 (1943).
—, and C. C. LITTLE: The incidence of adrenal cortical carcinoma in gonadectomized female mice of the extreme dilution strain. Cancer Res. **5**, 193, 203, 321 (1945).
— — The incidence of adrenal cortical carcinoma in gonadectomized male mice of the extreme dilution strain. Cancer Res. **5**, 211, 506 (1945).
— — Prevention of adrenal cortical carcinoma by diethylstilbestrol. Cancer Res. **6**, 491 (1946).
YEAKEL, E. H.: Medullary hyperplasia of the adrenal gland in aged wistar albino and gray norway rats. Arch. Path. (Chicago) **44**, 71 (1947).

e) Mamma

Spontane Brustdrüsengeschwülste mit alveolär-tubulärem Aufbau werden nach FISCHER und KÜHL (1958) u. a. bei der ***Maus*** häufig beobachtet, seltener dagegen Fibroadenome oder Fibrome, die aber bei Ratten häufiger gesehen werden. Bei Mäusestämmen mit einer hohen Mammacarcinomrate entstehen neben tubulär-alveolären Parenchymwucherungen häufig Hyperplasien der kleinen Ausführungsgänge. Während in Mäusestämmen mit hoher Tumorfrequenz sehr selten Plattenepithelmetaplasien der Mammadrüsen vorkommen, wird dies nach DUNN (1953) und FOULDS (1949, 1956) bei Mäusestämmen mit niedriger Tumorfrequenz besonders oft beobachtet. Nach Behandlung mit *oestrogenen* Hormonen traten bei verschiedenen Mäusestämmen vorwiegend acinöse Drüsenhyperplasien und cystische Erweiterungen der Drüsen und Ausführungsgänge auf. Diese Veränderungen werden mit steigendem Alter häufiger.

Cystische Veränderungen mit Drüsenwucherung bei der Maus und Ratte nach Oestrogenbehandlung wurden von zahlreichen Untersuchern beobachtet [BONSER (1936), LEWIS und GESCHICKTER (1936), PICCO (1936), GESCHICKTER (1939), GESCHICKTER und BYRNES (1942), EISEN (1944), COPELAND (1947), LACASSAGNE (1950), LOEB, BURNS, SUNTZEFF und MOSCOP (1937), NOBLE und CUTTS (1959)], es bestand aber bei den einzelnen Inzuchtstämmen eine verschiedene Anfälligkeit.

HEROLD und EFFKEMANN (1936) beobachteten nach Follikelhormonbehandlung in der Brustdrüse der *Ratte* Milchgangscysten und Veränderungen im Sinne der Mastopathie. PRIGOZINA (1951), PRIGOZINA und SHABAD (1950) sahen neben Mastopathie sogar präcanceröse Epithelwucherungen, ähnlich MORRIS (1953) nach Gonadotropininjektionen. GESCHICKTER (1941) fand nach Injektion von täglich 5 γ Oestrogen über 90—100 Tage ein buschiges Wachstum der Endknospen der Brustdrüse der Ratte. Nach Applikation höherer Dosen Oestrogen (200 γ Oestrogen täglich) stellte GESCHICKTER cystische Fibrose und Fibroadenome fest.

Fibroadenome wurden von COPELAND (1947), LEWIS und GESCHICKTER (1936) bei Ratten und Affen durch langdauernde hochdosierte Oestrogenbehandlung erzeugt.

Die Entstehung der Fibrome der Mamma der Ratte wird durch Behandlung mit Progesteron und Testosteron gehemmt [HEIMANN (1943), HUGGINS und MAINZER (1957), MOHS (1940)], ebenso durch Kastration [PICCO (1936)].

LIPSCHUTZ (1950) gelang es nicht, Fibrome beim Meerschweinchen zu erzeugen. Er fand nur vereinzelt metaplastische Epithelproliferationen [desgl. KLEIN (1938)], zu den gleichen Ergebnissen kamen LIPSCHUTZ (1950) bei weiblichen Cebus-Affen.

SABRAZÈS, LE CHUITON, GINESTE (1934) beschrieben nach Follikelhormonbehandlung bei Ratten Entwicklung von Schweißdrüsenadenomen im Bereich von Netzimplantationen. FLORENTIN und BINDER (1939) erzeugten auf die gleiche Weise eine Metaplasie der Talgdrüsen der Mamma beim Meerschweinchen. MOON, SIMPSON, LI und EVANS (1950) sahen nach langdauernder (über 400 Tage/16 Monate) Behandlung von Ratten mit *Wachstumshormon* (mit zunehmendem Alter der Tiere steigende Dosen von 0,6—3,0 mg täglich) Fibroadenome bei weiblichen, dagegen nie bei männlichen Ratten (11 von 15 Tieren hatten multiple Fibrome oder Fibroadenome, dagegen nur 3 von 15 Kontrollen); bei gleicher Behandlung am hypophysektomierten Tier sahen sie keine Tumoren der Mamma.

Literatur

e) Mamma

BONSER, G. M.: The effect of oestrone administration on the mammary glands of male mice of two strains differing greatly in their susceptibility to spontaneous mammary carcinoma. J. Path. Bact. **42**, 169 (1936).

COPELAND, M. M.: Newer aspects of benign tumors of breast. Arch. Surg. (Chicago) **55**, 590 (1947).

DUNN, T. B.: Morphology of mammary tumors in mice. In: F. HOMBURGER and W. H. FISHMAN (eds.). Physiopathology of cancer S. 123—148, New York: Hoeber-Harper Co. 1953.

EISEN, M. J.: The occurrence of benign and malignent mammary lesions in rats treatet with crystalline estrogene. Cancer Res. **2**, 632 (1944).

FISCHER, W., u. I. KÜHL: Geschwülste der Laboratoriumstiere. Dresden und Leipzig: Theodor Steinkopff 1958.

Florentin, P., et C. Binder: Métaplasie sébacée de la glande mammaire chez le cobaye folliculinisé. C. R. Soc. Biol. (Paris) **130**, 360 (1939).
Foulds, L.: Mammary tumours in hybrid mice: growth and progression of spontaneous tumours. Brit. J. Cancer **3**, 345 (1949).
— The histologic analysis of mammary tumors of mice. I. Scope of investigations and general principles of analysis. II. The histology of responsiveness and progression. The origin of tumors. III. Organoid tumors. IV. Secretion. J. nat. Cancer Inst. **17**, 701—802 (1956).
Geschickter, C. F.: Estrogenic mammary cancer in the rat. Radiology **33**, 439 (1939).
— Mammary carcinoma in the rat with metastasis induced by estrogen. Science **89**, 35 (1939).
— Corpus luteum studies. Progesterone therapy in chronic cystic mastitis. J. clin. Endocr. **1**, 147 (1941).
—, and E. W. Byrnes: Factors influencing the development and time of appearance of mammary cancer in the rat in response to estrogen. Arch. Path. (Chicago) **33**, 334—356 (1942).
Heiman, J.: Comparative effects of estrogen, testosterone and progesterone on benign mammary tumors of the rat. Cancer Res. **3**, 65 (1943).
Herold, L., u. G. Effkemann: Beziehungen des Follikelhormons zu pathophysiologischen Wachstumsvorgängen der Brustdrüse. I. Mitt. Brustdrüsenentwicklung unter gesteigerter Zufuhr von Follikelhormon bei der Ratte. Arch. Gynäk. **163**, 1, 85 (1936).
— — Beziehungen des Follikelhormons zu pathophysiologischen Wachstumsvorgängen der Brustdrüse. II. Mitt. Tierexperimentelle Untersuchungen über die Bedeutung einer langdauernden und vermehrten Follikelhormonwirkung in der Genese der Fibrosis Mammae cystica. Arch. Gynäk. **163**, 1, 94 (1936).
— — Beziehungen des Follikelhormons zu pathophysiologischen Wachstumsvorgängen der Brustdrüse. III. Mitt. Unterschiedliche Wirkung einer langdauernden Follikelhormonzufuhr auf die Brustdrüsenstruktur kastrierter und nichtkastrierter Ratten. Arch. Gynäk. **163**, 1, 309 (1936).
Huggins, C., and K. Mainzer: Hormonal influences on mammary tumors of the rat. II. Retardation of growth of a transplanted fibroadenoma in intact female rats by steroids in the androstane series. J. exp. Med. **105**, 485—500 (1957).
Klein, F.: Über den Einfluß von Follikulin auf einige Organe des Meerschweinchenbockes. Frankfurt. Z. Path. **51**, 2, 406 (1938).
Lacassagne, A.: Les cancers produits par des substances chimiques endogènes. Paris: Hermann & Co. 1950.
Lewis, D., and C. F. Geschickter: The demonstration of hormones in tumors. Ann. Surg. **104**, 787 (1936).
Lipschutz, A.: Steroid Hormones and Tumors. Baltimore: Williams & Wilkins Comp. 1950.
Loeb, L., E. L. Burns, V. Suntzeff and M. Moscop: Sexhormones and their relation to tumor production. Amer. J. Cancer **30**, 47 (1937).
Mohs, F. E.: Effect of estrogens and androgens on growth of mammary fibroma in rats. Proc. Soc. exp. Biol. (N. Y.) **43**, 270—272 (1940).
Moon, H. D., M. E. Simpson, Ch. H. Li and H. M. Evans: Neoplasms in rats treated with pituitary growth hormone. III. Reproductive organes. Cancer Res. **10**, 549 (1950).
Morris, H. P.: Influence of gonadotrophin on pyridoxine deficient and diet-restricted female mice. J. Nat. Cancer Inst. **14**, No. 3 (1953).
Noble, R. L., and J. H. Cutts: Mammary tumors of the rat. Cancer Res. **19**, 1125 (1959).
Picco, A.: Der Einfluß der Kastration auf die Entwicklung des Fibroadenoma mammae der Ratte. Tumori **22**, 231 (1936); Zbl. Path. **65**, 308 (1936).
Pierson, H.: Neubildung von mammaähnlichem Bau in den äußeren Magenschichten des Kaninchens bei langdauernder Behandlung mit Follikulin. Z. Krebsforsch. **48**, 3, 177 (1938); Zbl. Path. **73**, 214 (1939).
Prigozina, E. L.: Über exper. Krebs und präcancerale Veränderungen der Brustdrüsen, bei Ratten durch Synoestrol hervorgerufen (Über den exper. Krebs und präcanceröse Veränderungen der Milchdrüse bei der Ratte nach Synostrolbehandlung.) Arch. Path. **13**, 2, 46 (1951) (russisch); Berichte **11**, 194 (1952).
— u. L. M. Shabad: Experimentell durch wiederholte Schwangerschaft in den Milchdrüsen von Mäusen einer nichtkrebsigen Linie hervorgerufene Veränderungen. Arch. Path. (Chicago) **3**, 43 (1950); Arch. Geschwulstforsch. **4**, 1, 81 (1952).
Sabrazès, J., F. le Chuiton et G. Gineste: Hyperplasie des glandes tégumentaires et adénomatose sudoripare après injections de folliculine chez le rat blanc. C. R. Soc. Biol. (Paris) **117**, 30, 376 (1934).

f) Ovar

1944 gelang es erstmals Biskind und Biskind, durch *Implantation* von Ovarien in die Milz kastrierter Ratten Granulosazelltumoren zu erzeugen. Durch die

Implantation des Ovars in die Milz oder an eine andere Stelle im Bereich des Pfortadersystems, z. B. im Bereich des Pankreas, werden die im Ovar gebildeten Hormone direkt der Leber zugeleitet und dort weitgehend abgebaut. Wie die zahlreichen folgenden Untersuchungen zeigten, findet sich im Blut bei intakter Leberfunktion, z. B. bei Ratten nach der Leberpassage, kein Follikelhormon mehr.

Untersuchungen über den Follikelhormonabbau wurden von BISKIND und MARK (1939), BISKIND (1941), BISKIND und SHESLESNYAK (1942), BISKIND, PENCHARZ und BISKIND (1948),

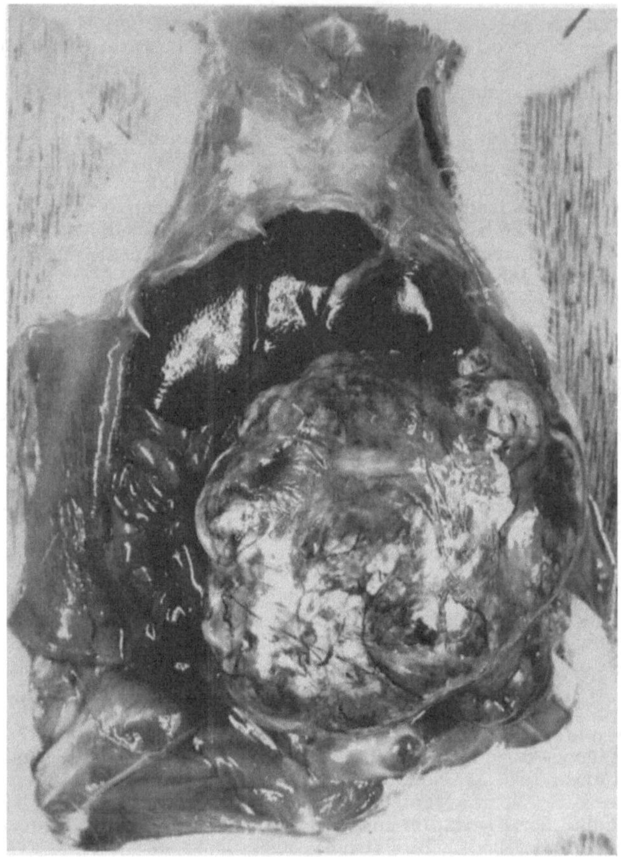

Abb. 17a. 619 Tage altes Ovartransplantat in der Milz. Großer, den Bauchraum zu $^2/_3$ ausfüllender Tumor

PINCUS und MARTIN (1940), SELYE (1941), GYÖRGY (1945), DE MEIO, RAKOFF, CANTAROW und PASCHKIS (1948), sowie LIPSCHUTZ (1950) durchgeführt.

Durch den Follikelhormonabbau in der Leber entsteht eine dauernde Unterbilanz an Follikelhormon im Blut und als Reaktion eine dauernde Mehrsekretion von gonadotropem Hormon. Durch diese Mehrstimulierung des transplantierten Ovars entsteht dann eine geschwulstartige Wucherung, die die verminderte Hormonproduktion ausgleicht. Die Größe der nach Transplantation auftretenden Ovartumoren zeigt sich insbesondere beim Vergleich mit der Milzgröße (Abb. 17a u. b).

Die Ovartumoren konnten auch von FURTH und SOBEL (1946, 1947) erzeugt werden, die bei den Tieren in der Leber eine sog. Hypervolämie, d. h. eine Blutfülle und Erweiterung der Gefäße fanden. Gleichartige Ovartumoren (Granulosazelltumoren und Luteome) wurden bei Ratten und Mäusen von FURTH (1946), FURTH und SOBEL (1947), LI und GARDNER (1947), TAKEWAKI (1949, 1950), LIPSCHUTZ (1950), VAN LANCKER und MAISIN (1950, 1953), LACOUR, OBERLING und GUÉRIN (1952), KLEIN (1952), PECKHAM und GREENE (1952), MÜHLBOCK (1952), TAKEWAKI, TAKASUGI und MAEKAWA (1952), BIELSCHOWSKY (1951), BIELSCHOWSKY und HALL (1953), BØE, TOGERSEN und ATTRAMADAL (1954), GARDNER (1954, 1955), KULLANDER (1954), ZULLI (1955), MARDONES und LIPSCHUTZ (1956), FELS (1956), MÜHLBOCK, VAN NIE und BOSCH (1958), RANZ (1960); bei Meerschweinchen von LIPSCHUTZ, PONCE DE LEON, WOYWOOD (1944), GAY (1944), IGLESIAS, MARDONES und LIPSCHUTZ (1953), MARDONES, IGLESIAS und LIPSCHUTZ (1955); bei Kaninchen von PECKHAM, GREENE und JEFFRIES

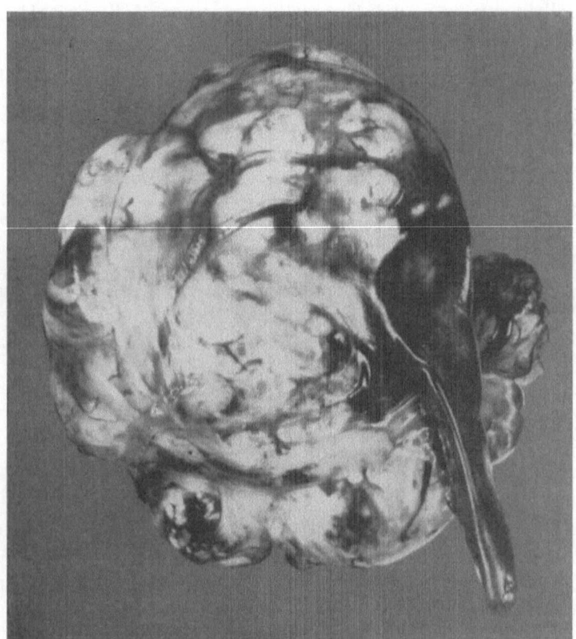

Abb. 17b. Der gleiche Tumor mit Milz

(1948), PECKHAM und GREENE (1952) beschrieben (nach Transplantation von Ovargewebe bei kastrierten Tieren in Milz oder Pankreas).

Eine Reihe Untersucher befaßte sich in der Folge mit der Frage der Genese des Ovartumors [FURTH (1946), LI und GARDNER (1950) u. a.]. HELLER und JUNGEK konnten 1947 zeigen, daß keine cyclische, sondern eine kontinuierliche Gonadotropin-Mehrsekretion nach der Transplantation des Ovars in die Milz erfolgt. Nach LIPSCHUTZ (1963) [LIPSCHUTZ und CERISOLA (1962), LIPSCHUTZ, PANASEVICH und ALVAREZ (1963)], die sich eingehend mit der Genese der Ovarialtumoren beschäftigte, „können Eierstocksgeschwülste durch experimentelle Eingriffe (subtotale Kastration, Eierstocksverpflanzung in die Milz) erzeugt werden, die die ovarialbedingte Steuerung der gonadotropen Funktion der Hypophyse stören. Der entstandene Ovarialtumor ist das Ergebnis einer Evolution, die sich bei der Maus über eine Zeitdauer von 10–12 Monaten erstreckt".

LI und GARDNER (1950) sahen auch Tumorentwicklung im Pankreas bei Mäusen. PECKHAM und GREENE (1952) beobachteten gleiche Tumoren nach Implantation des Ovars in die Milz des Kaninchens.

FURTH und SOBEL (1947) und LI (1948) sahen bei Mäusen von den Ovartumoren ausgehende *Metastasen* und MARDONES, IGLESIAS und LIPSCHUTZ (1955) beobachteten Metastasen in der Leber bei Meerschweinchen 58 Monate nach Implantation und berichten von fraglichen Metastasen in der Lunge bei Ovartumoren des Meerschweinchens, die durch gleiche Methodik erzeugt worden waren. In eigenen Versuchen fanden wir [RANZ (1960)] nie Metastasen, auch nicht bei Tieren, die über zwei Jahre alt geworden waren.

Die Ovartumoren entstehen auch nach Implantationen des Ovars in die Milz kastrierter Männchen, wie LI (1948) zeigen konnte. LI und GARDNER (1947, 1950), BISKIND, KORDAN und BISKIND (1950) fanden dagegen keine Tumoren, wenn nur einseitig kastriert wurde oder wenn die Maus mit Oestradiol oder Testosteron vorbehandelt wurde. Während eine Behandlung mit Oestrogen und Androgen die Entwicklung des Granulosazelltumors in der Milz hemmt [LI und GARDNER (1949)], fördern Androgen und Oestrogen das Wachstum des *spontan* auftretenden Granulosazelltumors und die Entwicklung seiner Malignität [IGLESIAS und MARDONES (1956)].

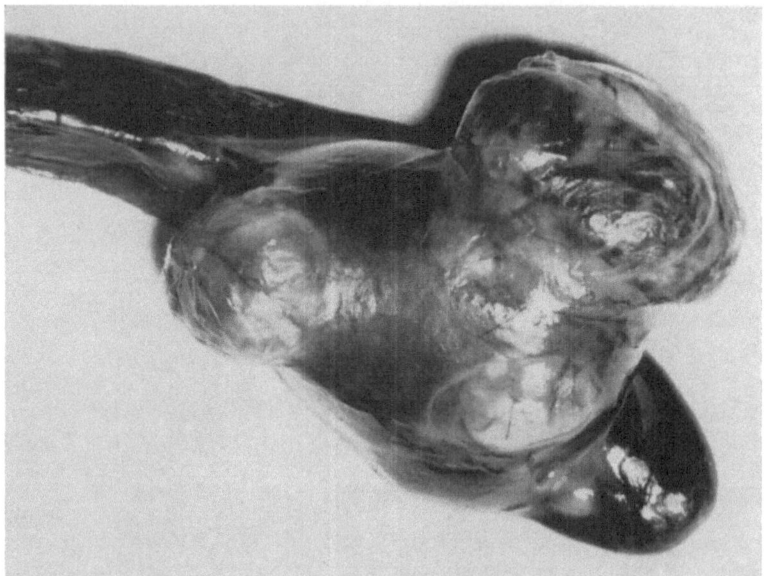

Abb. 18. Knolliger Ovarialtumor in der Milz, 407 Tage nach Implantation

Kastration fördert ebenfalls das Angehen des spontanen Granulosazelltumors [IGLESIAS, MARDONES (1956)]. Die meisten Untersucher sahen in gleicher Weise wie BISKIND und BISKIND (1949) keine Ovarialgeschwülste in der Milz, wenn durch Verwachsungen der Milz mit der Bauchwand eine Umgehung des Leberkreislaufes möglich war. DAVID, JAKOBOVITS, KOVACS und KORPASSY (1957) fanden nach Schädigung des Leberparenchyms durch Tetrachlorkohlenstoff ebenfalls eine Hemmung der Tumorentwicklung. Wir, DONTENWILL (1959) und RANZ (1960), beobachteten bei Goldhamstern, denen nach Kastration Ovargewebe in die Milz implantiert wurde, keine Tumorentstehung und führen dies auf den fehlenden oder unvollständigen Abbau des Follikelhormons in der Goldhamsterleber zurück.

BISKIND, KORDAN und BISKIND (1950) untersuchten die Wirkung der *Schwangerschaft* auf das in die Milz transplantierte Ovar und konnten zeigen, daß nach Entfernung des einen Ovars während der Schwangerschaft das andere in die Milz transplantierte Ovar neue Follikel und Corpora lutea bildet. Entfernt man am Ende der Gravidität das Ovar am normalen Orte, so entstehen nach BISKIND, KORDAN und BISKIND (1950) aus dem vorher in die Milz implantierten Ovar noch Tumoren. Das Alter des transplantierten Ovar spielt nach LI und GARDNER (1950) also keine wesentliche Rolle.

SILBERBERG und SILBERBERG und LEIDLER (1951) untersuchten den *Einfluß von Hypophysentransplantaten* auf das in die Milz implantierte Ovar. Sie konnten durch Hypophysenvorderlappenimplantation eine Förderung des Ovartransplantat-Wachstums erzeugen.

Nach MILLER und GARDNER (1954) hemmt Thyroxin das Wachstum des in der Milz entstandenen Granulosazelltumors ebenso wie eine Thiouracilbehandlung. Die Tumorentwicklung wird auch unterbunden durch Hypophysektomie [GARDNER (1958), KULLANDER (1956)] sowie durch Parahydroxypropiophenonbehandlung [BERNSTEIN und BISKIND (1952)]. ELY (1956, 1959) gelang es, durch antigonadotropes Serum die Tumorentwicklung zu hemmen.

MÜHLBOCK (1952) vergleicht die Entstehung des Ovartumors nach Transplantation in die Milz mit der Entstehung der Granulosazelltumoren nach Röntgenbestrahlung [BRAMBELL, PARKES und FIELDING (1927, 1928), BUTTERWORTH (1937)].

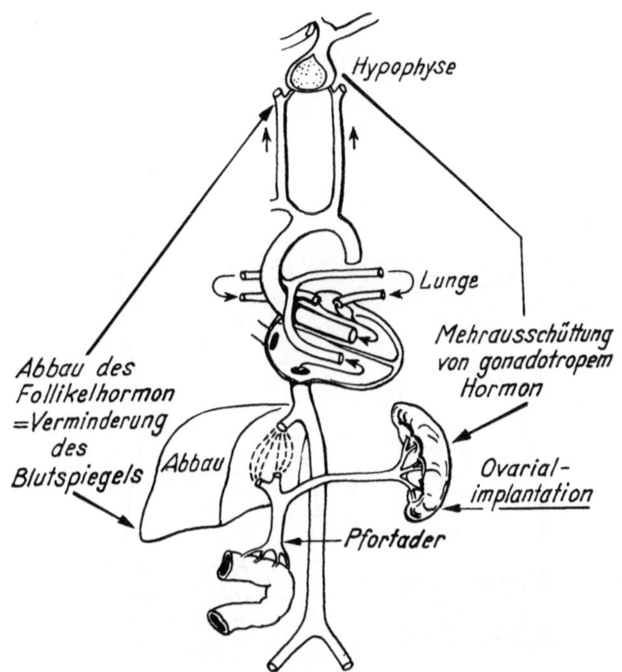

Abb. 19. Hormonsekretion des in die Milz transplantierten Ovarialgewebes

Granulosazelltumoren und Luteome nach Röntgenbestrahlung beschrieben außerdem FURTH und BUTTERWORTH (1936), FURTH und BOON (1947), FURTH (1949), LICK, KIRSCHBAUM und MIXER (1949), BALI und FURTH (1949), GARDNER (1950), KAPLAN (1950), FURTH und SOBEL (1947), KULLANDER (1953).

Während MÜHLBOCK (1952) durch Versuche beweisen konnte, daß durch die Störung der Follikelhormonproduktion bzw. durch den Follikelhormonabbau in der Leber (Abb. 19 zeigt die veränderten Verhältnisse des Follikelhormonabflusses in die Leber, die das Hormon weitgehend abbaut) über eine vermehrte Gonadotropinsekretion eine Stimulierung des Ovars in der Milz entsteht, nimmt er an, daß bei der Entstehung der Granulosazelltumoren nach Bestrahlung ähnliche Wirkungsmechanismen vorliegen (Abb. 20). Er glaubt, daß die Follikel durch die Röntgenbestrahlung zugrunde gehen und dann nur noch eine geringfügige Hormonproduktion aufrechterhalten werden kann. Wir haben die nach Bestrahlung zur Entstehung von Ovartumoren führenden Vorgänge in Abb. 20 schematisch wiedergegeben. Die daraus resultierende, von MILLER und PFEIFFER (1950) nachgewiesene Gonadotropinsekretion führt nach Ansicht von MÜHLBOCK (1952) zur Entstehung von Tumoren. Im Parabioseversuch mit 3 kastrierten Tieren konnte MÜHLBOCK (1952, 1953) [und TAKEWAKI (1953)] die Tumorentstehung aus dem Ovar in der Milz eines Tieres beschleunigen. JOHNSON und WITSCHI (1961) untersuchten die Veränderung der Ovarien bei Parabiose-Versuchen. Sie vereinigten kastrierte männliche oder weibliche Ratten des Holzmann-Stammes (Alter 30 Tage) mit hypophysektomierten Weibchen, mit Männchen mit Ovarialimplantaten und mit Weibchen, bei denen durch Testosteronimplantation (als Neugeborenes) ein Daueroestrus erzeugt worden war. Es entstanden in den Ovarien Granulosazelltumoren mit beachtlicher Oestrogenproduktion. Der kastrierte Partner liefert dauernd an den Parabionten Gonadotropine und löst so die Tumorbildung aus. Mühlbock (1952, 1953) konnte damit zeigen, daß

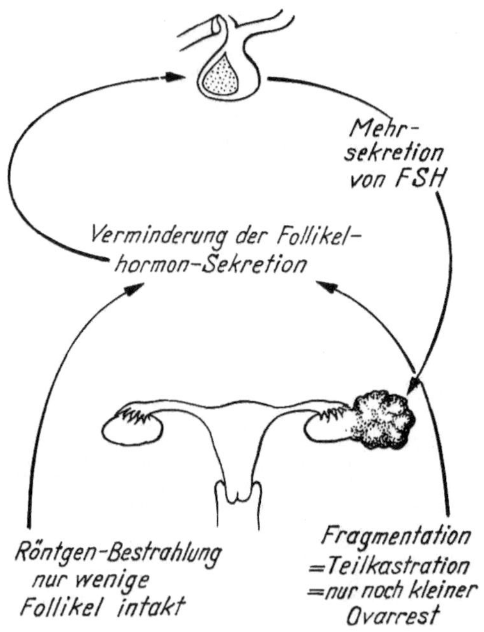

Abb. 20. Ovartumorentstehung durch Störung der Follikelhormonsekretion

offenbar das Maß der Gonadotropinsekretion wesentlich verantwortlich ist für die Zeitdauer der Tumorentstehung. Daß der Abbau der im Ovar gebildeten Hormone in der Leber letztlich die Tumorerzeugung veranlaßt, zeigen die Versuche von van Wagenen und Gardner (1950, 1953) beim Rhesusaffen. Sie sahen keinerlei Tumorentstehung, da die Leber des Rhesusaffen das Follikelhormon nicht abbaut.

Eine exogene Zufuhr von Gonadotropin fördert nach Biskind, Bernstein und Gospe (1953) die Entstehung von Luteomen, die meist in den ersten Monaten (90. bis 127. Tag) gefunden werden, und von Granulosazelltumoren, die etwas später auftreten (126. bis 194. Tag).

Gardner (1955), Elliot und Husni (1957) sowie Dontenwill und Ranz (1960) sahen nach Implantation von Ovargewebe in den Hoden zwar Wachstum, aber keine Tumorentwicklung.

Die *morphologische Struktur* der Geschwülste ist nach den Untersuchungen von Biskind (1949), Butterworth (1937), Henderson (1942), Mühlbock (1952), Guthrie (1957), Greene (1957), Gardner (1958), Ranz (1960) sehr verschieden. Meist entstehen zuerst Luteome (Abb. 21) und später Granulosazelltumoren (Abb. 22, 24). Bei der Entwicklung von Granulosazelltumoren handelt es sich offenbar um eine Umdifferenzierung, d. h. um Differenzierungsstadien des gleichen Grundgewebes. Auf Abb. 24 sehen wir beide Zellarten nebeneinander.

Cortisoninjektion hemmt nach MARDONES und LIPSCHUTZ (1956) die Entwicklung von Tumoren, erzeugt aber mehr Luteome (ohne Cortison traten 75% Granulosazelltumoren und 25% Luteome nach 1 Jahr auf und mit Cortison nur 10% Granulosazelltumoren und häufiger Degenerationen). Die Entwicklung ist bei den einzelnen Tierspecies verschieden. Beim Meerschweinchen z. B. entstehen im Verlauf des ersten Jahres nur Luteome. Granulosazelltumoren

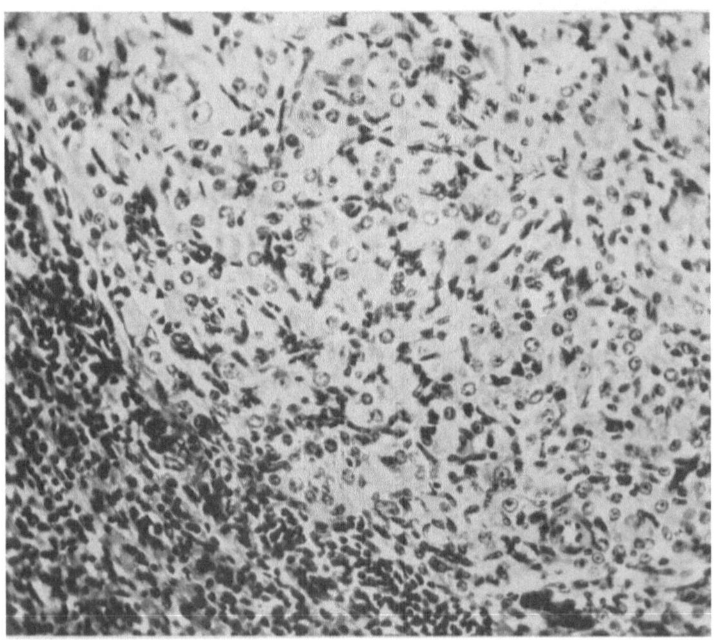

Abb. 21. Randpartie eines Luteoms. Rechts oben Milz. 182 Tage altes Implantat

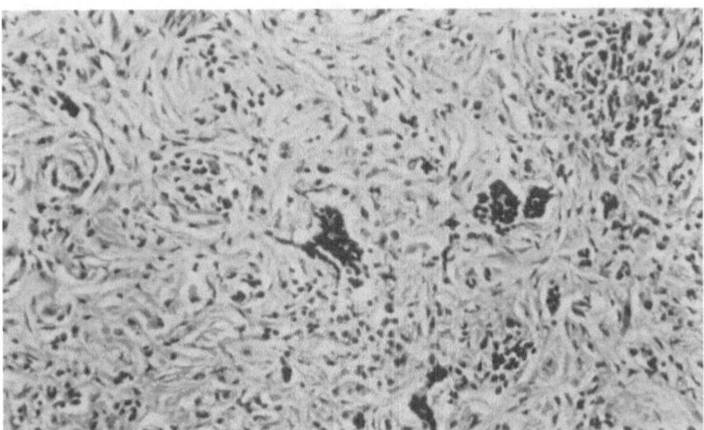

Abb. 22. Solide Granulosazellgruppen im Bindegewebe innerhalb der Milz. 288 Tage altes Implantat

werden erst sehr spät gesehen. Bestimmte Mäusestämme [GUTHRIE (1957)] zeigen vorwiegend Granulosazelltumoren. Transplantiert man den Ovartumor in den ersten Monaten auf andere Tiere, so ist er im Wachstum von den gleichen hormonellen Bedingungen abhängig [GREENE (1957) u. a.]. Transplantiert man ihn 1 Jahr nach der Implantation, so ist das Transplantat nicht mehr von den nach Kastration vorhandenen hormonalen Bedingungen abhängig [GREENE (1957)], es wächst auch beim nichtkastrierten Tier. Zwischen dem 9. und 12. Monat erreicht das Transplantat Autonomie.

Die Tumoren bei Meerschweinchen [MARDONES, IGLESIAS und LIPSCHUTZ (1955)] waren nicht transplantabel. Über erfolgreiche Transplantation bei Ratten und Mäusen berichten FURTH (1946), FURTH und SOBEL (1947), PECKHAM und GREENE (1952), FELS (1953), ZONDEK, LAUFER und TAMARI (1953), GARDNER (1955).

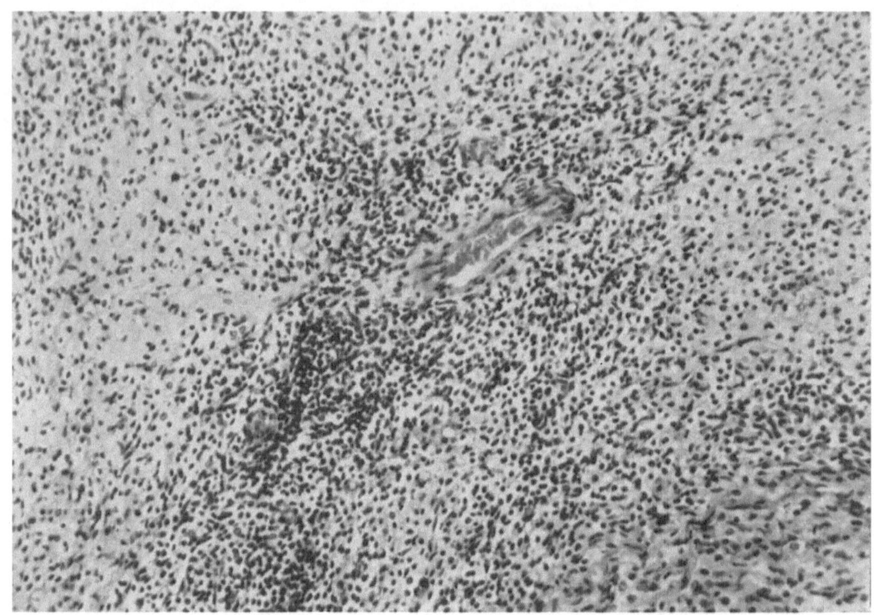

Abb. 23. Zellreiche fibromähnliche Strukturen in einem 407 Tage alten Implantat

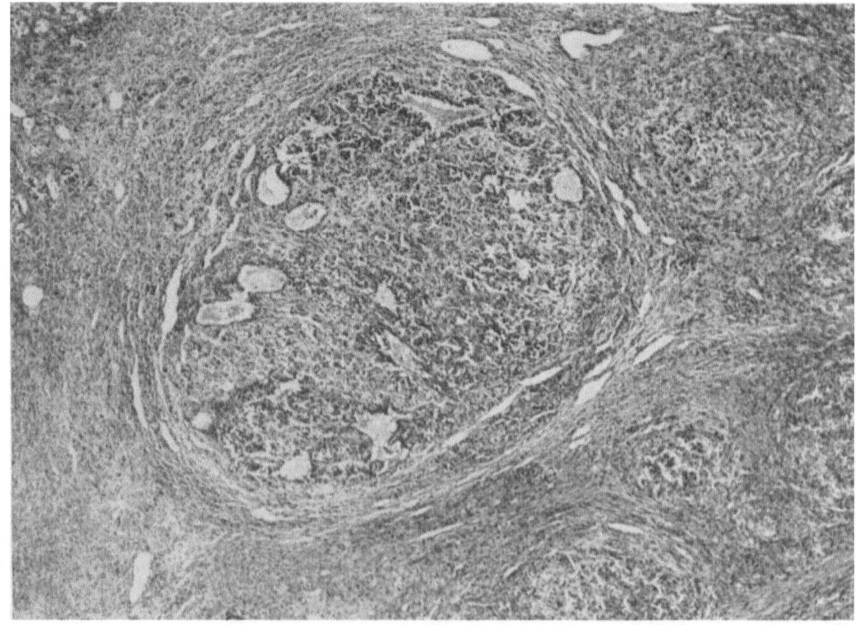

Abb. 24. Granulosazellknoten in einem Luteom. 292 Tage altes Implantat

Nach GARDNER (1958) produziert nur ein Teil der Geschwülste Hormone. Die tubulären Adenome und grobtrabeculären Granulosazelltumoren scheinen keine Hormone zu produzieren. GARDNER (1958) ist der Meinung, daß eine Tumorentwicklung nur bei Ovarien möglich ist, die durch Transplantation oder Röntgenbestrahlung geschädigt sind. Eine Ansicht, die sicher nicht zu Recht besteht, wie unsere eigenen Untersuchungen zeigen konnten [DONTENWILL und RANZ (1960)]. Die Hormonproduktion der Tumoren kann sich ändern mit oder ohne Änderung des morphologischen Bildes [MÜHLBOCK, VAN NIE und BOSCH (1958)]. Die Autonomie wird begünstigt, wenn die Tumorentwicklung unter ungünstigen Bedingungen steht. Daß die Tumoren Oestrogene bilden, ist an der Uterusmuskulatur und -schleimhaut erkennbar.

EVANS, SIMPSON und LI (1948), MOON, SIMPSON, LI und EVANS (1950) sahen nach langdauernder Behandlung mit *Wachstumshormon* (437 Tage, die Tiere erhielten mit zunehmendem Alter bis 3,0 mg Wachstumshormon täglich) bei 3 Ratten Granulosazelltumoren. CHAMPY (1937) beschreibt nach Follikelhormonbehandlung beim Meerschweinchen Cystadenome und LIPSCHUTZ (1950, 1957) adenomatöse Knötchen des Ovar. Bei Mäusen des BALB Stammes fanden LIPSCHUTZ, IGLESIAS und SALINAS (1962) nach langdauernder Behandlung mit Progesteron (subcutane Pelotten von 15-Nor-Progesteron) Granulosazelltumoren der Ovarien.

Literatur

f) Ovar

BALI, T., and J. FURTH: Morphological and biological characteristics of X-Ray induced transplantable ovarian tumors. Cancer Res. **9**, 449—472 (1949).

BERNSTEIN, D. E., and G. R. BISKIND: Effect of parahydroxypropiophenone on experimental ovarian tumors in rats. Proceedings of the Society for Experimental Biol. and Med. **79**, 149 (1952).

BIELSCHOWSKY, F.: Neoplastic changes in grafted ovaries. A. R. Brit. Emp. Cancer Campgn. **29**, 242 (1951).

—, and W. H. HALL: The endocrine imbalance induced in female rats by autotransplantation of the ovary into the tail. Aust. J. exp. Biol. med. Sci. **31**, 85 (1953). See also: Proc. Univ. Otago Med. Sch. **1952**, 29, N. 3.

BISKIND, G. R., The inactivation of estradiol and estradiol benzoate in castrate female rats. Endocrinol. **28**, 894 (1941).

— D. E. BERNSTEIN and S. M. GOSPE: The effect of exogenous gonadotrophins on the development of experimental ovarian tumors in rats. Cancer Res. **13**, 216 (1953).

—, and M. S. BISKIND: Experimental ovarian tumors in rats. Amer. J. clin. Path. **19**, 501 (1949).

— B. KORDAN and M. S. BISKIND: Ovary transplanted to spleen in rats: the effect of unilateral castration, pregnancy, and subsequent castration. Cancer Res. **10**, 309—318 (1950).

—, and J. MARK: The inactivation of testosterone propionate and estrone in rats. Bull. Johns Hopk. Hosp. **65**, 212 (1939).

— R. PENCHARZ et M. S. BISKIND: The pathogenesis of intrasplenic ovarian tumors in rats. Acta Un. int. Cancr. **6**, 97 (1948).

BISKIND, M. S., and G. R. BISKIND: Development of tumors in the rat ovary after transplantation into the spleen. Proc. Soc. exp. Biol. (N. Y.) **55**, 176—179 (1944).

—, and M. C. SHESLESNYAK: Effect of vitamin B complex defiency on inactivation of ovarian estrogen in the liver. Endocrinology **30**, 819 (1942).

BØE, F., O. TOGERSEN and A. ATTRAMADAL: Tumours produced by intrasplenic or intrahepatic ovarian grafting. Acta endocr. (Kbh.) **17**, 42 (1954).

BRAMBELL, F. W. R., A. S. PARKES and U. FIELDING: Changes in the ovary of the mouse following exposure to X-rays. Proc. roy. Soc. B. **101**, 29, 95, 316 (1927); **102**, 385 (1928).

BUTTERWORTH, J. S.: Observation on the histogenesis of ovarian tumors produced in mice by X-rays. Amer. J. Cancer **31**, 85 (1937).

CHAMPY, CH.: Production de tumeurs ovariennes par la folliculine. C. R. Soc. Biol. (Paris) **125**, 634 (1937).

DAVID, M., A. JAKOBOVITS, K. KOVACS u. B. KORPASSY: Beiträge zur Pathogenese der experimentellen Ovargeschwülste. Z. Krebsforsch. **62**, 197 (1957).

DONTENWILL, W.: Vergleichende Untersuchungen an in die Milz implantierten endokrinen Drüsen. Verh. dtsch. Ges. Path. **43**, Mannheim 243 (1959).

— u. H. RANZ: Vergleichende Untersuchungen an Transplantaten endokriner Drüsen. Beitr. Path. Anat. **124**, 229—241 (1961).

ELLIOTT, P. W., and E. HUSNI: Ovarian transplants in abdominally placed testes of mice (Strain C 57). A.M.A. Arch. Path. **63**, 621 (1957).
ELY, A.: Effect of antigonadotrophic serum on recent intrasplenic ovarian implants of castrate mice. Endocrinology **59**, 83—92 (1956).
— Inhibition of tumor formation in ovarian splenic implants after gonadotrophic antiserum. Cancer Res. **19**, **37** (1959).
EVANS, H., M. SIMPSON and CH. H. LI: The gigantism produced in normal rats by injection of the pituitary growth hormone, body growth and organ changes. Growth **12**, 15 (1948).
FELS, E.: Injerto de ovario en ratas despuês de la castration y despuês de la ligadura ovarica. Rev. Soc. argent. Biol. **29**, 148 (1953).
— Aspectos morfológicos y funcionales de los tumores experimentales del ovario. Rev. argent. Endocr. **2**, 1 (1956).
FURTH, J.: Transplantability of induced granulosa cell tumors and of luteoma in mice. Secondary effects of these growths. Proc. Soc. exp. Biol. (N. Y.) **61**, 212—214 (1946).
— Relation of pregnancies to induction of ovarian tumors by X-rays. Proc. Soc. exp. Biol. (N. Y.) **71**, 274 (1949).
— Radiation neoplasia and endocrine systems. Proc. 12th Ann. Symp. Found Cancer Research, M. D. Anderson Tumor Clinic, Houston, Texas (in press).
—, and M. C. BOON: Induction of ovarian tumors in mice by X-rays. Cancer Res. **7**, 241 (1947).
—, and J. S. BUTTERWORTH: Neoplastic diseases occurring among mice subjected to general irradiation with X-rays. — II. Ovarian tumors and associated lesions. Amer. J. Cancer **28**, 66 (1936).
—, and H. SOBEL: Hypervolemia secondary to grafted granulosa-cell tumor. J. nat. Cancer Inst. **7**, 103—113 (1946).
— — Neoplastic transformation of granulosa cells in grafts of normal ovaries into spleens of gonadectomized mice. J. nat. Cancer Inst. 8, 7 (1947).
GARDNER, W. U.: Ovarian and lymphoid tumors in female mice subsequent to Roentgen-ray irradiation and hormone treatment. Proc. Soc. exp. Biol. (N. Y.) **75**, **434** (1950).
— Studies on ovarian and pituitary tumorigenesis. J. nat. Cancer Inst. **15**, **693** (1954).
— Development and growth of tumors in ovaries transplanted into the spleen. Cancer Res. **15**, 109 (1955).
— Some studies on ovarian tumorigenesis. Colloquia on Endocrinology (Ciba foundation) **12**, 153 (1958).
GAY: Zit. bei LIPSCHUTZ 1950.
GOTTSCHALK, R. G., and J. FURTH: Polycythemia with features of cushing's syndrome produced by luteomas. Acta haema. (Basel) **5**, 100—123 (1951).
GREENE, J. A.: The effect of hormone administration on the growth, morphology, secretion of a transplanted mouse granulosa-cell tumor. Cancer Res. **16**, 417, 421 (1956).
— Morphology and transplantability of ten ovarian neoplasms induced by intrasplenic ovarian grafting. Proc. Amer. Ass. Cancer Res. **2**, 111 (1956).
— Secretion and transplantability of ten mouse ovarian neoplasms induced by intrasplenic ovarian grafting. Cancer Res. **17**, 86—91 (1957).
GUTHRIE, M. J.: Tumorigenesis in intrasplenic ovaries in mice. Cancer **10**, No. 1, 190 (1957).
GYÖRGY, P.: Inactivation of estrone by liver. Assay method in vivo for dietary hepatic injury in rats. Proc. Soc. exp. Biol. (N. Y.) **60**, 344 (1945).
HELLER, C. G., and E. C. JUNGEK: Regulation of ovarian growth. Inhibition by estrogen or stimulation by gonadotrophins? Proc. Soc. exp. Biol. (N. Y.) **65**, 152 (1947).
HENDERSON, D.: Granulosa and theca cell tumors of the ovary. Amer. J. Obstet. Gynec. **43**, 194 (1942).
IGLESIAS, R., and E. MARDONES: Twenty generations of a transplantable spontaneous functional ovarian granulosa-cell tumor in the rat. Cancer **9**, 740 (1956).
— — The influence of the gonads and of certain steroid hormones on the growth of the spontaneous and transplantable ovarian tumor in AXC rats. Cancer Res. **16**, 756—760 (1956).
— —, and A. LIPSCHUTZ: Evolution of luteoma in intrasplenic ovarian grafts in the guinea-pig. Brit. J. Cancer **7**, 214 (1953).
— — — The hormonal background of ovarian experimental tumorigenesis in the guinea-pig. Brit. J. Cancer **7**, 221 (1953).
JOHNSON, D. C., and E. WITSCHI: Endocrinology of ovarian tumor formation in parabiotic rats. Cancer Res. **21**, 783—789 (1961).
KAPLAN, H. S.: Influence of ovarian function on incidence of radiation-induced ovarian tumors in mice. J. nat. Cancer Inst. **11**, 125—132 (1950).
KLEIN, M.: Ovarian tumorigenesis following intrasplenic transplantation of ovaries from weanling, young adult, and senile mice. J. nat. Cancer Inst. **12**, 877 (1952).
— Induction of ovarian neoplasms following intrasplenic transplantation of ovarian grafts to old castrated mice. J. nat. Cancer Inst. **14**, 77 (1953).

KULLANDER, S.: The frequency of ovarian tumours and of estrus in mice treated with Roentgen radiation and hormones. Acta radiol. (Stockh.) **40**, 479 (1953).
— Studies in castrated female rats with ovarian tissue transplanted to the spleen. Acta endocrinol. (scand) supl. **22** (1954).
— Studies in spayed rats with ovarian tissue autotransplanted to the spleen. III. Development from the age of six months to one year in animals operated one at three weeks and the effect of administration of estrogens and of hypophysectomy. Acta Endocrinol. scand, supl. 27, Vol. 22 (1956).
LACOUR, F., CH. OBERLING et M. GUÉRIN: Tumeurs par greffe intrasplénique de thyroïde chez des rats thyroïdectomisés. Bull. Ass. franç. Cancer **39**, 390 (1952).
LANCKER, J. VAN, et J. MAISIN: Le sort des greffes intraspléniques d'ovaires et testicules. Acta Un. int. Cancr. **7**, 354 (1950).
— — Le sort des greffes intraspléniques chez le rat castré. C. R. Soc. Biol. (Paris) **147**, 2053 (1953).
— Experimental studies on the pathogenesis of ovarian tumors in mice. Cancer Res. **7**, 549 (1947).
LI, M. H.: Malignant granulosa-cell tumor in an intrasplenic ovarian graft in a castrated male mouse. Amer. J. Obstet. Gynec. **55**, 316 (1948).
— Tumors in intrasplenic ovarian transplants in castrated mice. Science **105**, 13 (1947).
---, and W. U. GARDNER: Granulosa cell tumors in intrapancreatic ovarian grafts in castrated mice. Science **106**, 608 (1947).
— — Further studies on the pathogenesis of ovarian tumors in mice. Cancer Res. **9**, 35 (1949).
— — Influence of age of host and ovaries on tumorigenesis in intrasplenic and intrapancreatic ovarian grafts. Cancer Res. **10**, 162 (1950).
LICK, L., A. KIRSCHBAUM and H. W. MIXER: Mechanism of induction of ovarian tumors by X-rays. Cancer Res. **9**, 535—536 (1949).
LIPSCHUTZ, A.: Steroid hormones and tumors. Baltimore: The Williams & Wilkins Company 1950.
— Steroid homeostasis hypophysis and tumorigenesis. Cambridge: W. Heffer & Sons Ltd. 1957.
— Experimentelle Ovarialtumoren. Gynaecologia **156**, 93—115 (1963).
—, and H. CERISOLA: Ovarian tumours due to a functional imbalance of the hypophysis. Nature (Lond.) **193**, 145—147 (1962).
— R. IGLESIAS, and S. SALINAS: Ovarian tumours induced by a sterilizing steroid. Nature (Lond.) **196**, 946—947 (1962).
— V. I. PANASEVICH, and A. ALVAREZ: New experimental evidence of tumorigenic hormonal imbalances. Nature (Lond.) **202**, 503—504 (1964).
— H. PONCE DE LÉON, E. WOYWOOD and O. GAY: Intrasplenic ovarian grafts in the guinea pig and the problem of neoplastic reactions of the graft. Rev. Canad. Biol. **5**, 181 (1946); Nature (Lond.) **157**, 551 (1946); Bol. Soc. Biol. Santiago **2**, 36, 38 (1944).
MARDONES, E., R. IGLESIAS and A. LIPSCHUTZ: Granulosa cell tumors in intrasplenic ovarian grafts, with intrahepatic metastases, in guinea pigs at five years after grafting. Brit. J. Cancer **9**, 409—417 (1955).
—, and A. LIPSCHUTZ: On the influence of cortisone on the evolution of tumoural growth in intrasplenic ovarian grafts in two strains of mice. Brit. J. Cancer **10** (1956).
MEIO, R. H. DE, A. E. RAKOFF, A. CANTAROW and K. E. PASCHKIS: Mechanism of inactivation of α-estradiol by rat liver "in vitro". Endocrinology **43**, 97 (1948).
MILLER, O. J., and W. U. GARDNER: The role of thyroid function and food intake in experimental ovarian tumorigenesis in mice. Cancer Res. **14**, 220 (1954).
—, and C. A. PFEIFFER: Demonstration of increased gonadotrophic hormone production in castrated mice with intrasplenic ovarian grafts. Proc. Soc. exper. Biol. (N. Y.) **75**, 178—181 (1950).
MÜHLBOCK, O.: Ovarian tumours in mice in parabiotic union. Acta endocr. (Kbh.) **12**, 105 (1953).
— Neuere experimentelle Untersuchungen über die Genese der Ovarialtumoren. Geburtsh. und Frauenheilk. **12**, 289 (1952).
— R. VAN NIE and L. BOSCH: The production of oestrogene hormones by granulosa cell tumors in mice. Colloquia on Endocrinology (Ciba foundation) Vol. 12, 78 (1958).
PECKHAM, B. M., R. R. GREENE and M. E. JEFFRIES: Granulosa cell tumors in female rats and rabbits. Science **107**, 319 (1948).
— — Experimentally produced granulosa-cell tumors in rats. Cancer Res. **12**, 25 (1952).
— — Experimentally produced granulosa-cell tumors in rabbits. Cancer Res. **12**, 654—656 (1952).
PINCUS, G., and D. W. MARTIN: Liver damage and estrogen inactivation. Endocrinology **27**, 838 (1940).

RANZ, H.: Zur Histogenese der Granulosazelltumoren. Z. Krebsforsch. **63**, 460 (1960).
SELYE, H.: On the rôle of the liver in the detoxification of steroid hormones and artificial estrogens. J. Pharmacol. exp. Ther. **71**, 236 (1941).
SILBERBERG, M., R. SILBERBERG and H. V. LEIDLER: Effects of anterior hypophyseal transplants on intrasplenic ovarian grafts. Cancer Res. **11**, 624—628 (1951).
TAKEWAKI, K.: The behaviour of the rat ovary after transplantation into the spleen. Proc. Japan Acad. **25**, 25 (1949).
— Intrasplenic ovarian grafts in cryptorchidized rats. Proc. Japan Acad. **26**, 50 (1950).
— Stimulation of ovaries of normal barabionts joined with spayed partners bearing intrasplenic ovarian grafts. Jap. J. Zool. **11**, 35 (1953).
— N. TAKASUGI and K. MAEKAWA: Ovaries of rats with gonadectomized intrasplenic ovarian grafts. Proc. Japan Acad. **28**, 97 (1952).
WAGENEN, G. VAN, and W. U. GARDNER: Functional intrasplenic ovarian transplants in monkeys. Endocrinology **46**, 265 (1950).
— — Absence of hepatic inactivation of estrogen in the monkey. Yale J. Biol. Med. **25**, No. 6 (1953).
WOYWOOD: Zit. bei LIPSCHUTZ 1950.
ZONDEK, B., A. LAUFER and I. TAMARI: Transplantation of a granulosa cell tumor into the spleen of castrated rats, treated with gonadotrophin. Proc. Soc. exp. Biol. (N. Y.) **84**, 173 (1953).
ZULLI, P.: Influenza di un estratto di milza sullo soiluppo del trapianto intrasplenico di ovaio. Folia endocr. (Pisa) 8, 877 (1955).

g) Uterus

Schleimhautveränderungen

Nach langdauernder Behandlung von *Mäusen* mit Follikelhormon fanden LACASSAGNE (1935, 1936), LOEB, BURNS, SUNTZEFF und MOSKOP (1936), LOEB, SUNTZEFF und BURNS (1938), GARDNER und ALLEN (1939), GARDNER, ALLEN, SMITH und STRONG (1938), SUNTZEFF, BURNS, MOSKOP und LOEB (1938), ALLEN und GARDNER (1941) (LACASSAGNE injizierte täglich subcutan 30—50 γ Follikelhormon) Epithelproliferationen der Cervix mit z. T. invasivem Wachstum, Epidermisation der Schleimhaut, glandulärcystische Hyperplasie des Endometriums und Fibrose der Muskulatur. Bei den Endometriosen wurde z. T. ein Vordringen der Drüsen durch die Serosa beobachtet.

LOEB, SUNTZEFF, BURNS und MOSKOP (1936) sahen sogar Vordringen der Drüsenschläuche durch die Muskulatur bis in die Lymphgefäße und deuteten dies als krebsähnliches Verhalten. ALLEN und GARDNER (1941) beobachteten bei diesen Versuchen auch vereinzelt metastasierende Carcinome und bezeichnen die proliferierenden Epithelveränderungen als Präcancerosen. Tiefes Eindringen von Drüsenschläuchen bzw. starke Epithelproliferation wurde auch von PFEIFFER (1939) bei experimenteller Erzeugung eines verlängerten Oestrus beobachtet. KREKELS (1936) erreichte bei follikelhormonbehandelten Mäusen unter 42 Tieren dreimal ausgeprägte Epithelzapfenbildung und führte diese auf den Daueroestrus zurück, der zu einer Sekretstauung führt.

Bei ähnlichen Versuchen, d. h. nach chronischer Follikelhormonbehandlung über Monate, wurden Epithelproliferationen mit Metaplasien bei *Ratten und Mäusen*, aber keine Carcinome der Cervix oder des Corpus uteri, beobachtet [KAUFMANN und STEINKAMM (1936), KAUFMANN (1937), KAUFMANN und MÜLLER (1950), NELSON (1939), ZONDEK (1937), HEROLD und EFFKEMANN (1937), MIGLIAVACCA (1936, 1937)]. Das Auftreten von Metaplasien der Uterusschleimhaut durch Oestrogene wird gefördert durch gleichzeitigen Vitamin A-Mangel [REITER (1965)]. Hyperkeratosen der Portioschleimhaut nach Oestrogenbehandlung beobachtete THIERY (1963) bei Mäusen, Carcinome konnte er nicht erzeugen. Beim *Kaninchen* sahen LACASSAGNE (1935), ZONDEK (1936), PIERSON (1934, 1937, 1938, 1940) und HOFBAUER (1939) nach Oestrogenbehandlung z. T. invasive metaplastische Wucherungen der Drüsen der Uterusschleimhaut mit Eindringen in die Muskulatur, stellenweise sogar metaplastische Knochenbildung, nie aber beobachteten sie Metastasen der Wucherungen der Uterusschleimhaut.

Ähnliche Beobachtungen wurden von PIERSON (1936, 1938) auch nach Prolaninjektion beschrieben. Endometriosen nach Prolaninjektion beobachteten auch ZALESKI (1937) und LIPSCHUTZ (1950) beim Kaninchen.

Beim *Meerschweinchen* sahen NELSON (1937, 1939), DESSAU (1937, 1938), LIPSCHUTZ (1950), KLEIN (1938) Metaplasien der Uterusschleimhaut mit Polypenbildung [BLANDAU (1949)], Eindringen der Uterusschleimhaut in die Uteruswand, Epidermisierung der Cervix und glanduläre Proliferation der Schleimhaut (Abb. 25, 26).

Diese Polypen der Korpusschleimhaut entstehen schon nach 3monatiger kontinuierlicher Behandlung mit Oestrogen (Gesamtdosis von 30—40 μg oder Pelotten) und hängen oft bis in

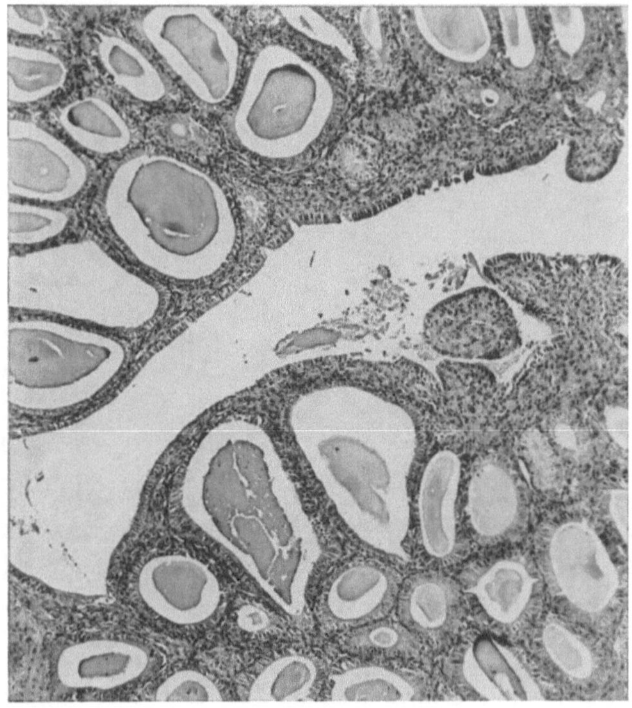

Abb. 25. Glandulär cystische Hyperplasie der Korpusschleimhaut mit Eindringen der Drüsenschläuche in die Uteruswand (Meerschweinchen, Behandlung 6 Monate 25 Tage, jeden 2. Tag 1,5 mg Cyren B)

die Vagina [LIPSCHUTZ (1950), BELLOLIO (1938), LIPSCHUTZ, VARGAS, JEDLICKY und BELLOLIO (1940), BRUZZONE (1942), BARAHONA (1949)]. Die Drüsen können auch bis über die Serosa wuchern [LIPSCHUTZ (1950, 1957), RIESKO (1947)].

Die Dosis zur Erzeugung von Metaplasien und polypösen Schleimhautwucherungen ist nach LIPSCHUTZ (1950) und RIESKO (1947) bei Meerschweinchen wesentlich niedriger als die zur Erreichung von Fibroiden. (In drei Monaten kontinuierliche Dosis von 30—40 μg täglich). OVERHOLSER und NELSON (1936) konnten beim Rhesus-*Affen* nach 6—24monatiger Behandlung mit 36400—73400 Ratteneinheiten Oestrogen lediglich Epitheleinsprossung am Uterus, aber, ebenso wie PFEIFFER und ALLEN (1948), keine Carcinome nachweisen.

HISAW und LENDRUM (1936) beobachteten nach Oestrogenbehandlung beim Affen Metaplasie der Cervixdrüsen. Nach Oestrogenbehandlung von Rhesus-Affen sahen ZUCKERMAN (1940), PFEIFFER und ALLEN (1948) keine Metaplasie im Endometrium, sondern nur in der Cervix und glandulär-cystische Hyperplasien der Korpusschleimhaut. Bei Cebus-Affen fanden

Iglesias und Lipschutz (1947), Awad (1946) Metaplasie der Fundusschleimhaut bei 3 von 9 Tieren, die 513 Tage mit Oestrogen behandelt wurden. Bei *Octon degu* (Nager) traten auch nach 8monatiger Behandlung mit Oestrogenen keine Metaplasien auf und kein Einwachsen der hyperplastischen und papillomatös gewucherten Drüsen [Lipschutz (1950)].

Bei den einzelnen Tierspecies finden sich also recht unterschiedliche Befunde, sowohl an der Cervix und Korpusschleimhaut als auch an der Uterusmuskulatur (s. Tab. 2).

Auch bei Tieren, bei denen nach früher Kastration Nebennieren- und Hypophysengeschwülste auftraten [Christy, Dickie, Alkinson und Woolley (1951),

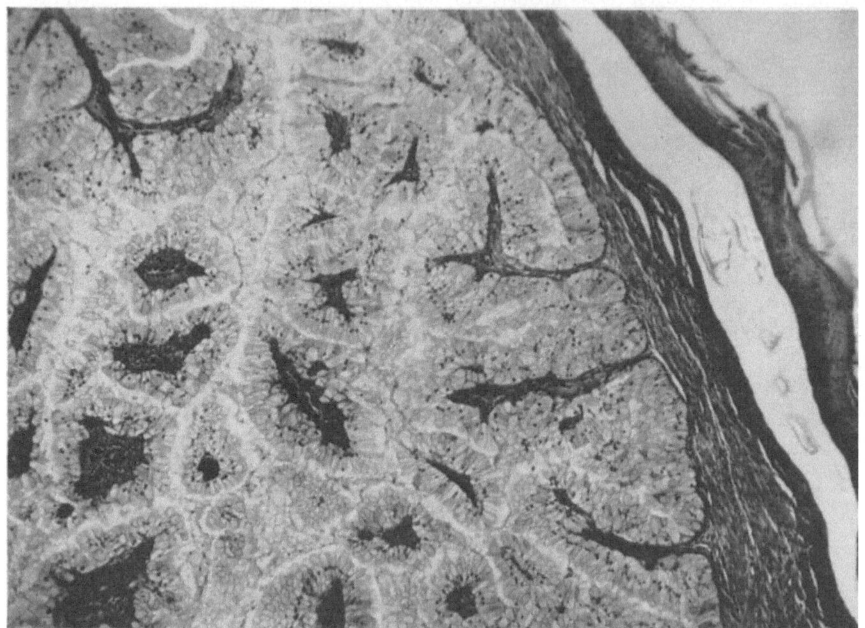

Abb. 26. Hochgradige Hyperplasie der Cervixschleimhaut bei gleichartiger Behandlung

Lit. bei Nebennieren], sahen die Untersucher hyperplastische Schleimhautveränderungen des Uterus und Endometriosen, die durch eine verstärkte Follikelhormonsekretion der Nebennierengeschwülste verursacht werden. Busse und Hoevener (1934) beobachteten nach Implantation von Hypophysenvorderlappengewebe beim Meerschweinchen keine präcancerösen Veränderungen der Portio, wie dies früher (1930) Hofbauer berichtet hatte.

Nach *subtotaler Kastration*, sog. Ovarfragmentation, entstanden beim *Meerschweinchen* durch den veränderten Cyclus neben Fibromyomen polypöse Schleimhautwucherungen, Endometriosen und adenomatöse Wucherungen des Wolffschen Ganges [Bruzzone und Lipschutz (1954), Cruz (1936)]. Beim Rhesus-Affen zeigte die Ovarfragmentation dagegen keinen Effekt [Dahl-Iversen und Hamburger und Jorgensen (1942)]. Bei der Ovarfragmentation kommt es nach Lipschutz (1950, 1957) zu einer Mehrproduktion gonadotropen Hormons durch die verminderte Oestrogenproduktion des Ovarrestes. Eine Transplantation von Hypophysenvorderlappengewebe eines solchen Tieres zeigt nach Lipschutz (1936, 1957) eine stärkere Wachstumsanregung auf den Uterus der infantilen Maus als normales Hypophysenvorderlappengewebe. Eine squamöse Hyperplasie der Uterusschleimhaut kann nach Bo (1957) bei der Maus schon nach einer 27—39 Tage dauernden

Tabelle 2. *Veränderungen an der Uterusschleimhaut und Muskulatur bei Hormonbehandlung oder Störung der Hormonsekretion*

Tierart	Art der Behandlung	Morphologische Veränderungen
Maus	Kontinuierliche Follikelhormonbehandlung	Proliferation der Cervix und Korpusschleimhaut mit Eindringen in die Muskulatur. Epithelmetaplasien. Endometriosen
	Frühzeitige Kastration, die zu Nebennierenrindenadenomen führt	Ähnliche Veränderungen wie bei Follikelhormonbehandlung
	Langdauernde Behandlung mit Wachstumshormon	Fibrose des Uterus
Ratte	Kontinuierliche Follikelhormonbehandlung	Proliferation der Cervix und Korpusschleimhaut mit Eindringen in die Wand, Epithelmetaplasien und Endometriosen. Myome des Uterus
Meerschweinchen (domestiziert)	Kontinuierliche Follikelhormonbehandlung oder subtotale Kastration bzw. Ovarfragmentation	Polypöse Schleimhautwucherungen an der Cervix und am Corpus uteri mit Einwachsen in die Wand. Epithelmetaplasien. Endometriosen *Multiple Fibrome und Myome bzw. Fibromyome* im Uterus und *im Bereich der Bauchhöhlenserosa* mit z.T. invasivem Wachstum
Meerschweinchen (nicht domestiziert)	Kontinuierliche Follikelhormonbehandlung	*Keine Myome*
Octon degu (Nager)	Kontinuierliche Follikelhormonbehandlung	Keine Metaplasien, kein Einwachsen der hyperplastischen Schleimhaut in die Uteruswand. *Keine Myome*
Kaninchen	Kontinuierliche Follikelhormonbehandlung	Hyperplasie und Einwuchern der Drüsen in die Uteruswand. Endometriosen. Myome des Uterus
Affe	Kontinuierliche Follikelhormonbehandlung	Epitheleinsprossung an der Uterusschleimhaut. Metaplasie der Cervixschleimhaut. *Keine Myome*
	Subtotale Kastration	*Keine Myome*

Oestrogenbehandlung beobachtet werden (2 mg Oestroldipropionat pro Woche).

ZITZELSPERGER (1941) beschrieb bei Ratten adenomartige Wucherungen des Uterus bei sog. *Scheinschwangerschaft*, Veränderungen, die später als Deciduome bei Scheinschwangerschaft vorwiegend als Folge der hormonell bedingten Deciduawucherung beschrieben wurden. [OLSEN, VELARDO, HISAW, DAWSON und BRAVERMAN (1951), VELARDO und HISAW (1951), PECKHAM (1947), PECKHAM, GREEN (1948), ERSHOFF und DEUEL (1943), ASTWOOD und GREEP (1938), SELYE, BORDUAS und MASSON (1942).] Die Entstehung der Deciduome bei der Scheinschwangerschaft wird durch Oestradiol-3-17β und Dimethylstilboestrol gehemmt [STONE und EMMENS (1964)].

Myome und Fibrome

Über hormonell bedingte Wucherungen bzw. Hyperplasien der Uterusmuskulatur und des Bindegewebes im Sinne von Myomen, Fibromen oder Myofibromen berichten bei Ratten, Kaninchen und Meerschweinchen LACASSAGNE (1935, 1936), CESA (1936), LIPSCHUTZ (1950, 1957), NELSON (1937, 1939), BARKS und OVERHOLSER (1938), MORICARD und CAUCHOIX (1938), MORICARD (1952), CAUCHOIX

(1939). Alle diese Untersucher nehmen an, daß durch die kontinuierliche Oestrogenzufuhr eine verstärkte Wachstumsanregung der Uterusmuskulatur hervorgerufen wird [LIPSCHUTZ und VARGAS (1941), PFEIFFER (1949)]. LIPSCHUTZ (1950), der sich in ausführlichen Untersuchungen besonders am Meerschweinchen (Abb. 26, 27) mit der Genese der Fibrome, Myome und Fibromyome, bzw. den sog. Fibroids des Uterus und der Serosa der Bauchhöhle beschäftigte, fand diese Geschwülste vorwiegend bei weiblichen, aber auch bei männlichen Tieren nach kontinuierlicher Behandlung mit Oestrogen (3—5 Monate täglich Injektionen von 10—30 μg Oestrogen). Bei weiblichen Tieren treten die Fibrome oder Myome im Uterus, der

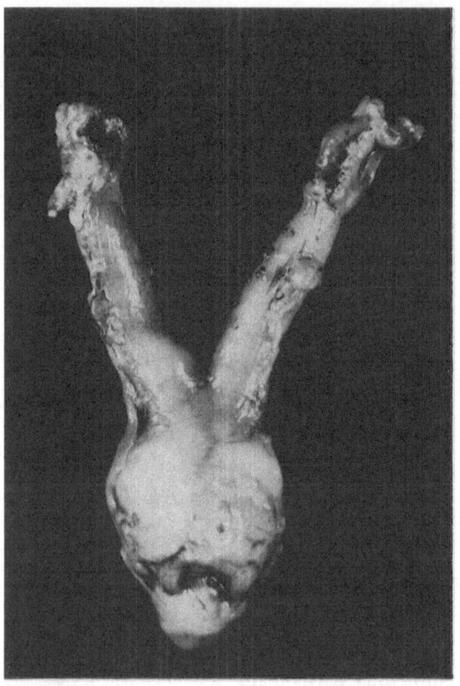

Abb. 27. Multiple kleine subseröse Fibromyome des Uterus. Starke Auftreibung der Cervix. Behandlung 6 Monate, 25 Tage, jeden 2. Tag 1,5 mg Cyren B

Bauchhöhlenserosa, besonders in der Umgebung von Magen, Pankreas und Milz auf, bei männlichen Tieren vorwiegend in der Serosa, in Magen-, Pankreas- und Milznähe (z. B. 38 Injektionen von insgesamt 320 μg Stilboestrol in 88 Tagen). Zum Teil wurde auch eine diffuse Fibrose der Bauchhöhlenserosa beobachtet.

Histologisch handelt es sich nach LIPSCHUTZ (1950) um Fibrome, Myome und Kombinationsgeschwülste (Abb. 28, 30), mit reichlich kollagenem Bindegewebe sowie vereinzelt Fettgewebsinseln.

Die Fibrome bzw. Myome entstanden auch nach Teilkastration bzw. Ovarfragmentation, nach denen beide Phasen des Cyclus verlängert sind [BRUZZONE und LIPSCHUTZ (1954)]. Der Uterus ist dabei oft 10mal so groß [LIPSCHUTZ (1950)] und zeigt polypöse Schleimhautwucherungen mit invasivem Wachstum der Drüsen. Leiomyome nach hormoneller Fehlsteuerung durch Teilkastration der Ratte sah auch PFEIFFER (1949). Intra- und extragenitale Fibrome und Myome wurden außerdem beschrieben von WOODRUFF (1941), PERLOFF und KURZROCK (1941), MOSINGER (1946, 1947), DUCUING (1946), NADEL (1949, 1950), MORATO (1941), VON WATTENWYL (1941, 1944), BRUZZONE (1943), BRUZZONE, ELGUETA, IGLESIAS und LIPSCHUTZ (1948), LIPSCHUTZ und IGLESIAS (1938), LIPSCHUTZ, IGLESIAS und VARGAS (1940),

VARGAS (1942), BIMES (1945), SAMMARTINO und HERRERA (1940), ELGUETA, IGLESIAS und BRUZZONE (1948), und LIPSCHUTZ (1942).

Die Fibrome wuchsen auch nach Oestrogenbehandlung bei hypophysektomierten Meerschweinchen [VARGAS (1943), LIPSCHUTZ (1950, 1957)] und entstanden nur nach kontinuierlicher, nicht aber bei cyclischer Injektion in Intervallen, wie Abb. 31 schematisch erkennen läßt.

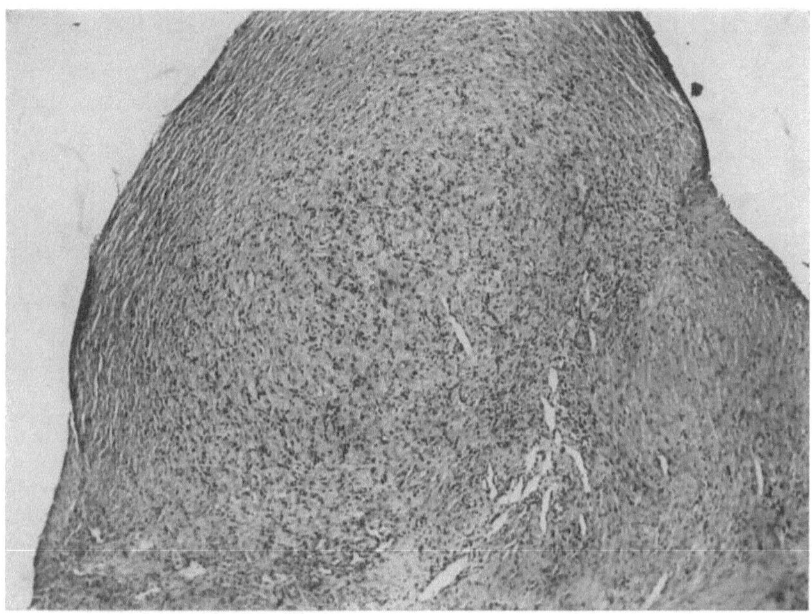

Abb. 28. Subseröses Myom. Fibro-Behandlung wie Abb. 27

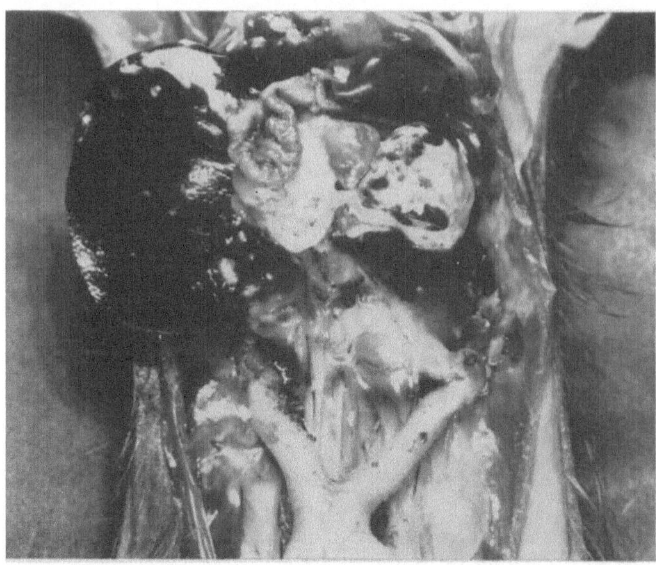

Abb. 29. Multiple, zum Teil miteinander verwachsene Fibromyome der Serosa zwischen Leber, Magen, Pankreas und Milz. Zuckergußartiger Überzug der Leber und Milz. Behandlung 6 Monate, 25 Tage, jeden 2. Tag 1,5 mg Cyren B

[LIPSCHUTZ (1950, 1957) — 3 Injektionen à 20—80 μg Oestradiol, dann Unterbrechung von 2—3 Wochen — erzeugt keine Fibrome oder Fibromyome.] Invasives Wachstum der Fibromyome in die Zwerchfellmuskulatur oder Bauchwandmuskulatur sahen LIPSCHUTZ (1950), VON WATTENWYL (1944) und MOSINGER (1946). MOSINGER spricht sogar von Fibrosarkomen, eine Bezeichnung, die LIPSCHUTZ (1950) ablehnt, da nach seiner Ansicht die Wucherungen nicht metastasieren und nicht transplantabel sind.

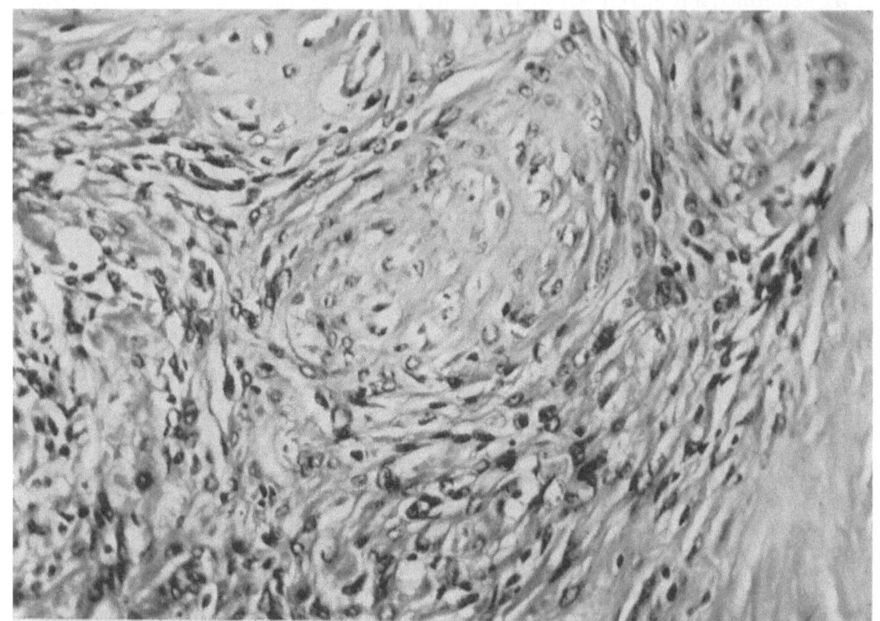

Abb. 30. Zum Teil hyalinisiertes Fibromyom der Serosa (parapankreatisch)

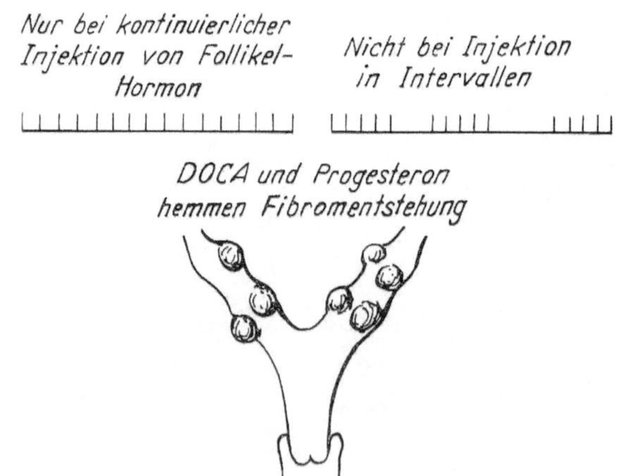

Abb. 31. Fibrom- und Myomentstehung nach Follikelhormonbehandlung

Bei Kaninchen beobachtete HORNING (1942) die gleichen Uterusgeschwülste nach Instillation von Oestradiol-benzoat-Pelotten.

Bei nicht domestizierten Meerschweinchen fand IGLESIAS [s. LIPSCHUTZ (1950)] nach 7 monatiger Oestradiolbehandlung keine Fibrome, und FEBRES (1944) beobachtete beim Octon degu nach 11 monatiger Behandlung, ebenso wie IGLESIAS und LIPSCHUTZ (1947) beim Cebus-Affen, keine Fibrome. Auch beim Rhesus-Affen sahen VARGAS (1943), ENGLE, KRAKOVER und HAAGENSEN (1943), PFEIFFER und ALLEN (1948) keine Fibromyome des Uterus nach Oestrogenbehandlung.

Das Auftreten von Myomen und Fibromen sowohl im Uterus als auch in der Serosa ist offenbar vom Genotyp der Tierspecies abhängig. Eine knotige oder diffuse Wucherung der Serosa zeigt nur das Hausmeerschweinchen.

Desoxycorticosteron und Progesteron hemmen durch ihren anti-luteinisierenden Effekt die Wirkung des Oestrogens am Uterus, d. h. die Entstehung von Fibromyomen nach Oestrogenbehandlung [LIPSCHUTZ und VARGAS (1939, 1941), LIPSCHUTZ, VARGAS und NUNEZ (1941), LIPSCHUTZ und ZANARTU (1942), LIPSCHUTZ, LUCO und ZANARTU (1942), LIPSCHUTZ und MAASS (1944), HERTZ, LARSEN und TULLNER (1947), BRUZZONE, FUENZALIDA, IGLESIAS und LIPSCHUTZ (1951), LIPSCHUTZ, MARDONES, IGLESIAS, FUENZALIDA und BRUZZONE (1952), MARDONES, IGLESIAS und LIPSCHUTZ (1953)].

Auch Testosteron hemmt die proliferative Oestrogenwirkung am Uterus [KORENCHEVSKY und DENNISON (1935), VERA (1942), JADRIJEVIĆ, MARDONES und LIPSCHUTZ (1956)].

MOSINGER sah 1949 nach langdauernder Behandlung von Meerschweinchen mit *Oestradiol* und *Diäthylstilboestrol* Hyperplasien der glatten Muskulatur, aber nicht nur im Uterus, sondern auch im Verdauungstrakt. Nach kombinierter Behandlung mit Oestrogen und Testosteron fanden BACON (1951) und KIRKMAN (1957) im Uterus Fibromyome. MOON, SIMPSON, LI und EVANS (1950) beobachteten neben Luteomen Fibromyome des Uterus nach langdauernder Behandlung mit Wachstumshormon bei Mäusen.

Cylindrische Adenome der Ovarien beschrieb CHAMPY (1937) nach Follikulinbehandlung, und KORENCHEVSKY (1935) fand Hyperplasie der Vorsteherdrüse bei kastrierten und mit Testosteron behandelten Ratten.

Literatur

g) Uterus

ALLEN, E., and W. U. GARDNER: Cancer of the cervix of the uterus in hybrid mice following long-continued administration of estrogen. Cancer Res. **1**, 359—366 (1941).

ASTWOOD, E. B., and R. O. GREEP: A corpus luteum-stimulating substance in the rat placenta. Proc. Soc. exp. Biol. (N. Y.) **38**, 713 (1938).

AWAD, T.: Proliferación atípica de las mucosas mullerianas en un antropoide del nuevo mundo. Tesis Univ. de Chile 1946 (Public. Dep. Med. Exp. No. 48).

BACON, R. L.: Leiomyomas of the uterus in the hamster following treatment with diethylstilbestrol and testosterone. Anat. Rec. **109**, 265 (1951).

BARAHONA, M.: Aspectos cuantitativos del control de la función gonadotrófica de la hipófisis por el estrógeno, y su importancia para la patología. Tesis Univ. de Chile 1949 (Public. Dep. Med. Exp. No. 70).

BARKS, O. L., and M. D. OVERHOLSER: Hyperplasia and hypertrophy of the uterine musculature in ovariectomized rats following estrone injections. Anat. Rec. **70**, 401 (1938).

BELLOLIO, P.: Estudio comparativo sobre la axión histerotrofíca y tumorígena del benzoato y diproprionato de estradiol. Tesis Univ. de Chile 1938.

BÎMES, M.: Recherches sur la fibromyomatose experimentale. Paris: Vigot 1945 (quoted from DUCUING 1946, and MOSINGER 1946).

BO, W. J.: The origin and development of estrogen-induced uterine metaplasie. A.M.A. Arch. Path. **64**, 595 (1957).

BLANDAU, R. J.: Experimental production of endometrial polyps in the guinea pig. Cancer Res. **9**, 526 (1949).

BRUZZONE, S.: Esterificaión y facultad tumorígena de un estrógena sintético (stilbestrol). Tesis. Univ. de Chile 1942.

— Producción de fibromas abdominales por estrógenos en animales impúberes. Bol. Soc. Biol. Santiago **1**, 12 (1943).

— H. ELGUETA, R. IGLESIAS and A. LIPSCHUTZ: Oestrogen-induced fibroids of the thoracic serosa. Brit. J. Cancer **2**, 267 (1948).

— F. FUENZALIDA, R. IGLESIAS and A. LIPSCHUTZ: Antifibromatogenic action of steroids with special reference to pregnenolones. In: A. WHITE ed., Steroids in Experimental and Clinical Practice. p. 72. Philadelphia: The Blakiston Co. 1951.

—, and A. LIPSCHUTZ: Tumorigenesis induced in the guinea-pig by ovarian fragmentation. Brit. J. Cancer **8**, 613 (1954); See also 6th Int. Cancer Congr. (São Paulo) 1954, p. 170.

BÜNGELER, W., u. W. DONTENWILL: Hormonell ausgelöste geschwulstartige Hyperplasien, hyperplasiogene Geschwülste und ihre Verhaltensweisen. Dtsch. med. Wschr. **1959**, 1885.

Burrows, H., and E. Horning: Oestrogen and neoplasia. Oxford: Blackwell 1952.

Busse, O., u. A. Hoevener: Ein Beitrag zur Frage des Zusammenhanges zwischen Hypophyse und Genitalcarcinom. Zbl. Gynäk. **1934**, 1218.

Cesa, I.: Wirkung des Follikel und Corpus Luteum Hormon auf die Cervixdrüsen. C. R. Soc. Biol. (Paris) **25**, 1237 (1936).

Chauchoix, J.: Hormone folliculaire et fibromatose. Paris: Vigot 1939.

Champy, Chr.: Experimentelle Eierstocksgeschwülste mittels Follikulin. C. R. Soc. Biol. (Paris), 125, 634 (1937); Zbl. allg. Path. path. Anat. **69**, 60 (1937).

Christy, N. P., M. Dickie, W. B. Alkinson and G. W. Woolley: Über die Pathogenese von Uterus-(Schleimhaut-)Läsionen jungfräulicher und gonadektomierter Mäuse, die Nebennierenrinden- und Hypophysengeschwülste besitzen. Cancer Res. **11**, 413 (1951).

Clifton, K. H.: Problems in experimental tumorigenesis of the pituitary gland, gonads, adrenal cortices and mammary glands: a review. Cancer Res. **19**, 2 (1959).

Cruz, H.: Hiperplasia quístico-glandular del endometrio consecutiva a fragmentación ovárica. Bol. Soc. chil. Obstet. Ginec. **1**, 194 (1936).

Dahl-Iversen, E., Ch. Hamburger and H. Jorgensen: Cystic glandular hyperplasia etc. in rhesus monkeys. Acta obstet. gynec. scand. **21**, 315 (1942).

Dessau, F.: Chronische Wirkungen oestrogener Stoffe am Meerschweinchenuterus. Arch. int. Pharmacodyn. **55**, 402 (1937).

— Fortgesetzte Untersuchungen über chronische Oestronwirkungen am Meerschweinchenuterus. Arch. int. Pharmacodyn. **58**, 344 (1938).

Ducuing, J. Le fibro-myome utérin. Cie, Paris: Masson 1946.

Elgueta, H. R., R. Iglesias y S. Bruzzone: Fibromas de la serosa torácica inducidos por el estrógeno. Bol. Soc. Biol. Santiago **6**, 36 (1948).

Engle, E. T., C. Krakower and C. D. Haagensen: Estrogen administration to aged female monkeys with no resultant tumors. Cancer Res. **3**, 858 (1943).

Ershoff, B. F., and H. J. Deuel: Prolongation of pseudopregnancy by induction of deciduomata in the rat. Proc. Soc. exp. Biol. (N. Y.) **54**, 167 (1943).

Febres, L.: Acciones tóxicas comparativas de los estrógenos en los roedores. Tesis Univ. de Chile 1944 (Public. Dep. Med. Exp. No. 34).

Fischer, W., u. I. Kühl: Geschwülste der Laboratoriumsnagetiere. Dresden u. Leipzig: Theodor Steinkopff 1958.

Gardner, W. U., and E. Allen: Malignand and nonmalignand uterine vaginal lesions in mice receiving estrogen and androgens simultaneously. Yale J. Biol. & Med. **12**, 213 (1939).

— — G. M. Smith and L. C. Strong: Zervixcarcinom bei Mäusen, die Oestrogen erhielten. J. Amer. med. Ass. **110**, 15 (1938).

Herold, L., u. G. Effkemann: Zur Frage der Epithelmetaplasie der Zervix-Korpusschleimhaut nach Zufuhr von Follikelhormon bei nichtkastrierten und kastrierten Ratten. Zbl. Gynäk. **2**, 27 (1937).

Hertz, R., C. D. Larsen and W. Tullner: Inhibition of estrogen-induced tissue growth with progesterone. J. nat. Cancer Inst. **8**, 123 (1947).

Hisaw, F. L., and F. C. Lendrum: Squamous metaplasia in the cervical glands of the monkey following oestrin administration. Endocrinology **20**, 228 (1936).

Hofbauer, J.: Kausale Faktoren der genitalen präkancerösen Veränderungen. Zbl. Gynäk. **54**, 2393 (1930).

— Hormonal gynaecological pathology and its clinical aspects. J. Obst. Gynaec. Brit. Emp. **46**, 232 (1939).

Horning, E. S.: Quoted from annual report 1941—1942 of the imperial Cancer Research Fund. London 1942, p. 8.

Iglesias, R., and A. Lipschutz: Effects of prolonged oestrogen administration in female new world monkeys, with observations on a pericardial neoplasm. J. Endocr. **5**, 88 (1947).

Jadrijević, D., E. Mardones and A. Lipschutz: Antifibromatogenic activity of 19-nor-17α-ethynyltestosterone. Proc. Soc. exp. Biol. (N. Y.) **91**, 38 (1956).

Kaufmann, C: Über die Wirkung fortgesetzter Zufuhr unphysiologischer Mengen Follikelhormon auf das Genitale weiblicher Ratten. Mschr. Geburtsh. Gynäk. **105**, 188 (1937).

—, u. H. A. Müller: Bemerkung zu der Arbeit von Butenandt: Zur physiologischen Bedeutung des Follikelhormons und der östrogenen Wirkstoffe für die Genese des Brustdrüsenkrebses und die Therapie des Prostata-Carcinoms. Dtsch. med. Wschr. **75**, 1409 (1950). Zusammenfassung.

— H. Müller, A. Butenandt u. H. Friedrich-Freksa: Experimentelle Bedeutung des Follikelhormons für die Carcinomentstehung. Z. Krebsforsch. **56**, 482 (1949).

— u. E. Steinkamm: Über die Wirkung fortgesetzter Zufuhr unphysiologischer Mengen Follikelhormon auf das Genitale weiblicher Ratten. Arch. Gynäk. **162**, 553 (1936).

Kirkman, H.: Steroid Tumorigenesis. Cancer (Chic.) **10**, 754 (1957).

KIRSCHBAUM, A.: The role of hormones in cancer: Laboratory animals. Cancer Res. **17**, 432 (1957).
— F. D. LAWRASON, H. S. KAPLAN and J. J. BITTNER: Influence of breeding on induction of mammary cancer with methylcholanthrene in strain Dba female mice. Proc. Soc. exp. Biol. (N. Y.) **55**, 141 (1944).
KLEIN, F.: Über den Einfluß von Follikulin auf einige Organe des Meerschweinchenbockes. Frankfurt. Z. Path. **51**, 406 (1938).
KONEFF, A. A., H. D. MOON, M. E. SIMPSON, CH. H. LI and H. M. EVANS: Über Geschwülste bei Ratten, die mit hypophysärem Wachstumshormon behandelt wurden. Cancer Res. **11**, 113 (1951).
KORENCHEVSKY, V., and M. DENNISON: Histological changes in the organs of rats injected with oestrone alone or simultaneously with oestrone and testicular hormone. J. Path. Bact. **41**, 323 (1935).
KREKELS, A.: Einfluß hoher Follikelhormondosen auf chronisch arsenvergiftete Mäuse. Frankfurt. Z. Path. 49, H. 3 (1936); Zbl. allg. Path. path. Anat. **66**, 160 (1936/37).
LACASSAGNE, A.: Modifications progressives de la structure du conduit tubo-utérin chez des lapines soumises à partir de la naissance, à des injections répétées d'oestrone (folliculine). C. R. Soc. Biol. (Paris) **120**, 685 (1935).
— Modifications progressives de l'utérus de la Souris sous l'action prolongée de l'oestrone. C. R. Soc. Biol. (Paris) **120**, 1156 (1935).
— Tumeurs malignes apparues au cours d'un traitement hormonal combiné, chez des souris appartenant à des lignées réfractaires au cancer spontané. C. R. Soc. Biol. (Paris) **121**, 607 (1936).
— Les cancers produits par des substances chimiques endogènes. Paris: Hermann Cie. 1950.
LIPSCHUTZ, A.: Croissance atypique et destructive des glandes utérines après des interventions ovariennes expérimentales. C. R. Acad. Sci. (Paris) **203**, 1025 (1936).
— Préhypophyse et ovaire chez le cobaye avec troubles expérimentaux du cycle sexuel. Arch. Biol. (Liège) **47**, 181 (1936).
— Induction and prevention of abdominal fibroids by steroid hormones, and their bearing on growth and development. Cold Spr. Harb. Symp. quant. Biol. **10**, 79 (1942).
— Steroid hormones and tumors. Baltimore: The Williams & Wilkins Company 1950.
— Experimentelle Forschung über endokrine Störungen und Geschwulstbildung. Münch. med. Wschr. **97**, 1007, 1023 (1955).
— Steroid homeostasis hypophysis and tumorigenesis. Cambridge: Heffer & Sons, Ltd. 1957.
—, et R. IGLESIAS: Multiples tumeurs utérines et extragénitales provoquées par le benzoate d'oestradiol. C. R. Soc. Biol. (Paris) **129**, 519 (1938).
— —, and L. VARGAS: Uterine and extrauterine localizations of experimental fibroids induced in guinea pig by prolonged administration of estrogens. Proc. Soc. exp. Biol. (N. Y.) **45**, 788 (1940).
— J. LUCO and J. ZAÑARTU: Quantitative aspects of the antifibromatogenic action of synthetic desoxycorticosterone acetate. Cancer Res. **2**, 200 (1942).
—, and M. MAASS: Progesterone treatment of uterine and other abdominal fibroids induced in the guinea pig by alpha-estradiol. Cancer Res. **4**, 18 (1944).
— E. MARDONES, R. IGLESIAS, F. FUENZALIDA and E. BRUZZONE: Comparative antifibromatogenic action of cortical steroids. Science **116**, 448 (1952).
— — Prevention of experimental uterine and extrauterine fibroids by testosterone and progesterone. Endocrinology **28**, 669 (1941); O. Ruz, Lancet **2**, 867 (1939).
— — Structure and origin of uterine and extragenital fibroids induced experimentally in the guinea pig by prolonged administration of estrogens. Cancer Res. **1**, 236 (1941).
— L. VARGAS, A. JEDLICKY and P. BELLOLIO: The minimum quantity of estrogen required to induce atypical epithelial growth of the uterine mucosa in the guinea pig. Amer. J. Cancer **39**, 185 (1940).
— —, and C. NUÑEZ: Comparative antitumoral action of desoxycorticosterone acetate and testosterone propionate. Proc. Soc. exp. Biol. (N. Y.) **48**, 271 (1941).
—, and J. ZAÑARTU: Anti-fibromatogenic action of a natural cortical hormone (dehydrocorticosterone of Kendall). Endocrinology **31**, 192 (1942).
LOEB, L., E. L. BURNS, V. SUNTZEFF and M. MOSKOP: Carcinoma-like proliferations in vagina, cervix and uterus of mouse treated with estrogenic hormones. Proc. Soc. exp. Biol. (N.Y.) **35**, 320 (1936).
— V. SUNTZEFF and E. L. BURNS: The effects of age and estrogen on the stroma of vagina, cervix and uterus in the mouse. Science 88, 432 (1938).
— — — Growth processes induced by estrogenic hormones in the uterus of the mouse. Amer. J. Cancer **34**, 413 (1938).
MARDONES, E., R. IGLESIAS and A. LIPSCHUTZ: Comparative antifibromatogenic action of progesterone and Δ^{11}-dehydroprogesterone. Experientia (Basel) **9**, 303 (1953).

MIGLIAVACCA, A.: Inkretogene heterotype Epithelwucherungen im Uterus. Arch. Gynäk. **162**, 595 (1936).
— Beiträge und Beobachtungen für neue Richtlinien bei der Untersuchung der Beziehungen zwischen Geschlechtshormonen und Geschwulstentwicklung. Tumori 11, F. 2, 246 (1937); Zbl. allg. Path. path. Anat. **68**, 188 (1937).
MOON, H. D. Geschwülste bei Ratten nach Behandlung mit Wachstumshormon des Hypophysenvorderlappens. II. Nebennieren. Cancer Res. **10**, 364 (1950).
— Rattengeschwülste nach Behandlung mit Hypophysenwachstumshormon. III. Fortpflanzungsorgane. Cancer Res. **10**, 549 (1950).
— Hypophysenwachstumshormon-Behandlung bei Ratten-Neoplasmen. V. Nichtvorhandensein von Neoplasmen bei hypophysektomierten Ratten. Cancer Res. **11**, 535 (1951).
— M. E. SIMPSON, CH. H. LI and H. M. EVANS: Neoplasmen bei mit Hypophysenwachstumshormon behandelten Ratten. I. Lungen- und lymphatische Gewebe. Cancer Res. **10**, 297 (1950).
— — — — Rattengeschwülste nach Behandlung mit Hypophysenwachstumshormon. III. Fortpflanzungsorgane. Cancer Res. **10**, 183 (1951/52).
MORATÓ, J.: Adenofibromyomata in the uterus of a guinea pig after extreme partial castration. Endocrinology **29**, 619 (1941).
MORICARD, R., et J. CAUCHOIX: Réalisation de volumineux fibromes chez la femelle de cobaye par l'injection de benzoate de dihydrofolliculine. C. R. Soc. Biol. (Paris) **129**, 556 (1938).
— Fibromatose experimentale. Maroc. méd. No. **330**, 31 (1952).
MOSINGER, M.: Le problème du cancer et son évolution récente. Paris: Masson & Cie. 1946.
— Cancers, tumeurs, bénignes et processus prolifératifs hyperplastiques et kystiques d'origine hormonale et cancérigène synthétique, chez le cobaye et le rat. Essais de transmission de la carcinorésistance du cobaye. Fol. anat. (Coimbra) **22**, No. 8 (1947).
— Sur les tumeurs oestrogènes et dyméthylbenzanthracéniques chez le Rat et le Cobaye. C. R. Ass. Anat. **55**, 285—291 (1949).
NADEL, E. M.: Fibroids in a guinea (family 13) after partial castration. J. nat. Cancer Inst. **9**, 271 (1949).
— Histopathologie von durch Oestrogene induzierten Tumoren bei Meerschweinchen. J. nat. Cancer Inst. **10**, 1043 (1950).
NELSON, W. O.: Endometrial and myometrial changes, including fibromyomatous nodules, induced in the uterus of the guinea pig by the prolonged administration of estrogenic hormone. Anat. Rec. **68**, 99 (1937).
— Atypical uterine growths produced by prolonged administration of estrogenic hormones. Endocrinology **24**, 50 (1939).
OLSEN, A. G., J. T. VELARDO, A. B. HISAW, A. B. DAWSON and L. E. BRAVERMAN: Prolongation of pseudopregnancy associated with the presence of deciduomata. Anat. Rec. **111**, **44** (1951).
OVERHOLSER, M. D., and W. O. NELSON: Migration of nuclei in uterine epithelium of monkey following prolonged estrin injections. Proc. Soc. exp. Biol. (N. Y.) **34** (1936).
PECKHAM, B. M.: Die Erzeugung sekundärer Deciduomata bei der kastrierten und bei der stillenden Ratte. Endocrinology **41**, 277 (1947).
—, and R. R. GREENE: Prolongation of pseudopregnancy by deciduomata in the rat. Proc. Soc. exp. Biol. (N. Y.) **69**, 417 (1948).
PERLOFF, W. H., and R. KURZROK: Production of uterine tumors in the guinea pig by local implantation of estrogen pellets. Proc. Soc. exp. Biol. (N. Y.) **46**, 262 (1941).
PFEIFFER, C. A.: The effects of an experimentally induced endocrine imbalance in female mice., Anat. Rec. **75**, 465 (1939).
— Development of leiomyomas in female rats with an endocrine imbalance. Cancer Res. **9** 277 (1949).
—, and E. ALLEN: Attempts to produce cancer in Rhesus monkeys with carcinogenic hydrocarbons and estrogens. Cancer Res. 8, 97 (1948).
PIERSON, H.: Experimentelle Erzeugung von Uterusgeschwülsten bei Kaninchen durch Ovarialhormone. Z. Krebsforsch. **41**, H. 2, 103 (1934).
— Experimentelle Erzeugung von Uterusgeschwülsten bei Kaninchen durch Prolan. Z. Krebsforsch. **45**, 28 (1936); ref.: Zbl. allg. Path. path. Anat. **67**, Nr. 11, 396 (1937).
— Weitere Follikulinversuche. Perforierende Plattenepithelwucherungen im Uterus des Kaninchens mit Knorpel- und Knochenbefunden. Z. Krebsforsch. **47**, H. 1, 1 (1937); Zbl. allg. Path. path. Anat. **70**, 66 (1938).
— Neue Follikulinversuche. Erzeugung von Neubildungen in- und außerhalb des Uterus von Kaninchen. Z. Krebsforsch. **46**, H. 3, 109 (1937); Zbl. allg. Path. path. Anat. **69**, 67 (1937).
— Experimentell erzeugtes infiltrierendes Adenom im Uterus des Kaninchens durch Hypophysenvorderlappenextrakt. Z. Krebsforsch. **47**, H. 2, 166 (1938); Zbl. allg. Path. path. Anat. **70**, 66 (1938).

Pierson, H.: Metaplastisch entstandene Knochenbildungen neben infiltrierenden Epithelwucherungen im Uterus des Kaninchens durch Follikelhormon. Z. Krebsforsch. **47**, H. 4, 336 (1938).
— The influence of various hormones on tumour development in the uterus of the rabbit. Acta Unio Int. Cancer **5**, 152 (1940).
Reiter, R. J.: Estrogen-induced uterine metaplasia in rats given oral supplements of vitamin A. Experientia (Basel) **21**, 207 (1965).
Riesco, A.: On the bearing of time on the neoplastic action of small quantities of α-estradiol in the endometrium of guinea pigs. Brit. J. Cancer **1**, 166 (1947); Bol. Soc. Biol. Santiago **4**, 4 (1947).
Sammartino, R., and R. G. Herrera: Los tumores producidos por estrógenos en cobayos. Rev. méd. latino-am. **25**, 976 (1940).
Selye, H., A. Borduas and G. Masson: Studies concerning the hormonal control of deciduomata and metrial glands. Anat. Rec. **82**, 199 (1942).
Stone, G. M., and C. W. Emmens: The action of oestradiol and dimethylstilboestrol on early pregnancy and deciduoma formation in the mouse. J. Endocrin. **29**, 137—145 (1964).
— — The effect of oestrogens and anti-oestrogens on deciduoma formation in the rat. J. Endocrin. **29**, 147—157 (1964).
Suntzeff, V., E. L. Burns, M. Moskop and L. Loeb: On the proliferative changes taking place in the epithelium of vagina and cervix of mice with advancing age and under the influence of experimentally administered estrogenic hormones. Amer. J. Cancer **32**, 256 (1938).
Thiery, M.: Het experimentele carcinoma colli uteri. Bruxelles: Presses académiques Européennes S. C. 1963.
Vargas, L.: Fibrosis diseminada peritoneal inducida en el cobayo por estrógenos. Rev. chil. Hig. **4**, 277 (1942).
— Attempt to induce formation of fibroids with estrogen in the castrated female rhesus monkey. Bull. Johns Hopk. Hosp. **73**, 23 (1943).
— Experimental fibroids in hypophysectomized female guinea pigs. Cancer Res. **3**, 309 (1943).
Velardo, J. T., and F. L. Hisaw: Quantitative inhibition of progesterone by estrogens in development of deciduomata. Endocrinology **49**, 530 (1951).
— A. Dawson, A. Olsen and F. Hisaw: Sequence of histological changes in the uterus and vagina of the rat during prolongation of pseudopregnancy associated with the presence of deciduomata. Amer. J. Anat. **93**, II, (1953).
Vera, O.: La acción antifibromatógena comparativa de los andrógenos. Tesis Univ. de Chile (1942); Publ. Dep. Med. Exp. No. 10.
Wattenwyl, H. von: Die Erzeugung von mesenchymalen Tumoren mit Follikelhormon. Helv. med. Acta **8**, 187 (1941).
— Follikelhormonapplikation und die hormonale Tumorentstehung (Tierversuche). Basel: Schwabe 1944.
Woodruff, L. M.: Tumors produced by estradiol benzoate in the guinea pig. Cancer Res. **1**, 367 (1941).
Zaleski, W.: Experimentelle Endometriosis bei Kaninchenweibchen nach Prolaninjektionen. Zbl. Gynäk. **42**, 2426 (1937).
Zitzlsperger, S.: Geschwulstbildungen in der Uterusschleimhaut beim sterilisierten Kaninchen. Z. mikr.-anat. Forsch. **49**, H. 2, 273 (1941).
Zondek, B.: The effect of prolonged application of large doses of follicular hormone on the uterus of rabbits. J. exp. Med. **63**, 789 (1936).
— The effect of long-continued large doses of follicle hormone upon the uterus of the rat. Amer. J. Obstet. Gynec. **33**, 979 (1937).
Zuckerman, S.: The histogenesis of tissues sensitive to oestrogens. Biol. Rev. **15**, 231 (1940).

h) Hoden, Nebenhoden

Nach langdauernder (etwa 60—70 Wochen) Follikelhormonbehandlung beobachteten erstmals Burrows (1935, 1936, 1949, 1952) und Gardner (1937) neben Veränderungen der Brustdrüse Hypertrophie der interstitiellen Zellen des Hodens bei verschiedenen *Mäuse*stämmen. Die unterschiedliche Häufigkeit der Hodentumoren bei verschiedenen Tierstämmen zeigt eine Übersicht von Gardner (1963).

Es wurden bei gleichartigen Versuchen in der Folgezeit von zahlreichen Untersuchern Hyperplasien der interstitiellen Zellen bzw. uni- und bilaterale Tumoren der Zwischenzellen des Hodens nach Oestrogenbehandlung von Mäusen beobachtet. Die durch langdauernde Follikelhormonbehandlung auftretende Homoistase

Auftreten von Hodenzwischenzelltumoren bei hybriden Mäusen nach Oestradiol und Oestron oder ihrer Ester sowie Stilboestrol über längere Zeitdauer

Stamm oder Gruppe	Behandlung					
	Zahl der Mäuse	Oestradiol, Oestron oder ihre Ester		Stilboestrol		
		Tumorzahl	durchschnittl. Alter bei Tumorentstehung	Zahl der Mäuse	Tumorzahl	durchschnittl. Alter bei Tumorentstehung
A × C57	47	1	350	10	1	468
C57 × A	53	6	495	12	3	411
A × C3H	55	6	486	14	2	434
C3H × A	70	7	413	11	4	399
C57 × CBA	43	—	(431)[1]	10	—	(561)[1]
CBA × C57	38	—	(427)[1]	10	—	(453)[1]

[1] Durchschnittliches Überlebensalter aller Mäuse in der Gruppe.

der Hypophyse führt, wie Abb. 32 zeigt, zu einer Wucherung der Hodenzwischenzellen [HOOKER, GARDNER, PFEIFFER (1940), BONSER und ROBSON (1940), SHIMKIN, GRADY, ANDERVONT (1941), SAMSONOFF (1941), GARDNER (1937, 1941, 1943, 1950, 1958), HOOKER und PFEIFFER (1942), BONSER (1942, 1944), GARDNER und BODDAERT (1950), BIELSCHOWSKY und HALL (1954), JONES (1955), HUSEBY (1958)]. Diese Tumoren traten bei bis zu 50% der Mäuse auf und zeigten z. T. Metastasen. Bei diesen Leydigschen Zwischenzelltumoren des Hodens wurde vermehrt follikelstimulierendes Gonadotropin des Hypophysenvorderlappens im Harn ausgeschieden. Ähnliche Tumoren konnten von PFEIFFER und HOOKER (1943) auch durch Injektion von Serum schwangerer Pferde erzeugt werden.

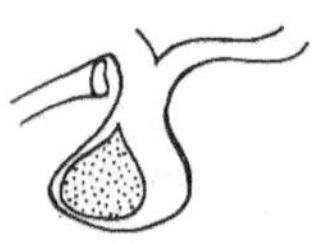

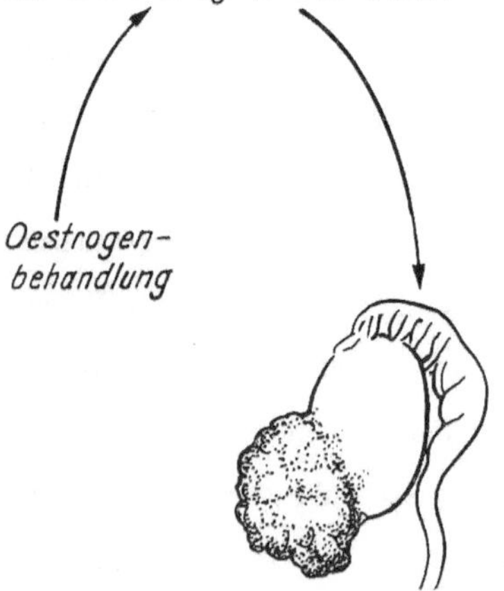

Abb. 32. Hodenzwischenzelltumorentstehung durch Homoistase der Hypophyse

TWOMBLY, MEISEL und STOUT (1949) konnten zeigen, daß die gleichen Tumoren sekundär durch eine chronische hormonale Stimulierung der Hypophyse hervorgerufen werden können. Sie implantierten Hoden infantiler *Ratten* in die Milz.

Da die Steroidhormone des transplantierten Hodens in der Leber inaktiviert werden [BISKIND und BISKIND (1943)], kommt es nach der Transplantation in die Leber nicht zu einer Hemmung der Gonadotropinsekretion der Hypophyse.

Aus den Transplantaten entstanden bei weiblichen und männlichen kastrierten Tieren in der Milz Leydig-Zell-Tumoren, teilweise von erheblicher Größe. Gleichartige Hyperplasien von Zwischenzellen hatten schon 1945 BISKIND und BISKIND durch Heterotransplantation von infantilem Hodengewebe auf kastrierte Ratten erzeugt. Es entstanden innerhalb von 11 Monaten große Tumoren, vorwiegend aus interstitiellen Zellen bestehend. Zum Teil sahen diese Untersucher auch granulosazelltumor- oder arrhenoblastomähnliche Bilder. LI, PFEIFFER und GARDNER (1947) beobachteten ebenfalls Hyperplasien der interstitiellen Zellen, sprechen aber nicht von Tumoren. Auch wir [DONTENWILL und RANZ (1960)] beobachteten nach Heterotransplantation von Hodengewebe in die Milz der kastrierten Ratte

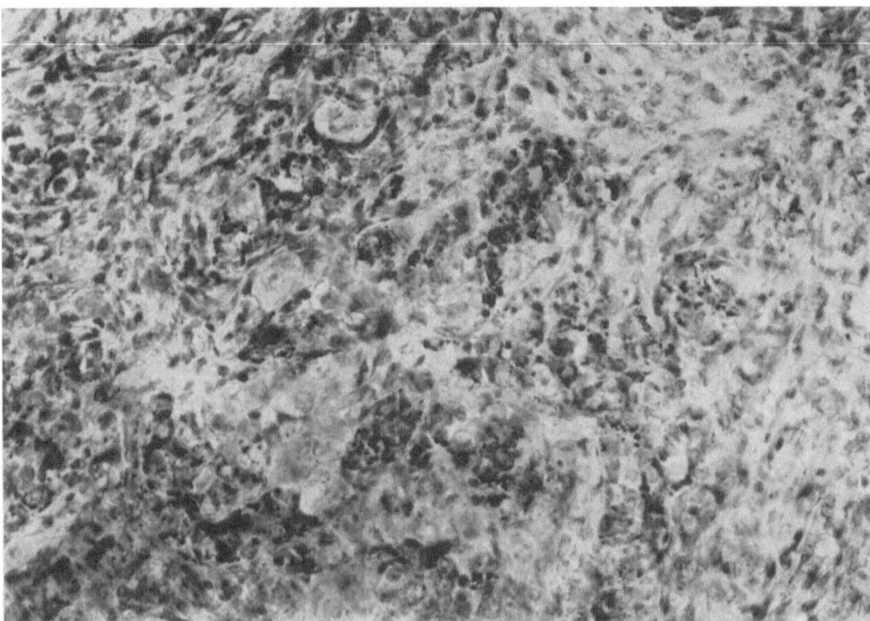

Abb. 33. Arrhenoblastomähnliche knotige Zwischenzellwucherung am Rande eines tubulären Hodenregenerates mit Lipoidablagerungen in den protoplasmareichen Zellen, 11 Monate, 14 Tage nach Transplantation von embryonalem Hodengewebe der Ratte

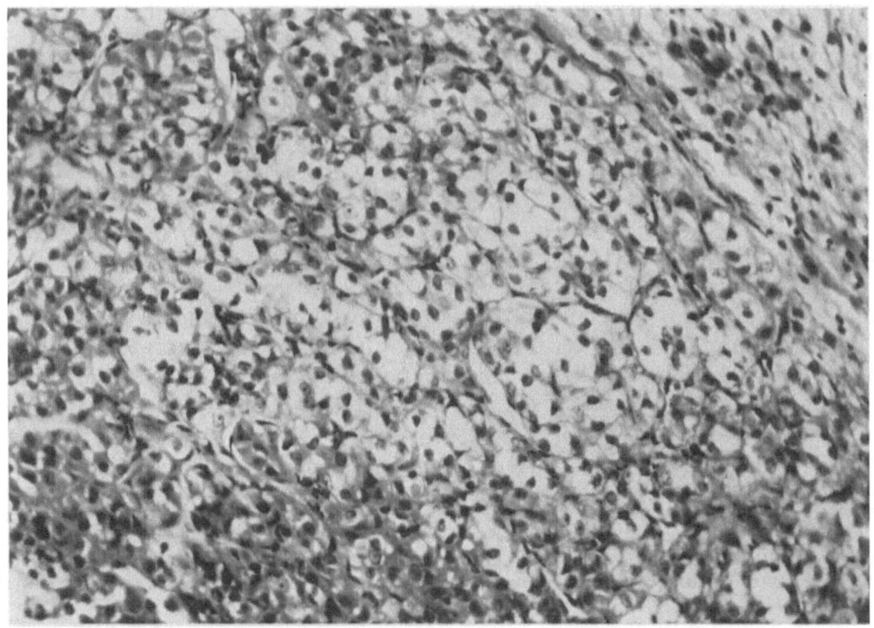

Abb. 34. Knotige Wucherung von Zwischenzellen am Rande eines tubulären Hodenregenerates, 10 Monate, 7 Tage nach Transplantation von embryonalem Hodengewebe bei Ratten

knotige Hyperplasien von Zwischenzellen, insbesondere bei Transplantation von embryonalem Hodengewebe. Neben den von BISKIND und BISKIND (1945) beschriebenen arrhenoblastomähnlichen Hodenzwischenzellregeneraten (Abb. 33) sahen wir interstitielle (Abb. 35b) und diffuse (Abb. 34) Wucherungen von Zwischenzellen neben z. T. hodenähnlichen Regeneraten (Abb. 35). Das embryonale Hodengewebe (gewonnen von 21 Tage alten Embryonen) zeigte eine wesentlich stärkere Regenerationsfähigkeit als das implantierte Hodengewebe ausgewachsener Ratten. Die Versuche zeigen, daß sowohl die durch Hormonbehandlung erzeugten Zwischenzelltumoren des Hodens wie auch die Hyperplasien der transplantierten Zwischenzellen durch eine hormonelle Mehrstimulierung von seiten der Hypophyse entstehen.

Daß die Hyperplasien der Hodenzwischenzellen in der Milz keine so großen Ausmaße annehmen wie beim Ovar, liegt wohl daran, daß die vorher weit auseinanderliegenden Hodenzwischenzellen nun nach dem Untergang der Hodenkanälchen sehr dicht liegen und deswegen die Regenerate im Vergleich zum Ovar ebenfalls als groß bezeichnet werden können. Unklar bleibt, wie unsere Versuche zeigen, weshalb embryonales Hodengewebe gut, embryonales Ovargewebe schlecht regeneriert und sich dieses Verhalten beim Ovar- und Hodengewebe erwachsener Tiere gerade umkehrt [DONTENWILL und RANZ (1961)]. Hier spielt neben der Stimulierung sicher auch die Ansprechbarkeit des Gewebes eine wesentliche Rolle.

GARDNER, PFEIFFER, TRENTIN und WOLSTENHOLME (1953) konnten zeigen, daß die Wirkung der oestrogenen Hormone auf die interstitiellen Zellen des Hodens nur über das gonadotrope Hormon (ICSH) der Hypophyse entsteht. Antigonadotropes Serum unterbindet die Oestrogenwirkung auf den Hoden [ELY (1953)].

Eine Überproduktion von ICSH kann aber auch durch einen erzeugten beiderseitigen langdauernden *Kryptorchismus* – d. h. durch eine operative Hodenverlagerung in die Bauchhöhle – entstehen, bei dem es zu ähnlichen Hypophysenveränderungen wie nach Kastration [MARTINS (1936), BIELSCHOWSKY und HALL (1954)] kommt.

Wucherungen der interstitiellen Zellen beschreiben BIELSCHOWSKY und HALL (1954) bei Ratten nach maximal 20monatigem Kryptorchismus und LIPSCHUTZ (1924, 1950) im Rest des Hodens, der nach Kastration in der Bauchhöhle zurückgeblieben war. Nach WEILL (1955) regt auch der einseitige Kryptorchismus die interstitiellen Zellen des anderen Hoden an, ein Vorgang, den wir auch bei einseitiger Entfernung anderer paarig angelegter innersekretorischer Drüsen kennen. Nach BIELSCHOWSKY und HALL (1954) wird die Tumorgenese im Bereich der interstitiellen Zellen durch den Kryptorchismus gefördert, da dieser die zur Mehrstimulierung notwendige endokrine Korrelationsstörung schafft.

Die interstitiellen Tumoren des Hodens konnten durch laufende *Hormoninjektionen*, wie auch durch Einführen von Hormonpelotten, erzeugt werden. GARDNER und BODDAERT (1950) stellten keine sichere genetische Abhängigkeit der Leistungsfähigkeit der Hodentumoren fest. TRENTIN und GARDNER (1958) nehmen auf Grund ihrer Untersuchungen an, daß die bei einzelnen Tierstämmen verschiedene Empfänglichkeit für die Induktion von Hodentumoren vom Hoden selbst bestimmt wird, also auch hier eine organgebundene genetische Abhängigkeit. Die Empfänglichkeit ist anders als bei den Mammatumoren; Mäuse des C3H-Stammes sind resistent.

Die Tumoren lassen sich nach BONSER (1944) bei bestimmten Stämmen ohne Follikelhormonbehandlung transplantieren, andere Stämme zeigen aber nach GARDNER (1958) erst nach langer Schlummerperiode Wachstum bei gleichzeitiger Follikelhormonbehandlung, sie sind also offenbar in ihrem Angehen von bestimmten hormonalen Ausgangssituationen abhängig. KLEIN und HELLSTRÖM (1962) transplantierten durch Diäthylstilboestrol erzeugte Leydig-Zelltumoren auf oestrogenbehandelte Mäuse und konnten dabei die Oestrogenabhängigkeit der Tumoren nachweisen.

Am transplantierten Geschwulstgewebe von induzierten Hodentumoren haben DOMINGUEZ, SAMUELS und HUSEBY (1958) ausgedehnte Untersuchungen über die

Biosynthese der Hormone vorgenommen. Sie konnten zeigen, daß die interstitiellen Tumoren erhebliche Mengen androgener Hormone bilden. Die Hormonproduktion kann sich bei mehrmaliger Transplantation ändern.

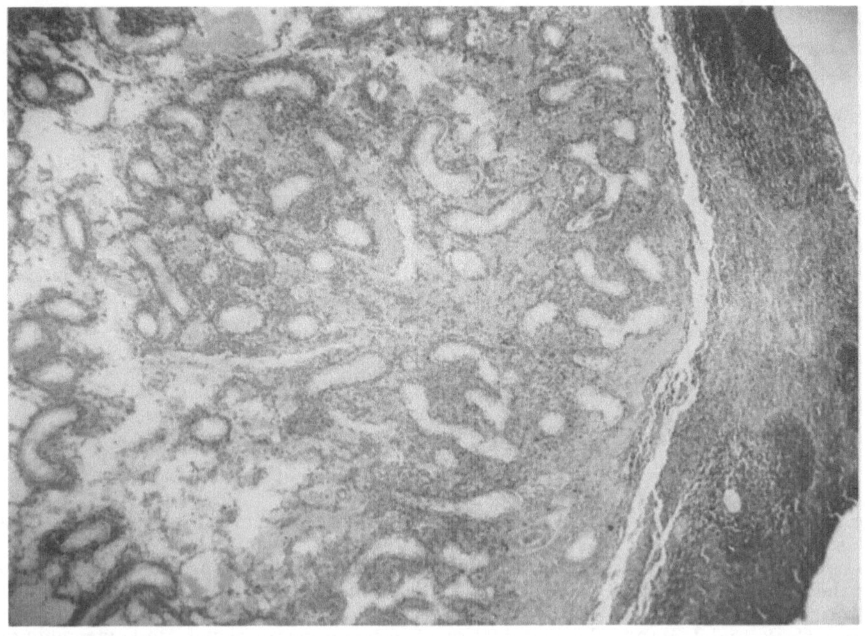

a

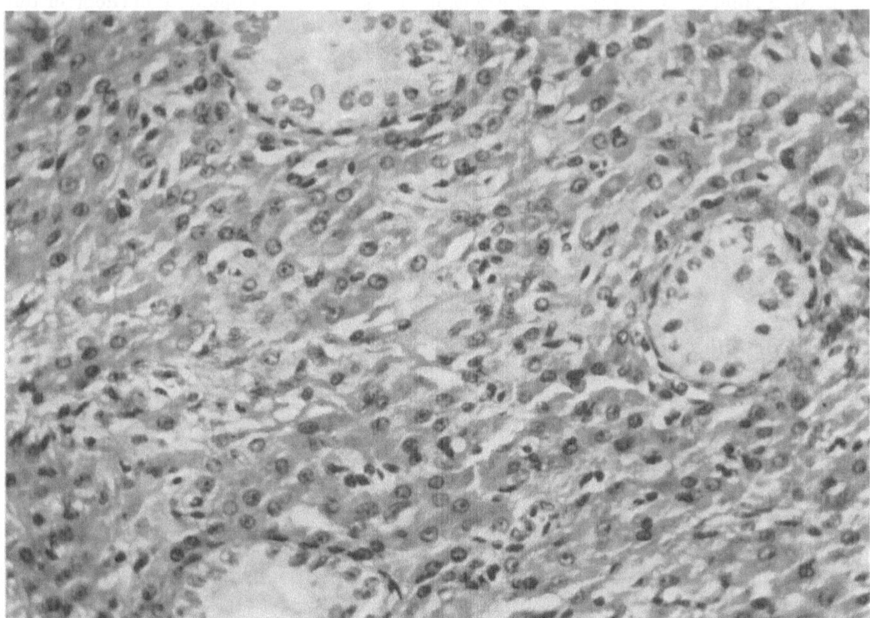

b

Abb. 35a u. b. Etwa haselnußgroßes Hodenregenerat a) mit starker intertubulärer Zwischenzellwucherung b) 10 Monate, 7 Tage nach Transplantation von embryonalem Hodengewebe der Ratte

SIMPSON und VAN WAGENEN (1954) beschrieben bei Affen, die laufend mit Gonadotropin behandelt wurden, Hyperplasien der interstitiellen Zellen mit Auftreten von peritubulären Knötchen. Zum Teil zeigten diese Zellen das typische Bild der Leydigschen Zwischenzellen. BACON sah 1952, KIRKMAN 1957 bei gleichzeitiger Behandlung von Goldhamstern mit Diäthylstilboestrol und Testosteron, nicht dagegen nach Behandlung mit Stilboestrol allein, Tumoren, die vom Bindegewebe des Nebenhodens und der Muskulatur des Samenstranges ausgingen.

BERN (1949) fand nach Oestrogenbehandlung bei männlichen Kaninchen Fibrome des Nebenhodens und KOREF, LIPSCHUTZ und VARGAS (1939), JEDLICKY, LIPSCHUTZ und VARGAS (1939) beobachteten Fibromyome beim Meerschweinchen nach Ligatur des Ductus deferens. Epithelproliferationen (Blase, Samenblase usw.) nach langdauernder Follikelhormonbehandlung hat bereits 1934—1937 LACASSAGNE (s. Monographie, 1950) bei Mäusen beschrieben.

Bei Ratten ist die Reaktion auf Oestrogenbehandlung unterschiedlich. GESCHICKTER und BYRNES (1942) gelang es nicht, einen Wachstumsreiz auf die Hoden auszuüben, sie beobachteten sogar Hodenatrophie. Bei einzelnen Rattenstämmen traten Hyperplasien der Zwischenzellen spontan auf. Die Untersuchungen zeigen also, daß bei der Auslösung von Hodengeschwülsten genetische Faktoren wesentliche Voraussetzung sind.

Literatur

h) Hoden

BACON, R. L.: Tumors of the epididymis in hamsters treated with diethylstilbestrol and testosteron propionate. Anat. Rec. **112**, 305 (1952).

BERN, H. A.: Some effects of long-continued estrogen treatment on male dutch rabbits. Cancer Res. **9**, 65 (1949).

BIELSCHOWSKY, E., and W. H. HALL: Experimentally induced hyper- and neo-plastic changes in the testis of rats. Proc. Univ. Otago med. Sch. **32**, 16 (1954). See also: A. R. Brit. Emp. Cancer Campgn. **32**, 352 (1954).

BISKIND, G. R., and J. MARK: The inactivation of testosterone propionate and extrone in rats. Bull. Johns Hopk. Hosp. **65**, 212 (1939).

BISKIND, M. S., and G. R. BISKIND: Inactivation of testosterone propionate in the liver during vitamin B complex deficiency. Alteration of the estrogen-androgen equilibrium. Endocrinology **32**, 97 (1943).

— — Tumor of rat testis produced by heterotransplantation of infantile testis to spleen of adult castrate. Proc. Soc. exp. Biol. (N. Y.) **59**, 4—8 (1945).

BONSER, G. M.: Malignant tumors of the interstitial cells of the testis in strong A mice treated with triphenylethylene. J. Path. Bact. **54**, 149 (1942).

— Mammary and testicular tumours in male mice of various strains following oestrogen treatment. J. Path. Bact. **56**, 15 (1944).

—, and J. M. ROBSON: The effects of prolonged oestrogen administration upon male mice of various strains: development of testicular tumors in the strong of a strain. J. Path. Bact. **51**, 9—22 (1940).

BURROWS, H.: Changes induced in the interstitial tissue of the testis of the mouse by certain oestrogens. J. Path. Bact. **41**, 218 (1935).

— A comparison of the changes induced by some pure oestrogenic compounds in the mammae and testes of mice. J. Path. Bact. **42**, 161 (1936).

— Biological actions of sex hormones. Sec. ed. Cambridge: Univ. Press (1949).

—, and E. HORNING: Oestrogen and neoplasia. Oxford: Blackwell 1952.

DOMINGUEZ, O. V., L. T. SAMUELS and R. A. HUSEBY: Steroid biosynthesis in induced testicular interstitial cell tumors of mice. In: G. E. W. WOLSTENHOLME and M. O'CONNOR (eds.),Ciba Found Coll. Endocr. **12**, 231—38 (1958).

DONTENWILL, W.: Vergleichende Untersuchungen an in die Milz implantierten endokrinen Drüsen. Verh. dtsch. Ges. Path. **43**, 243 (1959).

—, u. H. RANZ: Vergleichende Untersuchungen an Transplantaten endokriner Drüsen. Im Beitr. Path. Anat. **124**, 229—241 (1961).

ELY, C. A.: Effect of antigonadotrophic serum on testes of A-strain mice treated with estrogen. Proc. Soc. exp. Biol. (N. Y.) **84**, 501—505 (1953).

GARDNER, W. U.: Hypertrophy of interstitial cells in the testes of mice receiving estrogenic hormones. Anat. Rec. **68**, 339 (1937).

— Interstitielle Tumoren nach langdauernder Behandlung mit Triphenylethylen. Cancer Res. **1**, 345 (1941).

GARDNER, W. U.: Testicular tumors in mice of several strains receiving triphenylethylene. Cancer Res. 3, 92 (1943).
— Zwischenzelltumoren bei Bastardmäusen, die mit Tri-p-anisyl-chloräthylen behandelt wurden. Arch. Path. (Chicago) 50, 750 (1950).
— Testicular tumorigenesis. In: G. E. W. WOLSTENHOLME and M. O'CONNOR (eds.), Ciba Found. Coll. Endocr. 12, 239—249 (1958).
— Genetic aspects of hormonal influences on cancer. Ann. N. Y. Acad. Sci. 71, 1092—1099 (1958).
—, and J. BODDAERT: Testicular interstitial cell tumors in hybrid mice given tri-p-anisylchloraethylene. Arch. Path. (Chicago) 50, 750 (1950).
— C. A. PFEIFFER, J. J. TRENTIN and J. T. WOLSTENHOLME: Hormonal factors in experimental carcinogenesis. Physiopathology of Cancer. New York: Hoeber-Harper 1953.
GESCHICKTER, C. F., and E. W. BYRNES: Factors influencing the development and time of appearance of mammary cancer in the rat in response to estrogen. Arch. Path. (Chicago) 33, 334 (1942).
HOOKER, C. W., W. U. GARDNER and C. A. PFEIFFER: Testicular tumors in mice receiving estrogens. J. Amer. med. Ass. 115, 443 (1940).
— and A. PFEIFFER: The morphology and development of testicular tumors in mice of a strain receiving estrogens. Cancer Res. 2, 759 (1942).
HUSEBY, R. A.: Interstitial cell tumors of the mouse testis: studies of tumorigenesis, dependency and hormone production. In: G. E. W. WOLSTENHOLME and M. O'CONNOR (eds.). Ciba Found. Coll. Endocr. 12, 216—230 (1958).
JEDLICKY, A., A. LIPSCHUTZ et L. VARGAS: La spécificité sexuelle de la réaction tumorale conjonctive vis-à-vis de l'hormone folliculaire. (17-caprylate et 17-benzoate-3-n-butyrate d'oestradiol). C. R. Soc. Biol. (Paris) 130, 1466 (1939).
JONES, A.: Experimental production of interstitial cell tumors. Brit. J. Cancer 9, 640—645 (1955).
KIRKMAN, H.: Steroid hormon and tumorigenesis. Cancer (Philad.) 10, 754 (1957).
KLEIN, G., u. K. E. HELLSTRÖM: Transplantationsstudien an Oestrogen-induzierten Leydig-Zelltumoren der Maus. J. nat. Cancer Inst. 28, 99—115 (1962).
KOREF, O., A. LIPSCHUTZ et L. VARGAS: Spécificité sexuelle et tumorigenèse. C. R. Soc. Biol, (Paris) 130, 303 (1939).
LACASSAGNE, A.: Modifications de l'épithélium vésical chez la souris atteinte de rétention urinaire à la suite d'injections d'oestrone. C. R. Soc. Biol. (Paris) 120, 833 (1935).
— Les cancers produits par des substances chimiques endogènes. Paris: Hermann 1950.
—, et A. RAYNAUD: Injection de testostérone dans la vésicule séminale du rat castré, pour accroître la sensibilité de ce test biologique de l'hormone male. C. R. Soc. Biol. (Paris) 126, 576 (1937).
— — Influence de l'hormone mâle et de l'hormone femelle sur la structure histologique du pénis de la souris. C. R. Soc. Biol. (Paris) 126, 868 (1937).
LI, M. H., C. A. PFEIFFER and W. U. GARDNER: Intrasplenic transplantation of testes in castrated mice. Proc. Soc. exp. Biol. (N. Y.) 64, 319 (1947).
LIPSCHUTZ, A.: On the hypertrophy of the interstitial cells in the testicle of the guinea pig under different experimental conditions. Proc. roy. Soc. B 93, 132; 94, 83 (1922).
— Internal secretions of the sex glands. Cambridge: Heffer & Sons, Ltd. Baltimore: Williams & Wilkins Comp. 1924.
— Steroid hormones and tumors. Baltimore: Williams & Wilkins Comp. 1950.
— Steroid homeostasis hypophysis and tumorigenesis. Cambridge: Heffer & Sons, Ltd. 1957.
MARTINS, TH.: Glandulas sexuaes e hypophyse anterior. Sao Paulo: Cia. Editora Nacional 1936.
PFEIFFER, C. A., and C. W. HOOKER: Testicular changes resembling early stages in the development of interstitial cell tumors in mice of the A strain after long continued injections of pregnant mare serum. Cancer Res. 3, 762—766 (1943).
SAMSONOFF, N.: Sur la production expérimentale du tumeurs de la glande interstitielle du testicule chez le rat. C. R. Soc. Biol. (Paris) 135, 922 (1941).
SHIMKIN, M. B., H. G. GRADY and H. B. ANDERVONT: Induction of testicular tumors and other effects of stilbestrol-cholesterol pellets in strain C mice. J. nat. Cancer Inst. 2, 65—80 (1941).
SIMPSON, M. E., and G. VAN WAGENEN: Persistent nodules in testis of the monkey associated with Leydig cell hyperplasia induced by gonadotrophins. Cancer Res. 14, 289—293 (1954).
TRENTIN, J., and W. U. GARDNER: Site of gene action in susceptibility to estrogen-induced testicular interstitial-cell tumors of mice. Cancer Res. 18, 1, 110 (1958).
TWOMBLY, G. H., D. MEISEL and A. P. STOUT: Leydig-cell tumors induced experimentally in the rat. Cancer (Philad.) 2, 884 (1949).
WEILL, CL.: Notions nouvelles sur la cryptorchidie expérimentale. Effect de la cryptorchidie unilatérale, chez le cobaye, sur le testicule ectopique et sur l'autre testicule. C. R. Soc. Biol. (Paris) 149, 183 (1955).

i) Prostata

PARKES und ZUCKERMAN (1935), ZUCKERMAN und PARKES (1936) sahen nach langdauernder täglicher Injektion von Oestron bei männlichen jungen *Affen* (Macacamulatta und Papio papio) eine Vergrößerung der Prostata bei Verminderung des Drüsengewebes und Vermehrung des fibromuskulären Gewebes. Es entstand dabei eine deutliche Harnabflußbehinderung.

Testosteron hemmt die durch Oestrogen hervorgerufene Prostatavergrößerung bei Affen [ZUCKERMAN und PARKES (1936)] ebenso wie gleichzeitige Behandlung mit Progesteron [DE JONGH, QUERIDO und STOLTE (1939)] oder Desoxycorticosteron [ACUÑA (1944)].

Beim Hund ist die sog. Altershypertrophie der Prostata seit langem bekannt. KOCH (1936) injizierte jüngeren *Hunden* in den ersten Lebensjahren Prolan, pro Woche 2mal 500 RE. Die Prostata noch nicht geschlechtsreifer Tiere blieb völlig unempfindlich, während bei Tieren, die älter als 7 Monate waren, schon von der zweiten Woche an erheblich verstärktes Wachstum eintrat.

Bei älteren Tieren mit Prostatahypertrophie konnte eine vermehrte Ausscheidung von hypophysärem Follikelreifungshormon nachgewiesen werden. RÖSSLE und ZAHLER (1938) konnten bei Hunden durch Zufuhr von Hodenextrakten Hypertrophie der Prostata bis zur Entstehung von Harnverhaltung nachweisen.

BÜHLER (1938) behandelte junge und ältere *Ratten* mit Progynon (Schering). Dabei ergab sich eine erhebliche Epithelwucherung der Drüsen. Nach Behandlung mit männlichem Keimdrüsenhormon beobachtete BÜHLER eine Proliferation des Interstitiums. Die eindeutigen Veränderungen sah er nach Behandlung mit weiblichen Geschlechtshormonen, er verglich die Bilder mit denen der menschlichen Prostatahypertrophie. RICHTER (1950) sah nach Prolan behandlung bei Ratten eine Vergrößerung der Prostata mit Wucherung der Drüsen, bei kastrierten-Ratten eine Wucherung des Interstitiums. BULLIARD und RAVINA (1937) beobachteten nach Testosteronbehandlung bei unreifen Ratten (6 Injektionen im Verlaufe von 15 Tagen) eine Vergrößerung der Präputialdrüse um das Sechsfache.

Gewichtsanstieg und Vergrößerung der Prostata, sog. fibromuskuläre und adenomatöse Hyperplasie, z. T. vorwiegend im Bereich des periutricularen Gewebes [LIPSCHUTZ (1950)], z. T. mit gleichzeitiger Metaplasie der Schleimhaut, beschrieben bei *Hunden, Affen, Mäusen, Meerschweinchen* und *Hamstern*. LACASSAGNE (1950), LACASSAGNE und VILLELA (1933), DAVID, FREUD und DE JONGH (1934), KORENCHEVSKY und DENINSON (1934), DE JONGH, KOK, VAN-DER WOERD (1938), BURROWS und KENNEWAY (1934), COURRIER und COHEN-SOLAL (1936), KOCH (1936), COURRIER und GROS (1937), CHAMPY und COUJARD (1937), BÜHLER (1938), CALEF (1939), DEANSLEY (1939), CHEVREL-BODEN und LEROY (1941), ACUÑA (1944), LERMANDA (1945), LIPSCHUTZ, YANINE, SCHWARZ, BRUZZONE, ACUÑA und SILBERMAN (1945), HORNING (1949), BURROWS (1949), BERN (1949), HORNING und WHITTICK (1954).

HORNING und WHITTICK (1954) fanden nach Oestrogenbehandlung von Goldhamstern bei drei Tieren fibromuskuläre Sarkome der Prostata.

Literatur

i) Prostata

ACUÑA, J.: El fibromioepitelioma periutricular inducido por estrógenos y su prevención por el acetato de desoxicorticosterona. Tesis Univ. de Chile (1944) (Public. Dep. Med. Exp. No. 28).

BERN, H. A.: Some effects of long continued estrogen treatment on male dutch rabbits. Cancer Res. **9**, 65 (1949).

BÜHLER, F.: Über den Einfluß verschiedener Hormone auf die Prostata der Ratte. Beitrag zur Frage der innersekretorischen Ätiologie der menschlichen Prostatahypertrophie. Z. ges. exp. Med. **104**, 249 (1938); Zbl. allg. Path. path. Anat. **72**, 326 (1939).

BULLIARD, H., u. A. RAVINA: Wirkung des männlichen Sexualhormons auf die Präputialdrüse. C. R. Soc. Biol. (Paris) **125**, 965 (1937); Zbl. allg. Path. path. Anat. **70**, 115 (1938).

BURROWS, H.: Biological actions of sex hormones. Sec. ed. Cambridge (Engl.): Univ. Press 1949.

—, and N. KENNEWAY: Amer. J. Cancer **70**, 48 (1934).

CALEF, C.: Experimentelle Untersuchungen über die Veränderungen einiger endokriner Drüsen, die mit einer Prostatahyper- oder Hypofunktion zusammenhängen. Scritti Med. in onore del Prof. M. DONATI del 25. anno di insegnamento. Vol. 50. Zbl. allg. Path. path. Anat. **72**, 326 (1939).

CHAMPY, CH., u. R. COUJARD: Die Wirkung der Sexualhormone auf die Vorsteherdrüse. C. R. Soc. Biol. (Paris) **125**, 632 (1937); Zbl. allg. Path. path. Anat. **70**, 115 (1938).

CHEVREL-BODEN, M. L., et D. LEROY: Étude histologique de l'appareil génital mâle du lapin soumis à la folliculinization prolongée. Ann. Endocr. (Paris) **2**, 226 (1941).

COURRIER, R., et G. COHEN-SOLAL: L'utricule prostatique chez le cobaye soumis à la folliculinication. C. R. Soc. Biol. (Paris) **121**, 903 (1936).

—, et G. GROS: Étude des rapports fonctionnels entre les hormones ovariennes chez les primates. C. R. Soc. Biol. (Paris) **125**, 746 (1937).

DEANESLY, R.: The uterus masculinus of the rabbit and its reactions to androgens and oestrogens. J. Endocr. **1**, 300 (1939).

HORNING, E. S.: Über die Wirkung von Kastration und Behandlung mit Stilboestrol auf Prostatatumoren der Mäuse. Brit. J. Cancer **3**, 211 (1949).

—, and J. W. WHITTICK: The histogenesis of stilboestrol-induced renal tumours in the male golden hamster. Brit. J. Cancer **8**, 451 (1954).

JONGH, S. E. DE, D. J. KOK and L. A. VAN-DER-WOERD: Paradoxe Wirkungen des Follikelhormons bei männlichen Tieren. II. Die Beeinflußbarkeit durch gonadotropes Hormon. Die Beziehungen zur Prostatahypertrophie. Arch. int. Pharmacodyn. **58**, 310 (1938).

— A. QUERIDO and L. A. M. STOLTE: Paradoxical effects of oestrone in male animals. IV. The inhibition of the paradoxical effect by progesterone. Arch. int. Pharmacodyn. **62**, 390 (1939).

KOCH, W.: Zur Ätiologie der Prostatahypertrophie. Münch. med. Wschr. **1936**, Nr. 37; Zbl. allg. Path. path. Anat. **67**, 57 (1937).

KORENCHEVSKY, V., and M. DENNISON: Histological changes in the organs of rats injected with oestrone alone or simultaneously with oestrone and testicular hormone. J. Path. Bact. **41**, 323 (1935).

LACASSAGNE, A.: Metaplasie epidermoïde de la prostata provoquée, chez la souris, par des injections. Répétées de fertes doses de folliculine. C. R. Soc. Biol. (Paris) **113**, 590 (1933).

— Les cancers produits par des substances chimiques endogénes. Paris: Hermann 1950.

—, et E. VILLELA: Processus histologique de la métaplasie epidermoïde des lobes prostatiques postérieurs, chez la souris male folliculinée. C. R. Soc. Biol. (Paris) **114**, 870 (1933).

LERMANDA, V.: El fibromioepitelioma periutricular experimental en presencia del testiculo. Tesis Univ. de Chile 1945 (Public. Dep. Med. Exp. No. 44).

LIPSCHUTZ, A.: Steroid hormones and tumors. Baltimore: Williams & Wilkins Comp. 1950.

— Steroid homeostasis hypophysis and tumorigenesis. Cambridge: Heffer & Sons, Ltd. 1957.

— D. YANINE, J. SCHWARZ, S. BRUZZONE, J. ACUÑA and S. SILBERMAN: Induction and prevention of fibromyoepithelioma of the utricular bed in male guinea pigs. Cancer Res. **5**, 515 (1945).

PARKES, A. S., and S. ZUCKERMAN: Experimental hypoplasie of the prostata. Lancet **228**, 925 (1935); LACASSAGNE: C. R. Soc. Biol. (Paris) **113**, 590 (1933).

RICHTER, W. H.: Morphologisch-experimentelle Untersuchungen zum Problem der Prostatahypertrophie. II. Morphologisch-exper. Teil. Z. Urol. **43**, 185 (1950); 110 (1951).

RÖSSLE, R., u. H. ZAHLER: Experimentelle Untersuchungen über Hoden und Prostataveränderungen durch Zufuhr von Hodenwirkstoffen. Virchows Arch. path. Anat. **302**, H. 2/3 (1938).

ZUCKERMAN, S., and A. S. PARKES: Effect of sex hormones on the prostate of monkeys. Lancet **1936, I**, 242.

— — Inhibitory effect of testosterone propionate on experimental prostatic enlargement. Lancet **1936, II**, 1259.

k) Verschiedenes

QUERNER (1953), WRBA und QUERNER (1953) sahen bei Zahnkarpfen (Lebistes reticulatus) nach Behandlung mit Dehydroisoandrosteronacetat Proliferation des undifferenzierten Zwischengewebes im Kopfgebiet, andere Steroide zeigten diese Veränderungen nicht. GHADIALLY und WHITELEY (1952) beobachteten nach Testosteronbehandlung epitheliale Hyperplasie der Kiemen mit zum Teil papillomatösem Bau.

Literatur

k) Verschiedenes

GHADIALLY, F. N., and H. J. WHITELEY: Hormonally induced epithelial hyperplasia in the Goldfish (Carrasius auratus). Brit. J. Cancer **6**, 246 (1952).

QUERNER, H.: Zellwucherungen nach Applikation eines androgenen Wirkstoffes. Naturwissenschaften **1953**, 466.

WRBA, H., u. H. QUERNER: Auslösung spezifischer Wachstumsvorgänge bei Zahnkarpfen durch androgenes Steroidhormon. Z. Naturforsch. **11**, 5 (1956).

l) Tumoren beim Goldhamster nach Hormonbehandlung

Mit Absicht haben wir die nach Hormonbehandlung beim Goldhamster auftretenden Tumoren getrennt besprochen. Dafür wollen wir zwei Gründe anführen. Bisher nehmen die meisten Autoren bei den Versuchen mit Goldhamstern an, daß es sich um Versuche an einem genetisch einheitlichen Tiermaterial handelt, einzelne Beobachtungen zeigen aber, daß *möglicherweise auch beim Hamster verschiedene noch nicht abgrenzbare Stämme existieren.* So sahen z. B. FORTNER, GEORGE und STERNBERG (1960) bei Experimenten zur Erzeugung von Schilddrüsengeschwülsten (s. Schilddrüse) bei Hamstern von zwei verschiedenen Zuchten ganz unterschiedliche widersprechende Resultate und nahmen an, daß dafür genetische Unterschiede verantwortlich sind. In der gleichen Richtung sind möglicherweise auch die unterschiedlichen Ergebnisse der Arbeiten von KIRKMAN und ROBBINS (1956) einerseits und von RIVIÈRE, CHOUROULINKOV und GUERIN andererseits zu deuten, die bei Behandlung von Hamstern mit Testosteron (subcutante Pelotten von 100 mg Testosteronproprionat alle 6 Monate) sehr unterschiedliche Ergebnisse beobachteten. Während KIRKMAN und ROBBINS Tumoren der Nebenniere, Unterhautsarkome, Pankreascarcinome, Hepatome usw. fanden, beobachteten RIVIÈRE u. Mitarb. bei gleichen Versuchen nur bei einem Tier ein Uterusepitheliom. Der zweite Grund der getrennten Behandlung ist die von anderen Tumoren abweichende unterschiedliche biologische Verhaltensweise der hormonell erzeugten Hamstertumoren.

1952 beschrieben KIRKMAN und BACON Tumoren der Niere, die nach langdauernder Follikelhormonbehandlung bei kastrierten männlichen Goldhamstern auftraten. Die genannten Autoren behandelten kastrierte männliche Goldhamster mit Oestrogen bzw. Stilboestrol. Die Tiere erhielten 0,6 mg Oestrogen in 0,4 cm³ Sesamöl jeden zweiten Tag subcutan injiziert. Die Injektion wurde in der Regel zwischen dem 35. und 77. Lebenstag begonnen. Zum Teil erhielten die Tiere auch subcutane Hormon-Pelotten jeden 3. Monat. Es wurden von den Untersuchern verschiedene Oestrogene injiziert (Oestradiol, Stilboestrol, Äthyloestradiol, Fenocyklin). Tumoren traten nur bei Stilboestrol und Oestradiol auf. Die ersten Tumoren wurden nach 150 Tagen beobachtet. Bei einer Behandlung zwischen 150 und 199 Tagen traten 10% Geschwülste, bei einer Behandlung zwischen 200 und 249 Tagen 60% Geschwülste auf. Bei längerer Behandlung (über 250 Tage) traten bei 97% der Tiere Tumoren auf, wovon 45% eine Aussaat in die Bauchhöhle erkennen ließen. Alle kastrierten Tiere zeigten bis zum 415. Behandlungstag Tumoren und 17% davon Metastasen. Spontane Nierengeschwülste konnten die Untersucher nicht beobachten, insbesondere keine gleichartigen spontanen Nierentumoren.

HORNING (1954, 1956, 1958), HORNING und WHITTICK (1954) bestätigten diese Untersuchungen. Sie sahen bei einseitiger Nierenentfernung eine Beschleunigung des Tumorwachstums. Als Hormonpelotten wurden von ihnen subcutane Verabreichungen von je 20 mg Oestradiol verwandt. Wir selbst haben diese 20 mg Oestradiol in 180 mg Milchzucker gelöst. WARD, PUTCH, MCGREGOR und CHANG untersuchten (1964) mit markiertem Diethylstilboestrol (C14) die Resorption des Hormon bei verschiedenen Hormonpelotten. Die tägliche Hormonaufnahme schwankte zwischen 150 mg und 630 mg.

Die stärkste Ausbeute sahen wir [DONTENWILL und EDER (1957, 1958, 1959)] bei gleichartigen Versuchen nach Behandlung mit Cyren B (Diäthyldioxystilbenpropionat-Bayer, jeden 2. Tag 0,6 mg subcutan bis zu 18 Monate lang), insbesondere bei gleichzeitigerEntfernung der einen Niere. Alle einseitig nephrektomierten Tiere zeigten Tumoren, wenn sie über 8 Monate behandelt worden waren. Bei alleiniger Behandlung mit Cyren B sahen wir in 85% der Fälle Nierengeschwülste nach Behandlung von mindestens 8 Monaten. Bei Behandlung mit Cyren A (Diäthyldioxystilben-Bayer) beobachteten wir bei Tieren, die über 8 Monate behandelt wurden, in 48% der Fälle Tumoren. Die Oestrogene wirken nach KIRKMAN (1959) direkt auf die Niere, da Oestrogenpelotten in die Milz implantiert, keine tumorerzeugende Wirkung zeigen und auch bei hypophysektomierten Tieren

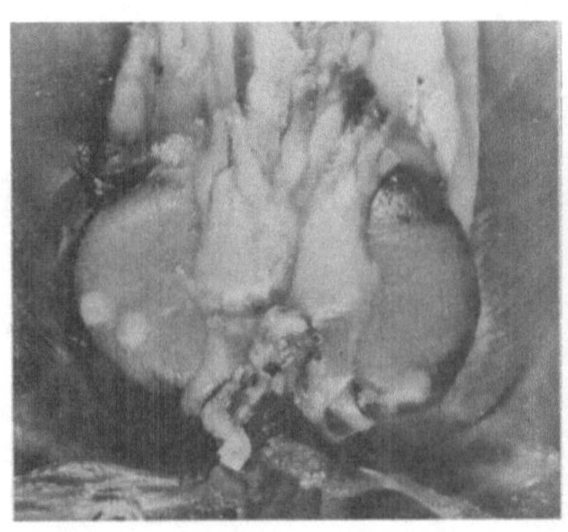
a

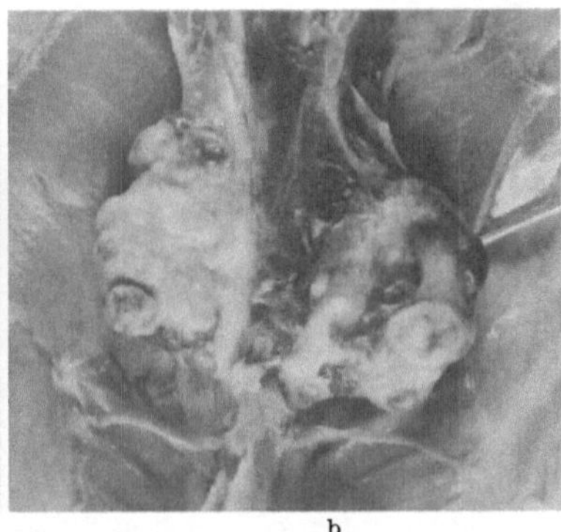
b

Abb. 36a. Einzelne bis stecknadelkopfgroße Tumoren beider Nieren. Behandlung 531 Tage Cyren A. (0,6 mg Cyren jeden 2. Tag)

Abb. 36b. Multiple höckerige Tumoren beider Nieren. Behandlung 531 Tage Cyren A. (0,6 mg Cyren jeden 2. Tag)

kein Tumor entstand. Bei gleichzeitiger Behandlung von kastrierten Hamstern mit einem Carcinogen und mit Follikelhormon (einmalige Injektion von etwa 0,2 cm^3 einer 10%igen öligen Benzpyrenlösung unter die Nierenkapsel einer Niere des Hamsters und gleichzeitige Behandlung mit den oben angeführten Hormondosen) sahen wir, DONTENWILL und RANZ (1960), nie die typischen Nierengeschwülste, die nach alleiniger Hormonbehandlung auftreten. Bei Behandlung mit Carcinogen und bei kombinierter Behandlung sahen wir Sarkome der Niere, die aber bei alleiniger Hormonbehandlung nie beobachtet wurden. Für die von KIRKMANN erstmals beschriebene typische geschwulstauslösende Wirkung des Oestradiols auf die Goldhamsterniere ist wie früher auch SCHÜMMELFEDER und GIMMY (1964) betonten, sicherlich nicht die chemische Ähnlichkeit mit den Cancerogenen verantwortlich zu machen, sondern die spezifische hormonelle Stoffwechselwirkung dieser Substanz, denn auch die oestrogenen Stilbene, die zu den cancerogenen Kohlenwasserstoffen keine strukturelle Beziehung besitzen, haben an der Niere des Goldhamsters den gleichen tumorauslösenden Effekt.

Bei inzwischen untersuchten Tieren (etwa 2000 Hamster) konnten wir nie Spontangeschwülste der Niere nachweisen, dagegen vereinzelt Sarkome u. a. der Extremitäten und Angiome der Milz, Adenocarcinome der Lunge, des Pankreas und der Leber. Die Nierentumorentstehung konnte weder durch Hepatektomie noch durch gleichzeitige Behandlung mit verschiedenen Carcinogenen wesentlich beeinflußt werden (gleichzeitige Behandlung mit Cyren B und mit Acetaminofluoren etwa 5 mg pro die oder mit Dimethylaminoazobenzol in gleicher Dosierung. Die Carcinogene wurden im Futter eingebacken).

Die Geschwülste der Nieren zeigen, wie bereits KIRKMAN (1957) und HORNING (1954, 1956, 1958) nachweisen konnten, ein eigenartiges Verhalten bei der *Trans-*

plantation. Transplantierte Tumoren wachsen nur bei kastrierten, gleichzeitig mit Follikelhormon behandelten Tieren. Sie wachsen sehr langsam, und nur bei hoch-

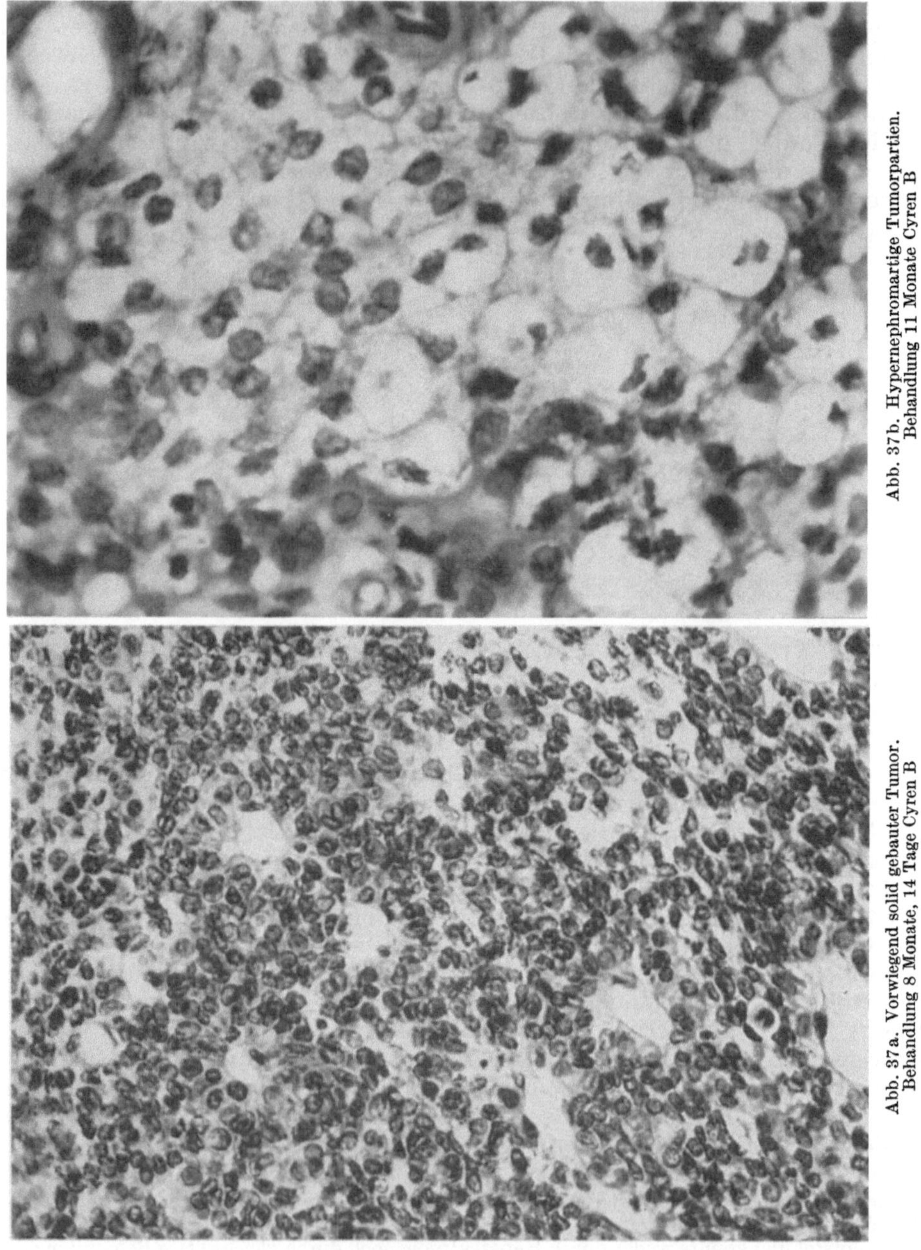

Abb. 37b. Hypernephromartige Tumorpartien. Behandlung 11 Monate Cyren B

Abb. 37a. Vorwiegend solid gebauter Tumor. Behandlung 8 Monate, 14 Tage Cyren B

dosierter Hormonbehandlung und gleichzeitiger Kastration konnten wir das Angehen der Geschwülste beschleunigen. Erst nach etwa 14 Passagen sah Kirkman (1957) eine unabhängige Wucherung des transplantierten Tumors, er spricht dann vom Übergang von der Abhängigkeit zur Autonomie.

Die Geschwülste zeigten eine recht unterschiedliche Struktur. Kleine Geschwülste bestanden meist aus solid angeordneten, zwischen den Tubuli gelagerten, ziemlich regelmäßig gebauten, ovalen Zellen (Abb. 39a u. b) in größeren

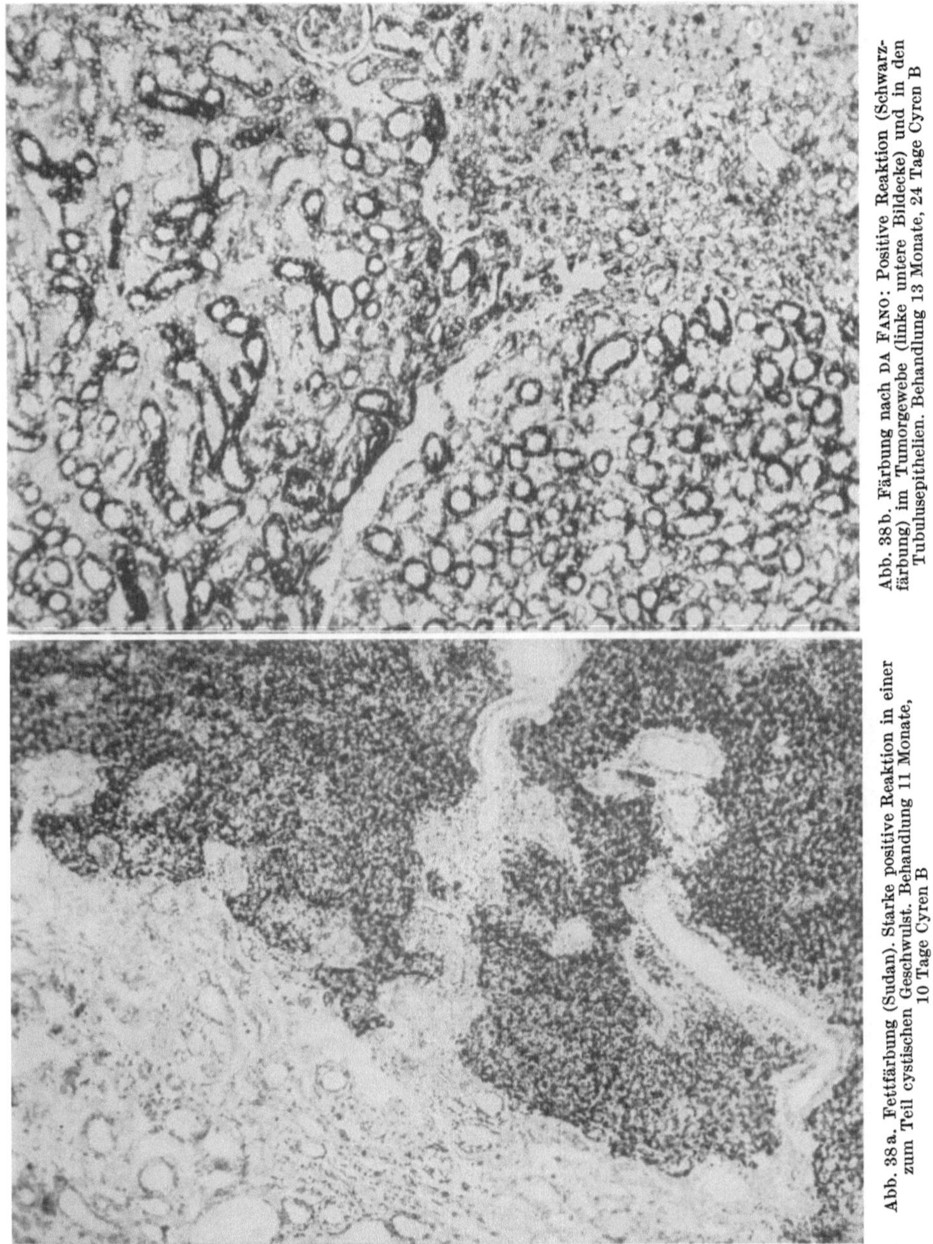

Abb. 38b. Färbung nach DA FANO: Positive Reaktion (Schwarzfärbung) im Tumorgewebe (linke untere Bildecke) und in den Tubulusepithelien. Behandlung 13 Monate, 24 Tage Cyren B

Abb. 38a. Fettfärbung (Sudan). Starke positive Reaktion in einer zum Teil cystischen Geschwulst. Behandlung 11 Monate, 10 Tage Cyren B

Geschwülsten fanden sich rosettenförmige, tubuläre und z. T. hypernephromartige Zellstrukturen. Diese protoplasmareichen Zellen enthalten reichlich doppelbrechende Lipoide (Abb. 38a). Die kleinen Tumorknoten wachsen zwischen den intakten Tubuli (Abb. 39a u. b), ein infiltratives Wachstum ist erst später erkennbar, und nur große Knoten zeigten nach blutigen Nekrosen und nach dem Durchbruch durch die Kapsel peritoneale und gelegentlich kleinste Absiedelungen in

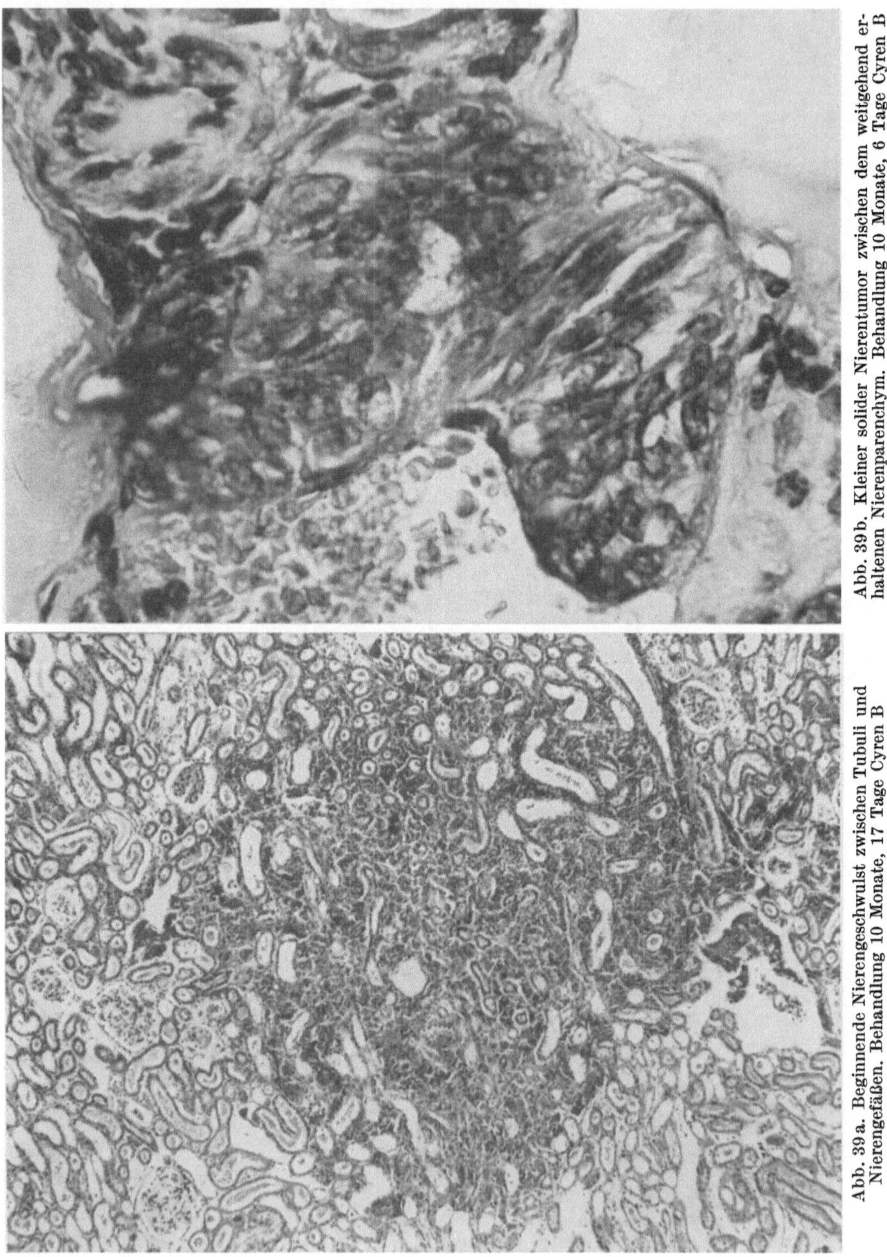

Abb. 39b. Kleiner solider Nierentumor zwischen dem weitgehend erhaltenen Nierenparenchym. Behandlung 10 Monate, 6 Tage Cyren B

Abb. 39a. Beginnende Nierengeschwulst zwischen Tubuli und Nierengefäßen. Behandlung 10 Monate, 17 Tage Cyren B

Lunge und Leber. Die Tumorzellen verhalten sich histochemisch (Da Fano-Reaktion) wie die Schaltstückepithelien und z. T. wie die Zellen des Hypernephroms beim Menschen (Abb. 38b) (FEYRTER), sie enthalten reichlich alkalische und saure Phosphatase. Bei den engen räumlichen Beziehungen, besonders der kleinen Nierengeschwülste zu den Schaltstückepithelien und auf Grund des bei der histochemischen Untersuchung gleichen Verhaltens, erscheint es uns sicher, daß sich die Nierengeschwülste aus dem intertubulären Keimlager der Schaltstückepithelien entwickeln. Autoradiographische Untersuchungen (mit H 3 Thymidin) während der Entstehung der Nierentumoren zeigen, daß die Zellvermehrung im Bereich der Schaltstückepithelien beginnt [DONTENWILL (1966)], die Tumoren also offenbar aus dem Schaltstückepithel entstehen. Diese Vorstellung wird auch von BOSCH (1963) geteilt.

In der Regel gehen die Geschwülste erst nach einer längeren Schlummerperiode an [HORNING (1958)]. Durch gleichzeitige Behandlung mit Desoxycorticosteron oder Progesteron konnte das Angehen der Transplantate gehemmt werden [KIRKMAN (1957)]. Uns [DONTENWILL und RANZ (1960)] gelang es durch gleichzeitige Wachstumshormonbehandlung nicht, das transplantierte Geschwulstgewebe zum Anwachsen zu bringen, obwohl der Wachstumseffekt an einer starken allgemeinen Gewichtszunahme der Tiere sichtbar wurde. Cortisonbehandlung fördert zwar nach KIRKMAN (1959) das Auftreten von Tumoren, kann aber allein das Wachstum der Transplantate nicht unterhalten.

KIRKMAN (1957) und wir sahen auch beim Wachstum eine deutliche Abhängigkeit vom Hormon. Nach Absetzen des Hormons fand KIRKMAN einen Rückgang der Tumoren. Nach einer Unterbrechung der Behandlung von 200 Tagen wuchsen diese erneut weiter. Ersetzte KIRKMAN (1957) die Oestrogengaben durch Testosteron, sah er zwar ein Weiterwachsen der Tumoren, aber kein Auftreten neuer Geschwülste. Wir beobachteten nach Unterbrechung der Hormonzufuhr eine Verkleinerung der Geschwulst bei der Kontrolle durch Laparotomie.

Eine Hormonbehandlung wirkt nur dann nach KIRKMAN (1957) nicht tumorerzeugend, wenn das Hormon in die Milz implantiert wird oder wenn beim hypophysektomierten Tier Hormon zugeführt wird. Bei gleichzeitiger Behandlung von Goldhamstern mit Oestrogen und Desoxycorticosteron bzw. Progesteron entstanden keine Tumoren. Cortison hatte dagegen keinen Effekt auf die Tumorentstehung.

KIRKMAN (1957) gelang es auch, Geschwülste bei weiblichen Tieren zu erzeugen unter folgenden Bedingungen:

1. Bei Ovarektomierten nach Behandlung durch Diäthylstilboestrol.
2. Bei Beginn der Behandlung am niedersten Punkte der Progesteronsekretion des Metoestrums.
3. Bei Behandlungsbeginn in den ersten 5 Tagen des Lebens.
4. Wenn die Hypophyse des Neugeborenen mit Androgen maskulinisiert (15 Tage) und dann eine Oestrogenbehandlung angeschlossen wurde.

Wenn die maskulinisierten Tiere einen Cyclus bekommen, genügt das endogene Oestrogen zur Tumorentstehung. In allen Versuchen konnten die gleichen Ergebnisse erzielt werden, es zeigte sich immer eine bestimmte Abhängigkeit des Tumors in Entstehung, Wachstum und Transplantation von einer bestimmten hormonalen Ausgangslage. Lediglich die Nephrektomie oder wie ISING 1956 zeigen konnte, die Unterbindung des Ureters, konnten durch eine gleichzeitige stärkere Proliferation des Nierengewebes die Tumorentstehung beschleunigen. Nach KIRKMAN (1959) erleichtert die traumatische Schädigung der Niere die Induktion von Tumoren, sie entstehen auch in Nierenfragmenten neugeborener Tiere.

Bei der Untersuchung des Tumorgewebes in bezug auf Atmung und Glykolyse zeigten die Geschwülste Werte, die für einen gutartigen Tumor sprechen [BÜNGELER und DONTENWILL (1959)].

Auch beim Wachstum des Nierentumors in der *Gewebekultur* fanden wir [DONTENWILL und WRBA (1959)], eine weitgehende Abhängigkeit von der hormonellen Stimulierung (Abb. 40a u. b). Bei mit wasserlöslichem Oestrogensulfat behandelten Gewebskulturen zeigt sich, ebenso wie bei Behandlung mit Serum follikelhormonbehandelter Goldhamster, eine Stimulierung der im Mittelstück der

Kultur liegenden Tumorzellen, während ohne Oestrogenzufuhr sich das aus Tumorzellen bestehende Mittelstück auflockert und allmählich degeneriert.

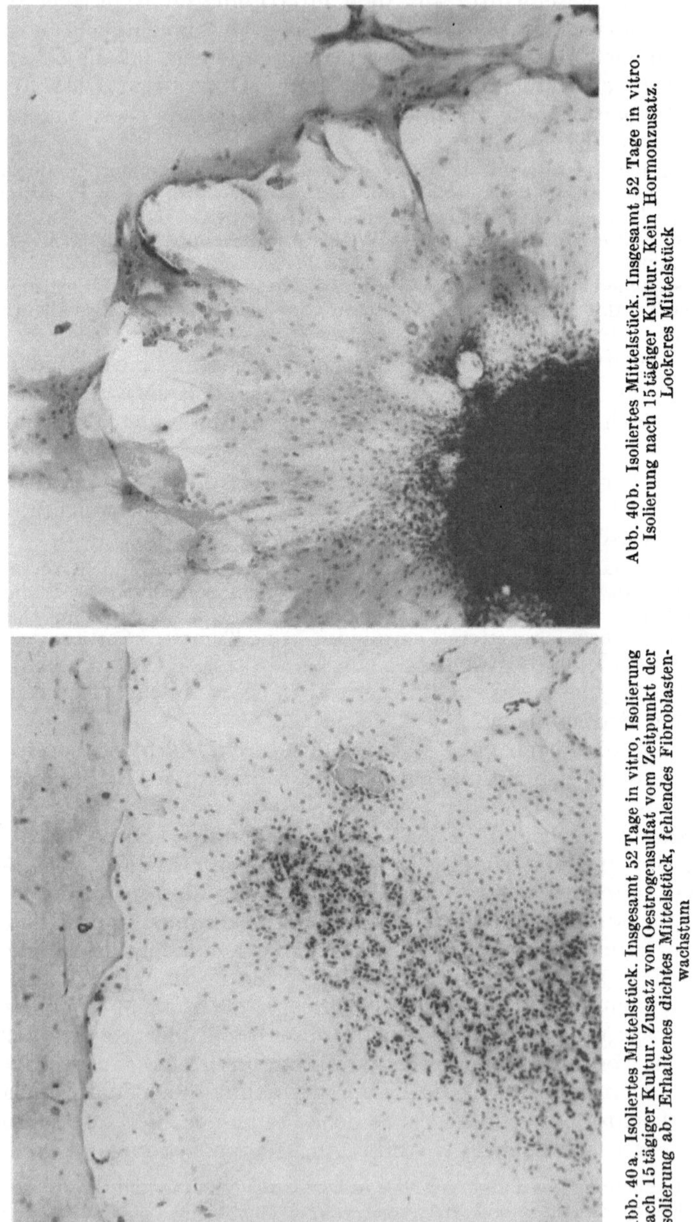

Abb. 40a. Isoliertes Mittelstück. Insgesamt 52 Tage in vitro, Isolierung nach 15tägiger Kultur. Zusatz von Oestrogensulfat vom Zeitpunkt der Isolierung ab. Erhaltenes dichtes Mittelstück, fehlendes Fibroblastenwachstum

Abb. 40b. Isoliertes Mittelstück. Insgesamt 52 Tage in vitro. Isolierung nach 15tägiger Kultur. Kein Hormonzusatz. Lockeres Mittelstück

KIRKMAN (1957) sah bei Behandlung von Goldhamstern mit Oestrogen und Androgen, nicht dagegen mit Oestrogen allein, Fibromyome des Uterus und Leiomyome bzw. Leiomyosarkome des Samenstranges. Die Tiere erhielten subcutane Implantate von Stilboestrolpellets à 20 mg und Testosteron-Proprionatpellets à 30 mg. Die tägliche Absorption von Stilboestrol betrug 0,11 mg und von Testosteronproprionat 0,15 mg. Die beiden Tumorarten sind also nur transplantabel bei gleichzeitiger Hormonbehandlung. KIRKMAN und ALGARD berichten 1965 über weitere Studien an dem hormonabhängigen Leiomyosarkom des Ductus deferens. Annähernd 100% der mit beiden Hormonen behandelten Hamster zeigten Leiomyosarkome mit fasciculärem Aufbau der Zellen. Hypophysektomie konnte die Entstehung der Tumoren nicht verhindern. Auch in der 60. Passage waren die Tumoren bei der Transplantation noch hormonabhängig. Die Latenzperiode nahm bei der Transplantation allmählich ab (von 200 zu 40 Tagen). Die Hormonabhängigkeit konnte in der Gewebekultur (Algard) nicht reproduziert werden. Die beim Hamster auch spontan auftretenden Basalzellenepitheliome sind in der Regel klein, bei Behandlung mit Oestrogen und Testosteron werden sie größer und manchmal metastasieren sie. Progesteron kann die Entstehung dieser Geschwülste nicht verhindern. KIRKMAN und ALGARD (1964) unterschieden drei Stadien bei der Entstehung der Basalzellepitheliome.

1. Das Wachstum der Haar-Matrix-Zellen in die Hautschichten und Hautpapillen mit Bildung von Knoten, die von Bindegewebslamellen umgeben werden. Diese Knötchen kommen normalerweise nur bei Männchen im Alter von 185 und mehr Tagen vor, nicht bei Weibchen. Sie erfordern das Vorhandensein von Androgen und werden durch Oestrogen verhindert.

2. Unter dem Einfluß von exogenem Androgen nehmen die Knötchen an Größe zu und verschmelzen durch die Wirkung von Androgen und Oestrogen zu größeren Knoten.

Das Chaetepitheliom (Basalzellepitheliom) metastasierte, war aber auch nach 21 Passagen immer noch hormonabhängig. Eine spezifische Hormonabhängigkeit des Gewebes wird zusammen mit der „hormonalen imbalance" als entscheidende Ursache angesehen [ALGARD, DODGE und KIRKMAN (1964)]. RIVIÈRE, CHOUROULINKOV und GUÉRIN (1960, 1961) sahen nach kombinierter Testosteron- und Oestrogenbehandlung von Goldhamstern (alle 5 Monate subcutane Pelotten von je 100 mg Testosteronproprionat und 25 mg Diäthylstilboestroldiproprionat) ebenfalls Tumoren der Muskulatur des Nebenhodens und des Uterus. Einzelne der z. T. als Leiomyosarkome bezeichneten Tumoren zeigten Metastasen in den Lungen. VASQUEZ-LOPEZ beschrieb 1944 ein metastasierendes Carcinom des Nebenhodens nach Oestrogenbehandlung.

Nach langdauernder Behandlung männlicher, z. T. kastrierter Goldhamster mit Follikelhormon (jeden 2. Tag 0,6 mg Cyren B subcutan) hatten wir nach etwa einem Jahr neben Nierentumoren [DONTENWILL und EDER (1958)] z. T. cystische Gallengangswucherungen beobachtet (Abb. 41).

Nach Oestrogenbehandlung bzw. Implantation von Hypophysentumoren haben bereits GARDNER, ALLEN und SMITH (1941) sowie FURTH, GADSDEN und UPTON (1952) Gallengangswucherungen und -erweiterungen beschrieben, bei deren Entstehung sie eine vermehrte Stimulierung der Hypophyse annahmen. Unsere anfängliche Vermutung, daß bei der hormonellen Dysregulation, die nach chronischer Follikelhormonbehandlung auftritt, eine vermehrte Ausschüttung von Wachstumshormon zu Gallengangswucherungen führt, konnte durch langdauernde Behandlung mit STH bei Goldhamstern nicht bestätigt werden [DONTENWILL und RANZ; tgl. 1 mg STH über 4 Monate (1960)].

Gallengangswucherungen konnten wir [DONTENWILL und MOHR (1961)] auch nach Fütterung von Acetaminofluoren (tgl. 5 mg im Futter eingebacken über etwa 10—12 Monate) beobachten. Wir nehmen deswegen an, daß beide Stoffe (Cyren B und Acetaminofluoren) am gleichen Zellsystem angreifen. Die Tab. 3 läßt deutlich erkennen, daß die Veränderungen nur beim Hamster auftreten und bei gleichartiger Behandlung von Hamstern und Ratten völlig verschiedenartige Zellproliferationen beobachtet werden. Bei kombinierter Behandlung mit Cyren B und

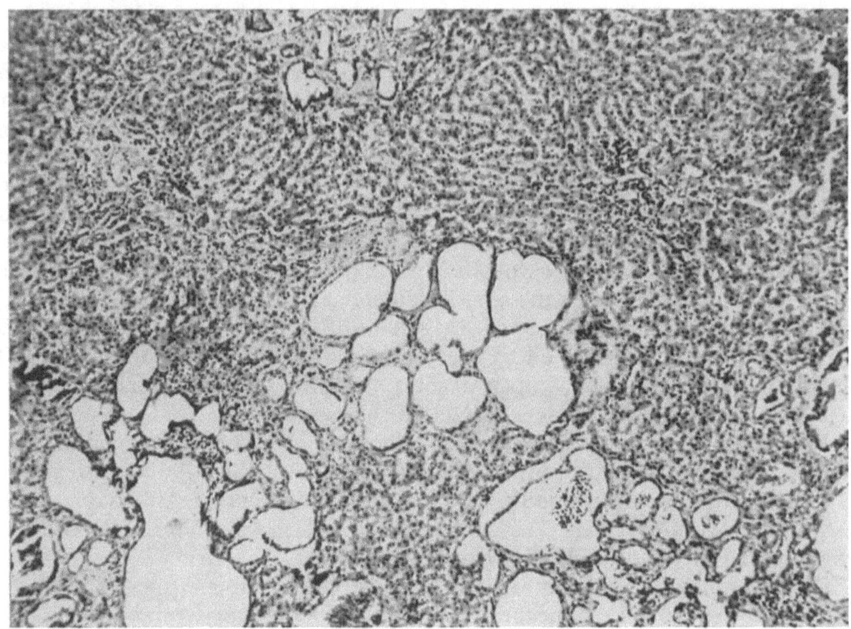

Abb. 41. Einzelne cystische Gallengangswucherungen nach Behandlung von Goldhamstern mit Cyren B (jeden 2. Tag 0,6 mg 14 Monate lang)

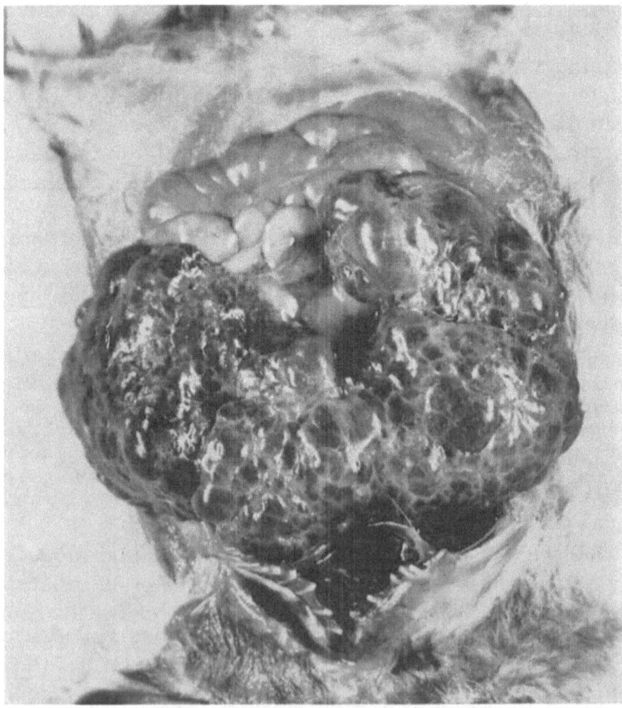

Abb. 42a

Acetaminofluoren (jeden 2. Tag 0,6 mg Cyren B subcutan und täglich etwa 5 mg Acetaminofluoren im Futter eingebacken), treten Veränderungen auf, die fast einem Cystadenopapillom glichen. Die Leber war maximal vergrößert und bestand in der Regel nur noch aus dichtstehenden, cystisch erweiterten Gallengängen, die

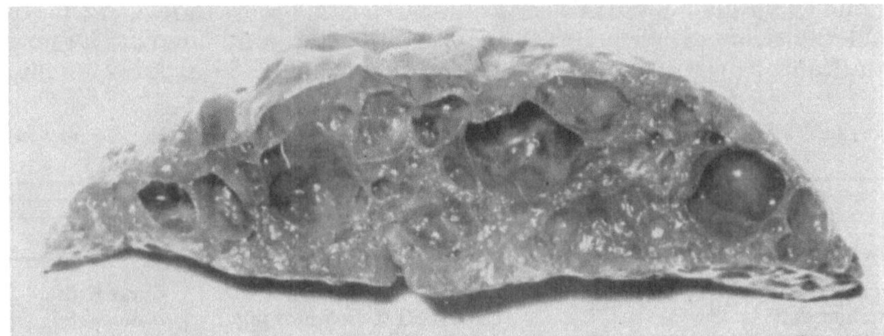

Abb. 42 b

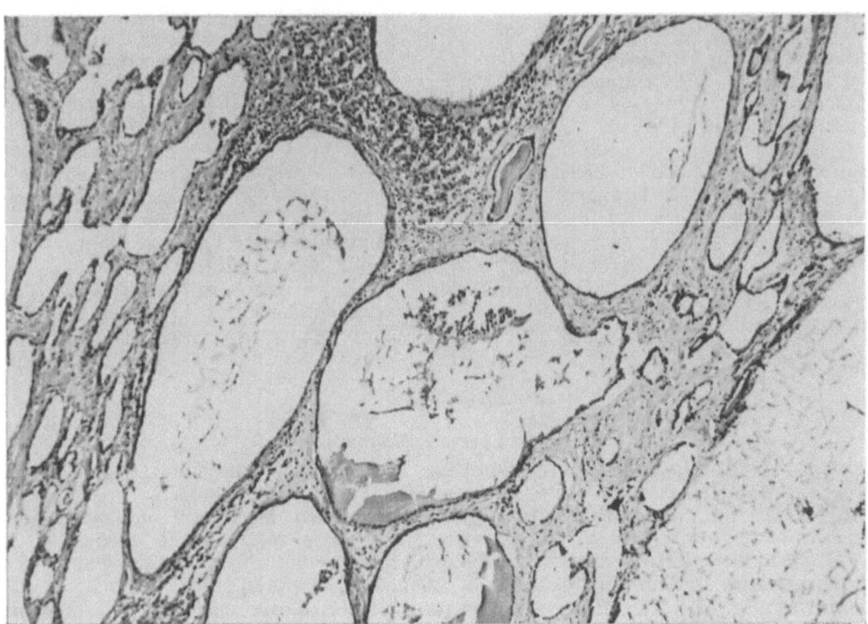

Abb. 42 c

Abb. 42a—c. Grobcystische Leberdystrophie mit Bildung von cystopapillären Gallengangswucherungen. Behandlung 10 Monate jeden 2. Tag 0,6 mg Cyren B und täglich im Futter 5 mg Acetaminofluoren

adenomartig nebeneinander gelagert waren. Die Leber füllte den ganzen Bauchraum aus (Abb. 42a—c), das Leberparenchym selbst war hochgradig vermindert (Abb. 42c). Testosteronbehandlung (2 mg Testosteronproprionat pro Woche) hemmt die Entstehung von Cysten der Gallengänge. Auch bei kombinierter Behandlung von Goldhamstern mit Cyren bzw. Testosteron und Diäthylnitrosamin sahen wir ähnliche Ergebnisse, d. h. das Follikelhormon fördert die bei der Carcinogenwirkung auftretende Cystenbildung der Gallengänge. Testosteron hemmt diese Cystenbildung. Das Follikelhormon ist aber nicht in der Lage, die fehlende Carcinogenwirkung des Dimethylaminoazobenzols und Acetaminofluorens auf die Hamsterleber zu beeinflussen. Auch bei zusätzlicher Follikelhormonbehandlung erzeugten diese Carcinogene keine Lebertumoren. Die proliferationssteigernde Wirkung des Follikelhormons fehlt bei der durch Diäthylnitrosamin [DONTENWILL und MOHR (1961)] ausgelösten Carcinogenese am Bronchialepithel. Das Follikelhormon kann also nur dann kocarcinogen wirken, wenn es auch normalerweise am gleichen Gewebe proliferationsfördernd angreift. Es potenziert die am Gallengangssystem angreifende Wirkung, z. B. die des Acetaminofluorens.

Tabelle 3. *Vergleichende Wirkung von Hormonen und Carcinogenen auf die Ratten- und Hamsterleber*

← Ratte →		← Hamster →	
Ergebnisse aus der Literatur		Eigene Untersuchungen	
Eiweißarme Diät (Cirrhosediät)	Lebercirrhose	Cirrhosediät	ohne Erfolg
		STH-Behandlung	ohne Erfolg
Acetaminofluoren Diäthylnitrosamin Dimethylaminoazobenzol	Cirrhosen und Carcinome	CCl_4-Behandlung	Cirrhosen
		Dimethylaminoazobenzol	keine Cirrhosen
Acetaminofluoren oder Dimethyl aminoazobenzol + Follikelhormon	Förderung der Carcinomentstehung	Diäthylnitrosamin	schwerste Dystrophie Cirrhose m. Lebercarcinome (Bronchialcarcinome)
		Acetaminofluoren	Cirrhosen mit Gallengangscysten
Cyren B allein	keine Leberveränderungen	Cyren B	Cirrhosen mit Gallengangswucherungen Nierentumoren
		Acetaminofluoren + Cyren B	*Cystenleber* Nierentumoren
		Acetaminofluoren + Testosteron	Cirrhosen mit wenig Cysten

Literatur

l) Tumoren beim Goldhamster etc.

ALGARD, F. T.: Hormonal induzierte Tumoren. I. Geschwülste des Flank-Organs und der Niere des Hamsters in vivo. J. nat. Cancer Inst. **25**, 557—571 (1960).

— Characteristics of an androgen/estrogen-induced dependent leiomyosarcoma of the ductus deferens of the syrian hamster. II. In vitro. Cancer Res. **25**, 147—151 (1965).

— A. H. DODGE, and H. KIRKMAN: Development of the flank organ (scent gland) of the syrian hamster. I. Embryology. Amer. J. Anat. **114**, 435—455 (1964).

BIELSCHOWSKY, F., and E. S. HORNING: Aspects of endocrine carcinogenesis. Brit. med. Bull. **14**, 106 (1958).

BOSCH, L. A.: Estudios experimentales sobre oncogénesis: La accion del tetracloruro de carbono y estradiol en el desarrollo de los tumores renales malignos del hamster dorado. Archivo espanol de morfologia, tesis doctoral, Valencia 1964.

BÜNGELER, W., u. W. DONTENWILL: Hormonell ausgelöste geschwulstartige Hyperplasien, hyperplasiogene Geschwülste und ihre Verhaltensweisen. Dtsch. med. Wschr. **1959**, 1885.

DONTENWILL, W.: Experimentelle Erzeugung von Nieren- und Lebertumoren durch Follikelhormon. Verh. dtsch. Ges. Path. **42**, 457 (1958).

— Die endokrinen Regulationen hyperplastischer und maligner Gewebsproliferationen. Verh. dtsch. Ges. Path. 45. Tag. Münster 74 (1961).

— Die Bedeutung der Hormone für die Geschwulstentstehung. Zbl. Gynäk. **83**, 1704 (1961).

—, u. M. EDER: Neue Befunde über Geschwulstbildungen nach Follikelhormonbehandlung beim Goldhamster. Naturwissenschaften **1957**, 591.

— — Histogenese und biologische Verhaltensweise hormonell ausgelöster Geschwülste. Beitr. path. Anat. **120**, 270 (1959).

DONTENWILL, W., u. W. MOHR: Cystische Leberdystrophie beim Goldhamster im Experiment. Klin. Wschr. **1961**, 593.

— — Proliferationsfördernde und hemmende Wirkung der Geschlechtshormone bei Behandlung von Goldhamstern mit Carcinogenen. Z. Krebsforsch. **64**, 381 (1961).

— — Die unterschiedliche lungencarcinogene Wirkung des Diäthylnitrosamin bei Hamster und Ratte. Z. Krebsforsch. **64**, 499 (1962).

— — Experimentelle Erzeugung metastasierender Strumen nach Behandlung von Goldhamstern mit Tabakrauchkondensaten. Z. Krebsforsch. **65**, 69 (1962).

—, u. H. RANZ: Untersuchungen über die hormonale Abhängigkeit des durch Follikelhormon erzeugten Nierentumors des Goldhamsters bei der Transplantation. Klin. Wschr. **1960**, 828.

— — Experimentelle Untersuchungen zur Genese von Nierengeschwülsten beim Goldhamster. Beitr. path. Anat. **122**, 381 (1960).

—, u. H. WRBA: Das Wachstum des durch Oestrogene erzeugten Nierentumors beim Goldhamster in der Gewebekultur. Beitr. path. Anat. **121**, 301 (1959).

— — Die spezifische Wirkung von Oestrogensulfat auf Gewebekulturen eines hormoninduzierten Nierentumors beim Goldhamster. Klin. Wschr. **1959**, 727.

FORTNER, J. G., P. A. GEORGE, and S. S. STERNBERG: Induced and spontaneous thyroid cancer in the Syrian (golden) hamster. Endocrinology **66**, 364 (**1960**).

FURTH, J., E. L. GADSDEN and A. C. UPTON: Hyperplasia and cystic dilation of extrahepatic biliary tracts in mice bearing grafted pituitary growths. Cancer. Res. **12**, 739—743 (1952).

HORNING, E. S.: The influence of unilateral nephrectomy on the development of stilboestrol-induced renal tumours in the male hamster. Brit. J. Cancer **8**, 627 (1954).

— Endocrine factors involved in the induction, prevention and transplantation of kidney tumours in the male golden hamster. Z. Krebsforsch. **61**, 1 (1956).

— Observations on hormone-dependent renal tumours in the golden hamster. Brit. J. Cancer **10**, 678 (1956).

— Induction of pituitary tumors and melanomas in the golden hamster. In: G. E. W. WOLSTENHOLME and M. O'CONNOR (eds.); Ciba Found. Coll. Endocr. **12**, 22—29 (1958); London: J. & A. Churchill, Ltd. 1958.

—, and J. W. WHITTICK: The histogenesis of stilboestrol-induced renal tumours in the male golden hamster. Brit. J. Cancer **8**, 451 (1954).

ISING, U.: The effect of unilateral ureterectomy on the development of estrogen-induced renal tumours in male hamsters. Acta path. microbiol. scand. **39**, 188 (1956).

KIRKMAN, H.: Steroid tumorigenesis. Cancer (Philad.) **10**, 754 (1957).

— Estrogen-induced tumors of the kidney in the syrian hamster. National Cancer Institute Monograph. Nr. 1/1959.

—, and F. TH. ALGARD: Androgen-Estrogen-induced tumors. I. The flank organ(scent gland) chaetepithelioma of the syrian hamster. Cancer Res. **24**, 1569—1593 (1964).

— — Characteristics of an androgen/estrogen-induced dependent leiomyosarcoma of the ductus deferens of the syrian hamster. I. In vivo. Cancer Res. **25**, 141—145 (1965).

— — Malignant renal tumors in male hamsters (cricetus auratus) treated with estrogen. Cancer Res. **10**, 122 (1950).

—, and R. L. BACON: Estrogen-induced tumors of the kidney. I. Incidence of renal tumors of intact and gonadectomized male golden hamsters treated with diethylstilbestrol. J. nat. Cancer Inst. **13**, 745—755 (1952).

— — Estrogen-induced tumors of the kidney. II. Effect of dose, administration, type of estrogen, and age on the induction of renal tumors in intact male golden hamsters. J. nat. Cancer Inst. **13**, 757 (1952).

RIVIÈRE, M. R., I. CHOUROULINKOV et M. GUÉRIN: Actions hormonales experimentales de longue durée chez le hamster du poit de vue de leur effet cancerigene. Bull. Cancer (Franc.) **48**, 499 (1961); **47**, 557 (1960).

— — — Actions hormonales expérimentales de longue durée chez le hamster du point de vue de leur effet cancérigène. I. Etude de la Testostérone. Extrait Bull. Cancer **47**, 557—564 (1960).

— — — Actions hormonales experimentales de longue durée chez le hamster du point de vue de leur effet cancérigène. II. Etude de la testostérone associée à un oestrogène. Extrait Bull. Cancer **48**, 499—525 (1961).

SCHÜMMELFEDER, N., u. J. GIMMY: Zur Ätiologie und Pathogenese des Krebses. Münchn. Med. Wschr. **106**, 1—11 (1964).

VASQUEZ-LOPEZ, E.: The relation of the pituitary gland and related hypothalamic centres, in the hamster to prolonged treatment with oestrogens. J. Path. Bact. **56**, 1 (1944).

WARD, D. N., J. D. PUTCH, R. F. MCGREGOR, and J. P. CHANG: Estrogen-induced kidney tumors in the golden hamster. II. Diethylstilbestrol absorption and distribution in tissues. Cancer Res. **24**, 319—326 (1964).

II. Erzeugung bösartiger Geschwülste
(Carcinome und Sarkome)

Einleitung

Hormone werden nur von einzelnen Autoren als sog. Vollcarcinogene bezeichnet, d. h. als Stoffe, die allein, ohne Mithilfe anderer Faktoren in der Lage sind, Carcinome zu erzeugen. Von einem Vollcarcinogen können wir nur sprechen, wenn es carcinomauslösend ist, auch bei nicht krebsbelasteten Tierstämmen und ohne Mithilfe sog. Cocarcinogene.

Nach GARDNER (1957) unterscheiden sich Hormone von anderen Carcinogenen dadurch, daß sie

1. nur in bestimmten Organen Carcinome erzeugen,
2. daß die Hormonempfindlichkeit möglicherweise genetisch festgelegt ist.

Es zeigen sich also in bezug auf Carcinomhäufigkeit und Lokalisation starke Stammesunterschiede bei den einzelnen Tierarten, was besonders beim Mammacarcinom deutlich wird. Nach seiner Ansicht (GARDNER) ist das Follikelhormon unter den Hormonen der am meisten carcinogene Stoff. KIRSCHBAUM (1957) hält die carcinogene Potenz der Oestrogene für gesichert, während er die Androgene und die Nebennierenrindenhormone als nicht cancerogen bezeichnet. Nach seiner Ansicht ist das Zusammenwirken von Viren, chemischen Cancerogenen und Hormonen erwiesen, alleinige Tumorentstehung durch ein Hormon aber die Ausnahme. Die genetisch festgelegte Gewebsempfindlichkeit, die auch GARDNER (1957) annimmt, kann möglicherweise durch Hormone beeinflußt werden, d. h. offenbar ist das gestörte hormonelle Gleichgewicht, [s. auch LIPSCHUTZ (1950)], ein wesentlicher Faktor. Nach LACASSAGNE (1950) stellen die Hormone, wenn sie kontinuierlich wirken, endogene Gifte dar, die viel öfter Gelegenheit haben, wirksam zu werden, als die gelegentlich wirksamen exogenen chemischen Ursachen, die Krebs erzeugen. Bei allen Überlegungen wird der exakte Nachweis einer vollcarcinogenen Wirkung der Hormone, insbesondere der Oestrogene, immer davon abhängig sein, ob genetische Faktoren mitwirken und ob es sich bei den Neubildungen oder hormonell gesteuerten Gewebsproliferationen wirklich um biologisch bösartige Veränderungen handelt. Wenn eine genetische Disposition der Tierstämme oder der Organe bei hormoneller Einwirkung häufiger zur Carcinomentstehung führt, oder wenn ein überschüssiger Proliferationsreiz ein hormonell gesteuertes Organ oder Gewebe wuchern läßt, ist das nicht immer ein Beweis einer echten cancerogenen Wirkung, bzw. mit der Wirkung eines Vollcancerogens gleichzusetzen.

Bei der Wirkung der Hormone auf die Geschwülste müssen wir also immer unterscheiden zwischen der allein krebsauslösenden und der die Krebsentstehung oder das Krebswachstum fördernden oder hemmenden Wirkung der Hormone.

A. Durch Hormone allein

Im folgenden Abschnitt soll im wesentlichen die Wirkung der natürlichen Hormone, bzw. die Bedeutung endogen-hormoneller Faktoren für die Tumorentstehung und das Tumorwachstum besprochen werden.

BIELKA, BIERWOLF, GRAFFI und SCHRAMM (1966) haben ausführlich über Stilbenderivate berichtet, bei denen die „carcinogene Wirkung unmittelbar erfolgt und nicht auf indirektem Wege, wie etwa über die oestrogenen Eigenschaften der betreffenden Substanzen". Die Unterscheidung erscheint uns außerordentlich wichtig, wie wir bereits eingangs am Beispiel der Nierentumorenentstehung beim Goldhamster nach Behandlung mit Stilboestrol erwähnten. Für die geschwulstauslösende Wirkung des Stilboestrol auf die Goldhamsterniere und auf andere

Gewebe des Hamsters ist sicherlich die spezifische hormonelle Stoffwechselwirkung der Substanz ausschlaggebend [SCHÜMMELFEDER und GIMMY (1964)]. Beim Nierentumor des Goldhamsters handelt es sich außerdem, ebenso wie beim Leiomyosarkom um "dependent tumors" die in ihrer biologischen Verhaltensweise gegenüber den typischen Carcinomen und Sarkomen Unterschiede zeigen.

Die Frage, ob durch endogene Stoffwechselstörungen aus natürlichen Hormonen carcinogene Substanzen entstehen können, ist bisher noch nicht geklärt. Eine Reihe künstlicher Oestrogene [DANNENBERG (1963)] und krebserzeugender Amine haben das gleiche aromatische Grundskelet, unterscheiden sich aber durch ihre funktionellen Gruppen. Die Hydrozylgruppen bedingen oestrogene, die Aminogruppen carcinogene Wirkung. DANNENBERG (1963) konnte bei den den natürlichen Oestrogenen nahestehenden Aminoverbindungen nie oestrogene oder oestrushemmende Wirkung nachweisen. (Literatur über Stilbene im Kapitel BIELKA, BIERWOLF, GRAFFI und SCHRAMM.) Ob Hormone schwache Carcinogene [HADDOW, HARRIS, KOH und ROE (1948)] oder nur bedingte Carcinogene (BUTENANDT), bzw. cocarcinogene Substanzen sind, ist weiter umstritten, hängt aber von der Definition der angeführten Begriffe ab. Die krebsfördernde Wirkung der Hormone wäre auf mehreren Wegen denkbar.

1. Durch Proliferationssteigerung, bzw. Erhöhung des Zellumsatzes, ähnlich wie bei anderen Hyperplasiogenen oder Cocarcinogenen.

2. Durch Veränderung an der genetischen Substanz im Sinne von DANNENBERG (1963). Durch die proliferationsfördernde Wirkung entsteht eine Entspiralisierung, bzw. eine Auflockerung der DNS (puffing), die das Eindringen, bzw. Wirksamwerden carcinogener Noxen begünstigt. Die hormonelle Wirkung fördert die Reaktionsbereitschaft der Zelle zur malignen Transformation.

3. Steroide hemmen möglicherweise die Interferonbildung und begünstigen so das Angreifen von onkogenen Viren.

a) Uterus

LOEB, BURNS, SUNTZEFF und MOSKOP (1936) sahen carcinomähnliche Proliferation in der Vagina, der Cervix und im Uterus von Mäusen, die langdauernd mit Oestrogenen behandelt wurden. Sie bezeichnen diese Proliferationen als carcinomähnliche oder präcanceröse Veränderungen.

LACASSAGNE (1936, 1950) sah ein kleines Carcinom des Endometriums eines Uterushornes mit Epithelmetaplasie nach langdauernder Oestrogen- und Gonadotropinbehandlung. Über vereinzeltes Auftreten von Carcinomen bzw. Epitheliomen des Uterus berichtete bei der Maus PFEIFFER (1949) nach hormoneller Fehlsteuerung, hervorgerufen durch Teilkastration und LIPSCHUTZ (1957) (Epitheliom der Cervix) beim Meerschweinchen bei gleichartigen Versuchen. Epithelproliferationen an der Portio und am Endometrium mit Metaplasie und invasivem Wachstum bis zur Serosa, Myome und Endometriosen mit z. T. atypischen Zellbildern wurden nach Hormonbehandlung oder ovarieller Dysregulation von verschiedenen Untersuchern gesehen (s. Uterus, Ovar), aber nur selten [LOEB (1936) u. a.] als Carcinome, häufiger dagegen als präcanceröse Veränderungen gedeutet.

GARDNER, ALLEN, SMITH und STRONG (1938) sahen nach Oestrogenbehandlung bei einer Maus (C3H-Stamm, 10.500 internationale Einheiten Oestradiol-Benzoat in 319 Tagen) ein metastasierendes Cervixcarcinom, 11 weitere Mäuse dieser Versuchsreihe zeigten präcanceröse, invasive Epithelveränderungen an der Cervix.

SHABAD (1946, 1949) beobachtete Adenocarcinome des Corpus uteri nach über 5monatiger Oestrogenbehandlung kastrierter Ratten. KAUFMANN (1952) konnte bei eigenen Versuchen nach Follikelhormonbehandlung nie bösartige Geschwülste am Uterus von Mäusen nachweisen.

PAN und GARDNER (1948) sahen bei 4 von 10 mit Oestrogen (16,6 μg → 25 μg Oestradiol-Benzoat oder Stilboestrol wöchentlich bis 2 Jahre) behandelten Mäusen (C3H ♀ × PM ♂) Cervixcarcinome, bei anderen Stämmen 9 von 25 (PM ♀

× C3H ♂). Andere Tiere hatten invasive Epithelveränderungen. Bei dem PM-Stamm war aber schon früher von GARDNER und PAN (1948) spontanes Vorkommen von malignen Uterus- und Vaginaltumoren beobachtet worden. Über spontanes Auftreten von Cervixcarcinomen der Maus berichten auch FISCHER und KÜHL (1958). Bei 6 verschiedenen Mäusestämmen zeigten von 206 weiblichen Tieren 52 Cervixtumoren nach Oestrogenbehandlung von über einem Jahr [GARDNER (1947)].

Nach langdauernder Behandlung (bis 365 Tage) von Mäusen mit Stilboestrol (wöchentlich 0,25 mg in Öl) sahen GARDNER und FERRIGNO (1956) Adenome und Adenocarcinome des Uterus und bei zwei Tieren ein epidermoidales Cervixcarcinom. Außerdem wurden Granulosazelltumoren und Endometriosen beobachtet. Ausgedehnte Untersuchungen über Tumorentstehung im Uterus wurden von GARDNER (1959) beschrieben. Nach intravaginaler Instillation von 1—4 μg Stilboestrol entwickelten sich bei 3 von 21 Mäusen epidermoidale Carcinome der Vagina oder der Vaginalfornices und schmale epitheliale invasive Epithelveränderungen bei 5 Mäusen. Von 40 Mäusen des BC-Stammes, die mit Stilboestrolpelotten 260 Tage behandelt wurden, entwickelten sich bei 8 Tieren Carcinome und bei 12 Tieren invasive Epithelveränderungen. Bei 14 gleichartig behandelten Tieren eines anderen Stammes (CBA, A, C 57) entstanden keine Carcinome. Eine von 112 Kontrollmäusen hatte nach 401 Tagen ein Vaginalcarcinom. Bei 6 von 13 Mäusen, die mit Stilboestrol und Testosteronpelotten (zus.) behandelt wurden, fanden sich Epithelläsionen.

Invasive Epithelveränderungen fanden sich bei 15 von 37 Mäusen des BC-Stammes nach Behandlung mit Stilboestrol oder Oestradiol (16,6 μg wöchentlich). Eine unterschiedliche Wirkung von Oestradiol-Benzoat oder Stilboestrol konnte offenbar nicht nachgewiesen werden. 21 von 35 Mäusen, die in gleicher Weise mit Puder (enthaltend Urea, adipic acid, carbomethylcellulose acid) behandelt wurden, bekamen invasive Epithelveränderungen, bei 10 Tieren wurden Carcinome gefunden.

DUNN und GREEN (1963) injizierten neugeborenen weiblichen Mäusen 0,1 cm³ einer 2 %igen Lösung von Diäthylstilboestrol (in physiol. Kochsalzlösung). Bei 6 von 17 Mäusen fanden sie nach 13–26 Monaten 6 Uterus- bzw. Vaginalcarcinome und 1 Granulosazelltumor. Unter den vier nur mit Kochsalzlösung behandelten Kontrollen fand sich bei einem Tier ein Carcinom der Vagina und ein Granulosazelltumor.

VAN NIE, BENEDETTI und MÜHLBOCK (1961) beobachteten bei 26 von 42 weiblichen Mäusen (F1 Hybriden, C57BL × DBA) nach subcutaner Implantation von 1–2 mg Testosteronpropionat Carcinome des Uterus, bei denen z. T. Lungenmetastasen auftraten.

In eigenen Versuchen [DONTENWILL, MOHR und BERNHARD (1963)] konnten wir zeigen, daß die Follikelhormonanwendung nur dann zu Carcinomen am Uterus führt, wenn das Hormon direkt auf das Portioepithel wirkt. Während nach subcutaner Behandlung weiblicher Goldhamster mit Follikelhormon bei keinem der Tiere Vaginal- oder Portiocarcinome auftraten, fanden sich bei den durch intravaginale Anwendung von Hormonstyli (2,5 mm dicke Styli enthielten bei 8 mm Länge 40 mg Cyren-B – die Styli wurden alle 8 Wochen erneuert) behandelten Tieren bei über 50 % Carcinome der Portio und Vagina.

Literatur

DANNENBERG, H.: Über die endogene Krebsentstehung. Dtsch. med. Wschr. **83**, 1726—1732 (1958).

— Über Beziehungen zwischen Steroiden und krebserzeugenden Verbindungen. Z. Krebsforsch. **65**, 396—403 (1963).

FURTH, J.: Conditioned and autonomous neoplasms: a review. Cancer Res. **13**, 477 (1953).

GARDNER, W.: Hormones and carcinogenesis. Canad. Cancer Conf. **2**, 207 (1957).
HADDOW, A., R. J. HARRIS, G. A. R. KOH, and E. M. F. ROE: Phil. Trans. B **241**, 147 (1948).
KIRSCHBAUM, A.: The role of hormones in cancer: laboratory animals. Cancer Res. **17**, 432 (1957).
LACASSAGNE, A.: Les cancers produits par des substances chimiques endogènes. Paris: Hermann 1950.
LIPSCHUTZ, A.: Steroid hormones and tumours. Baltimore: Williams & Wilkins Comp. 1950
MAEYER-GUIGNARD, J. DE, and E. DE MAEYER: Effect of carcinogenic and noncarcinogenic hydrocarbons on interferon synthesis and virus plaque development. J. nat. Cancer Inst. **34**, 265—276 (1965).
SMART, K., and E. KILBOURNE: The influence of cortisone on experimental viral infection. J. exp. Med. **123**, 299 (1966).

(Uterus)

DONTENWILL, W., U. MOHR u. J. BERNHARD: Die unterschiedliche Wirkung des Follikelhormons auf die Portio- und Vaginalschleimhaut bei parenteraler und lokaler Applikation. Z. Krebsforsch. **65**, 303—308 (1963).
DUNN, TH. B., and A. W. GREEN: Cysts of the epididymis, cancer of the cervix granular cell myoblastoma and other lesions after estrogen injection in newborn mice. J. nat. Cancer Inst. **31**, 425—455 (1963).
FISCHER, W., u. I. KÜHL: Geschwülste der Laboratoriumsnagetiere. Dresden, Leipzig: Theodor Steinkopff 1958.
GARDNER, W. U.: studies on steroid hormones in experimental carcinogenesis. Recent Progr. Hormone Res. (Proc. Laurentian Horm. Confer.) **1**, 217 (1947).
— Hormonal aspects of experimental tumorigenesis. Advanc. Cancer Res. **1**, 173 (1953).
— Carcinoma of the uterine cervix and upper vagina: Induction under experimental conditions in mice. Ann. N. Y. Acad. of Sci. **75**, 543 (1959).
— Experimental induction of uterine cervical and vaginal cancer in mice. Cancer Res. **19**, II, 170 (1959).
— Role of steroids in cervical cancer. Proceedings of the second National Cancer Conference. American Cancer Society, Inc., National Cancer Institute of the U. S. Public Health Service, American Association for Cancer Research 1959.
— E. ALLEN, G. M. SMITH and L. C. STRONG: Carcinoma of the cervix of mice receiving estrogens. J. Amer. med. Ass. **110**, 1182 (1938).
—, and M. FERRIGNO: Unusual neoplastic lesions of the uterine horns of estrogen-treated mice. J. nat. Cancer Inst. **17**, 601 (1956).
—, and S. C. PAN: Malignant tumors of the uterus and vagina in untreated mice of the PM Stock. Cancer Res. **8**, 241—256 (1948).
— C. A. PFEIFFER, J.J. TRENTIN, and J. T. WOLSTENHOLME: Hormonal factors in experimental carcinogenesis. The Physiopathology of Cancer 225. New York: Paul B. Hoeber, Inc. 1953.
LACASSAGNE, A.: Tumeurs maligne apparues au cours d'un traitement hormonal combiné chez des souris appartenant à des lignées refractaires au cancer spontane. C. R. Soc. Biol. (Paris) **121**, 607 (1936).
— Les cancers produits par des substances chimiques endogènes. Paris: Hermann 1950.
LIPSCHUTZ, A.: Steroid hormones and tumors. Baltimore: Williams & Wilkins Comp. 1950.
— Steroid homeostasis hypophysis and tumorigenesis. Cambridge: Heffer & Sons, Ltd. 1957.
LOEB, L., E. L. BURNS, V. SUNTZEFF and M. MOSKOP: Carcinoma-like proliferations in vaginal cervix and uterus of mouse treated with estrogenic hormones. Proc. Soc. exp. Biol. (N. Y.) **35**, 320 (1936).
NIE, R. VAN, E. L. BENEDETTI, and O. MÜHLBOCK: A carcinogenic action of testosterone provoking uterine tumours in mice. Nature (Lond.) **192**, 1303—1305 (1961).
PAN, S. C., and W. U. GARDNER: Carcinomas of uterine cervix and vagina and estrogen-and-androgen treated hybrid mice. Cancer Res. **8**, 337 (1948).
PFEIFFER, C. A.: Adenocarcinoma in the uterus of an endocrine imbalance female rat. Cancer Res. **9**, 347 (1949).
SHABAD, L. M.: Trends in Cancer Research in USSR. Amer. Rev. Soviet Med. **4**, 166 (1946).
— Adeno-ca des corpus uteri nach hohen Dosen Oestrogen (5—5$^1/_2$ Mo.) bei der kastrierten Ratte. Sowjetwiss. **1949**, H. 4.

b) Verschiedenes

GARDNER, SMITH, STRONG und ALLEN (1936), LACASSAGNE (1937, 1939, 1950), BURNS, SUNTZEFF und LOEB (1938), COOK und KENNAWAY (1940), MOSINGER (1947, 1951) beschreiben *Sarkome* in der Nachbarschaft der Injektionsstellen bei Mäusen, die lange mit Oestrogenen behandelt wurden. LACASSAGNE glaubte an die Möglichkeit der carcinogenen Wirkung des ölhaltigen Lösungsmittels, aber auch nach Injektion von wäßrigem Oestrogen wurden von

BURNS, SUNTZEFF und LOEB (1938), BURROWS und HORNING (1947) Sarkome gesehen. BURNS u. a. (1938) beobachteten außerhalb der Injektionsstelle noch Sarkome in der Vagina und LACASSAGNE (1937, 1938) in der Wand der Harnblase. DUNNING, CURTIS und SEGALOFF (1947, 1953) sahen bei oestrogenbehandelten Ratten neben Blasensteinen auch *Blasencarcinome*, Mammacarcinome und Nebennierenrindenadenome und -carcinome. Die Tumorhäufigkeit war bei einzelnen Stämmen verschieden. HORNING (1958) beobachtete bei langdauernder Behandlung von weiblichen Ratten mit Testosteronproprionat (wöchentlich subcutan 0,5 mg Testosteronproprionat — mit zunehmendem Alter auf 2,5 mg wöchentlich ansteigend) *Thecazelltumoren* (ein Tumor hatte das Aussehen eines Spindelzellsarkoms) und hyperplastische Veränderungen des Uterus. Bei gleichbehandelten Hamstern sah er ein *Nebennierenrindenadenom* und ein *Carcinom*, aber Metastasen ließen sich nicht nachweisen.

RUDALI, DESORMEAUX und JULIAND (1956) beobachteten nach *Androgenbehandlung* (19 Monate) bei Mäusen maligne *Nierentumoren*. HOMBURGER, BORGES und TREGIER (1957) sahen *Uterussarkome* bei Mäusen (Swiss und BALB) nach Testosteronbehandlung. LACASSAGNE (1939) fand nach Testosteronbehandlung bei Mäusen in 37% subcutane Sarkome. Sarkome wurden auch von BURROWS (1945) nach Testosteroninjektion bei der Maus beobachtet.

GILMAN, GILBERT und SPENCE (1957) behandelten kastrierte, 6 Wochen alte weibliche Ratten mit *Progesteron* (Pelotten à 8—10 mg). Von 5 Tieren entwickelte sich bei einem Tier nach 696 Tagen Behandlung ein *Lebercarcinom*. Eine langdauernde Behandlung mit Oestrogen (8,3 μg wöchentlich subcutan) verhütet das Auftreten von Hepatomen in C3H-Mäusen. Sarkome des Unterhautgewebes bei der Maus sahen BISCHOFF und RUPP (1946) nach Behandlung mit synthetischem Progesteron.

Bei der Besprechung gutartiger hyperplastischer Veränderungen nach Hormonbehandlung bzw. hormoneller Dysregulation haben wir des besseren Verständnisses wegen auch die als bösartig oder maligne bezeichneten Tumoren erwähnt. Hier wollen wir aus diesen Kapiteln noch einmal die Tumoren herausstellen, bei denen auf Grund morphologischer oder biologischer Kriterien von einer Bösartigkeit im Sinne von Carcinomen und Sarkomen gesprochen wurde.

Bösartige Tumoren fanden neben gutartigen, z. T. adenomatösen Hyperplasien, zahlreiche Untersucher im *Hoden* (Zwischenzelltumoren) nach Oestrogenbehandlung und in der *Nebennierenrinde* nach Kastration. Bei beiden Tumoren handelt es sich um Veränderungen, bei denen sowohl die gutartigen wie auch die bösartigen bei bestimmten Mäusestämmen auftraten. Ihre Entstehung ist sicher an genetische Faktoren gebunden. Diese Tumoren gelang es nur bei bestimmten Tierstämmen im Experiment zu erzeugen. Zur Entstehung ist also eine genetisch kontrollierte Disposition nötig, die Hormonbehandlung ist nicht die allein auslösende Ursache (s. im Abschnitt I Ad u. I Ah).

Sarkomatöse Entartungen von Uterusmyomen nach Oestrogenbehandlung beschrieb lediglich MOSINGER (1946), während LIPSCHUTZ (1950) und andere die morphologischen Kriterien als nicht ausschlaggebend ansahen.

Die von VASQUEZ-LOPEZ (1944) beschriebenen Carcinome des *Nebenhodens* beim Hamster nach Oestrogenbehandlung konnten von anderen Untersuchern nicht bestätigt werden.

Über *Prostatasarkome* (fibromuskuläre) bei oestrogenbehandelten Hamstern berichteten BIELSCHOWSKY und HORNING (1958); diese wurden von anderen Untersuchern [KIRKMAN (1957), DONTENWILL und EDER (1959)] bei gleichen Versuchen nicht beobachtet.

Bei den von DONTENWILL und EDER (1959) nach Oestrogenbehandlung des Goldhamsters gefundenen *Lebercarcinomen* ist nicht sicher, ob die, bei gleichzeitig gefundener Lebercirrhose, ablaufenden regeneratorischen Prozesse wesentliche Ursachen sind, da nur bei etwa 5% der Cirrhosen Carcinome gefunden wurden. Das Follikelhormon ist hier sicher nicht als allein auslösende Ursache, sondern höchstens als cocarcinogener Faktor anzusehen.

MIRAND, REINHARD und GOLTZ (1953) beobachteten bei Mäusen des Marsh-Albinostammes nach 3monatelanger täglicher Behandlung mit Desoxycorticosteronacetat (0,2 mg auf 0,1 cm^3 Sesamöl) Entwicklung von *Fibrosarkomen* und *Myosarkomen*.

Literatur

(Verschiedenes)

BIELSCHOWSKY, F., and E. S. HORNING: Aspects of endocrine carcinogenesis. Brit. med. Bull. **14**, 106 (1958).

BISCHOFF, F., and D. RUPP: Cancer Res. **6**, 403 (1946).

BURNS, E. L., V. SUNTZEFF and L. LOEB: The development of sarcoma in mice injected with hormones or hormone-like substance. Amer. J. Cancer **32**, 534—544 (1938).

BURROWS, H.: Sarkome nach Testosteroninjektion. Biological action of sex hormones, S. 194. London: Cambridge University Press 1945.

BURROWS, H., and E. S. HORNING: Oestrogens and neoplasia. Brit. med. Bull. **4**, 390 (1947).
COOK, J., and E. L. KENNAWAY: Chemical compounds as carcinogenic agents. Amer. J. Cancer **39**, 381 (1940); **39**, 521 (1940).
DONTENWILL, W., u. M. EDER: Histogenese und biologische Verhaltensweise hormonell ausgelöster Geschwülste. Beitr. path. Anat. **120**, 270 (1959).
DUNNING, W. F., M. R. CURTIS and A. SEGALOFF: Strain differences in response to diethylstilbestrol and the induction of mammary gland and bladder cancer in the rat. Cancer Res. **7**, 511—521 (1947).
— — — Strain differences in response to estrone and the induction of mammary gland, adrenal and bladder cancer in rats. Cancer Res. **13**, 147—152 (1953).
GARDNER, W. U., G. M. SMITH, L. C. STRONG and E. ALLEN: Development of sarcoma in male mice receiving estrogenic hormones. Arch. Path. (Chicago) **21**, 504 (1936).
GILMAN, J., C. GILBERT and I. SPENCE: Primary cancer of the liver in rats after subcutaneous implantation of pellets of progesterone and testosterone propionate. Experientia (Basel) **13**, 4, 160 (1957).
HOMBURGER, F., P. BORGES and A. TREGIER: Uterussarkome bei Mäusen (Swiss and BALB) nach Testosteronbehandlung. Proc. Amer. Cancer Res. **2**, 215 (1957).
HORNING, E. S.: Carcinogenic action of androgens. Brit. J. Cancer **12**, 414 (1958).
KIRKMAN, H.: Steroid tumorigenesis. Cancer (Chic.) **10**, 754 (1957).
LACASSAGNE, A.: Sarcomes fusocellulaires apparus chez des souris longuement traitées par des hormones oestrogènes. C. R. Soc. Biol. (Paris) **126**, 190 (1937).
— Statistique des différents cancers constatés dans des lingnées selectionnées des souris, apres action prolongée d'hormones oestrogènes. Bull. Cancer **27**, 96 (1938).
— Les rapports entre les hormones sexuelles et la formation du cancer. Ergebn. Vit. Horm.-Forsch. **2**, 258 (1939).
— 37% der mit Testosteron behandelten Mäuse bekamen subcutane Sarkome. Bull. Ass. franç. Cancer **28**, 951 (1939); C. R. Soc. Biol. (Paris) **132**, 365 (1939).
— Les cancers produits par des substances chimiques endogènes. Paris: Hermann 1950.
LOEB, L., E. L. BURNS, V. SUNTZEFF and M. MOSKOP: Sex hormones and their relation to tumor production. Amer. J. Cancer **30**, 47 (1937).
MIRAND, E. A., M. C. REINHARD and H. L. GOLTZ: Development of sarcoma in marsh-albino mice following injection of desoxycorticosterone acetate in sesame oil. Proc. Soc. exp. Biol. (N. Y.) **83**, 14—17 (1953).
MOSINGER, M.: Le problème du cancer et son évolution récente. Paris: Masson et Cie. 1946.
— Über die Beziehungen zwischen den oestrogenen cancero- und anticancerogenen sklerogenen kolloido-cytogenen und karyoklastischen Effekten. C. R. Soc. Biol. (Paris) **141**, 298 (1947).
— Proliferative Prozesse bei den Nagern, ausgelöst durch synthetische Krebserzeuger und hormonale, namentlich oestrogene Substanzen. Bull. Ass. franç. Cancer **42**, 4 (1951); Arch. Geschwulstforsch. **3**, H. 3, 262 (1951).
RUDALI, G., B. DESORMEAUX et L. JULIAND: Nierentumoren nach Behandlung mit Androgen (19 Monate) bei Mäusen. Bull Ass. franç. Cancer **43**, 445 (1956).
VASQUEZ-LOPEZ, E.: The relation of the pituitary gland and related hypothalamic centres in the hamster to prolonged treatment with oestrogens. J. Path. Bact. **56**, 1 (1944).

B. Durch Hormone bei endogener Disposition

a) Mammacarcinom

BIELKA, BIERWOLF, GRAFFI und SCHRAMM (1966) haben im Abschnitt Mammacarcinom bereits darauf hingewiesen, daß es sich bei der Entstehung und Auslösung des Mammacarcinoms der Maus um ein komplexes, keineswegs geklärtes Geschehen handelt. Als wir diesen Beitrag abfaßten (1958–1960) war die Meinung vorherrschend, daß das Bittner-Virus den Carcinogeneseprozeß lediglich beschleunigt, aber nicht eigentlich Voraussetzung für die Carcinomenentstehung sei. Heute geht die allgemeine Auffassung dahin, daß die hormonelle Stimulierung der Brustdrüse bei bestimmter genetischer Konstitution, bzw. genetisch bestimmtem hormonellem Muster, eine Vorbedingung für die Wirkung des onkogenen Bittner-Virus darstellt. Das Bittner-Virus (s. ausführlich bei BIELKA, BIERWOLF, GRAFFI und SCHRAMM) ist nach BRYAN (1963) sowohl in Geweben männlicher wie auch weiblicher Mäuse und in der Milch während des ganzen Lebens nachweisbar. Dies gilt auch für Tiere, bei denen kein Mammacarcinom entsteht. Männliche Tiere entwickeln das virusinduzierte Mammacarcinom erst nach Vorbehandlung mit weiblichem Hormon, d. h. erst dann, wenn die männliche Brustdrüse durch die Hormonwirkung zur Proliferation angeregt wird, da dann für das Virus der geeignete, biologische Boden zur malignen Transformation vorhanden ist. Nach DeOme (1963) wird die spezifische Hormonempfindlichkeit durch die genetische Konstitution des Tieres bestimmt, wobei das Virus die proliferationsfördernde Wirkung vergrößert. Im Handbuchbeitrag über das Mammacarcinom der Maus haben Bielka, Bierwolf, Graffi und Schramm ausführlich über das Vorkommen

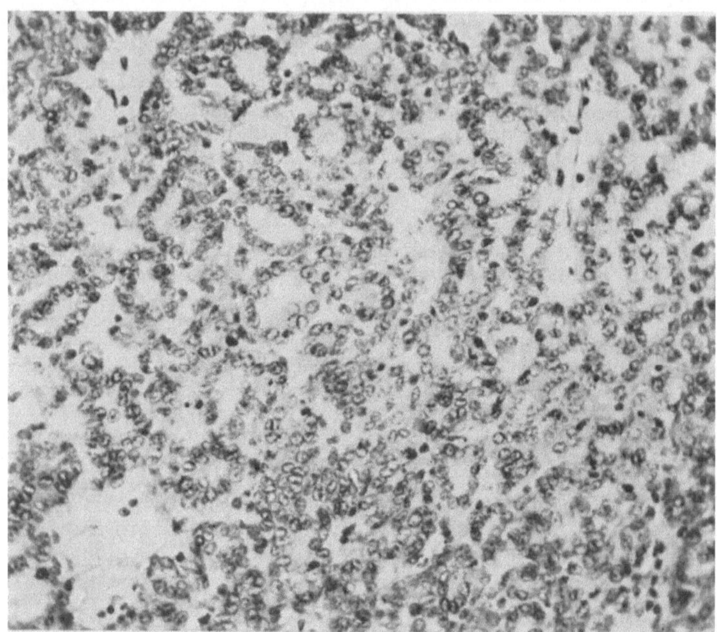

Abb. 43. Mammacarcinom der Maus. Stamm C 57. Typische Adenostruktur der mäßig polymorphen Zellen

und die Übertragungsweise des Milchfaktors oder Bittner-Virus gesprochen. Wir wollen uns hier weitgehend auf die Erörterung der Bedeutung der Hormone bei der Mammacarcinomentstehung beschränken.

Nachdem Loeb (1924) beobachtet hatte, daß nach Ovarektomie Mammacarcinome bei einem Mäusestamm mit einer Spontanrate von 60–70% nur noch in 9% auftraten und nach den Untersuchungen von Murray (1927, 1934), daß nach Kastration und Ovarimplantation bei Männchen die Carcinomrate von 0,39% auf 18,09% ansteigt, ist die Diskussion über die Bedeutung des Follikelhormons bei der Krebsentstehung nicht verstummt. Diese Beobachtungen wurden später von Cori (1927), Shimkin und Wyman (1945), Smith (1948), Woolley, Fekete und Little (1939, 1941) bestätigt. Während von anderen Hormonen nur vereinzelt und nicht überzeugend eine carcinogene Wirkung angenommen wird, handelt es sich beim Follikelhormon nach Ansicht mehrerer amerikanischer Autoren um ein Hormon mit echter cancerogener Wirkung. Sie wird vor allem am Beispiel des Mammacarcinoms demonstriert.

Bittner hat 1942 angenommen, daß beim Mammacarcinom der Maus drei Faktoren eine wesentliche kausale Rolle spielen:

1. Die genetisch bestimmte Anfälligkeit.
2. Der mütterliche Milch-Faktor (mammary tumor agent) und
3. das genetisch bestimmte hormonelle Verhältnis (Muster).

Die Ansprechbarkeit der einzelnen Tierstämme gegenüber dem Mammacarcinom-Virus, bzw. einer Hormonbehandlung ist außerordentlich unterschiedlich. Nach BITTNER (1942, 1948, 1952, 1953, 1954, 1955, 1956, 1958) ist der Milchfaktor für die Tumorentstehung nicht absolut notwendig. Zahlreiche Untersuchungen der letzten zwei Jahrzehnte haben den wesentlichen Einfluß des Follikelhormons für die Entstehung und das Wachstum des Mammacarcinoms bewiesen, es ist aber bis heute noch umstritten, ob das Follikelhormon auch ohne das Vorhandensein genetischer Faktoren carcinogen für die Mamma wirkt. Durch die Untersuchungen von KAUFMANN, MÜLLER, BUTENANDT und FRIEDRICH-FREKSA (1949), KAUFMANN und MÜLLER (1950) und BUTENANDT (1950) konnte gezeigt werden, daß sich durch die Follikelhormonbehandlung die genetisch bedingte Anfälligkeit oder Disposition für das Mammacarcinom erhöht, daß aber bei Mäusen ohne entsprechende genetische Disposition keine Geschwülste entstehen. Nie gelang es dagegen KAUFMANN und MÜLLER (1950) durch Follikelhormon oder Ovarialextrakte Uteruscarcinome zu erzeugen.

Viele Untersucher haben sich in der Folgezeit mit dem Problem der Carcinomentstehung in der Mamma befaßt und versucht, die Bedeutung der Hormone zu klären [BONSER (1935, 1936), BONSER, STICKLAND und CONNAL (1937), BURROWS (1936), LACASSAGNE (1936, 1937, 1950, 1951, 1955), GARDNER, SMITH, ALLEN und STRONG (1936), ROBSON und BONSER (1938), SUNTZEFF, KIRTZ, BLUMENTHAL und LOEB (1941), BIERICH und ROSENBOHM (1942)]. LACASSAGNE konnte 1932 erstmals berichten, daß eine langdauernde Injektion von Oestrogen bei Mäusestämmen, deren Weibchen spontane Mammacarcinome in einem hohen Prozentsatz zeigen, auch bei den männlichen Tieren dieser Stämme zur Mammacarcinomentstehung führt. SHIMKIN und WYMAN (1946) nahmen auf Grund ihrer Untersuchungen an, daß die Entwicklung des Brustdrüsenkrebses bei der Maus geschlechtsgebunden sei. Die Wirkung der Oestrogene beruht nach ihrer Ansicht entweder auf dem Verweiblichungseffekt mit Bildung und Wucherung von Brustdrüsengewebe und Krebsentstehung oder auf einem spezifischen stimulierenden Effekt auf das Brustdrüsengewebe. SUNTZEFF, BURNS, MOSKOP und LOEB (1936) beobachteten bei ihren Versuchen an verschiedenen Tierstämmen nicht nur eine starke Zunahme der Tumorrate der weiblichen Tiere, sondern auch eine sehr erhebliche Häufung von Carcinomen der Mamma bei den männlichen Tieren der gleichen Stämme. Durch Oestrogenbehandlung gelang es aber keineswegs, bei allen Tierstämmen Carcinome zu erzeugen, auch nicht, in der Mamma vorhandene Adenome und Fibrome in Carcinome umzuwandeln [WRIGHT, KLINCK und WOLFF (1940)].

LACASSAGNE diskutierte schon 1933, 1938 den Einfluß eines familiären Faktors auf die Entstehung des Mammacarcinoms der Maus. Heute wissen wir durch viele Untersuchungen, z. B. BOOT und MÜHLBOCK (1956), daß die Veranlagung zum Mammacarcinom erblich gebunden ist, besonders beim C3H-Stamm und wahrscheinlich auch beim JF-Stamm. Die spontane Häufigkeit ist sehr unterschiedlich, sie ist nach GRAFFI und BIELKA (1960) beim:

C3H-Stamm	sehr hoch
A-Stamm	hoch
White-lable-Stamm	mittel
C-Stamm	niedrig
JF-Stamm	sehr niedrig
C57-Stamm schwarz	sehr niedrig

Über die stammesabhängige Tumorhäufigkeit bei Maus und Ratte berichten BITTNER (1942), GARDNER, STRONG und SMITH (1940), GARDNER und STRONG (1940), GARDNER (1941). Mäuse des JK- und Js-Stammes waren resistent gegen die Entwicklung des Mammacarcinoms, [BITTNER (1958)]. Nach TWOMBLEY (1940) entstehen keine Carcinome bei männlichen Mäusen, wenn Mäusestämme mit geringer spontaner Tumorhäufigkeit (bei Weibchen) verwandt werden, bei gleichzeitigem Fehlen des sog. Bittnerschen Milchfaktors (Mammary turmor agent). Dagegen entstehen bei männlichen Tieren aus Stämmen mit einer hohen Tumorrate (bei weiblichen Tieren nach Oestrogenbehandlung) auch Carcinome ohne Anwesenheit des Milchfaktors [HESTON und DERINGER (1953)].

Mäuse mit einer ähnlichen genetischen Disposition wie C3H-Mäuse, d. h. C3Hf-Mäuse, zeigen auch Carcinome ohne Milchfaktor, aber erst in einem späteren Lebensabschnitt. Diese und andere Untersuchungen, HESTON (1945), HESTON, DERINGER und LEVILLAIN (1949), HESTON, DERINGER, DUNN und LEVILLAIN (1950) ergaben, daß der Milchfaktor den Carcinogeneseprozeß beschleunigt, daß sich aber auch Carcinome ohne Milchfaktor entwickeln können.

In zahlreichen Untersuchungen werden die Ergebnisse von BITTNER bestätigt [BITTNER (1946, 1947, 1948), BITTNER und HUSEBY (1945, 1950), ARMSTRONG (1948), DMOCHOWSKI (1948, 1949), DMOCHOWSKI und ORR (1949), HESTON, DERINGER und LEVILLAIN (1949), BURROWS (1949), PULLINGER (1949), MÜHLBOCK (1949), ANDERVONT und DUNN (1948, 1950), TRENTIN (1951), HESTON, DERINGER und DUNN (1956), ANDERVONT, DUNN und CANTER (1958), HOWARD, THELMA und HARRY (1958)], der zwischen genetisch bedingten Faktoren und dem Milchfaktor unterscheidet. Dabei zeigt sich immer wieder, daß anscheinend Tiere oder Tierstämme mit einem hohen Grad an Tumoranfälligkeit für Mammatumoren auch in Abwesenheit des Mammatumoragens (Milchfaktor) Geschwülste entwickeln, daß aber bestimmte Hormonbehandlung, insbesondere langdauernde Follikelhormonbehandlung, die Tumorrate erhöht und die gleichzeitige Anwesenheit des Milchfaktors ebenfalls die Häufigkeit der Tumorenentstehung stark beeinflußt. Bei nicht belasteten Tierstämmen konnten WRIGHT, KLINCK und WOLFF (1940) auch durch Oestrogengaben häufig auftretende Adenofibrome nicht in Carcinome umwandeln, obwohl ja, wie schon seit langem bekannt ist, diese Adenofibrome durch hormonelle Stimulierung der Mamma entstehen und durch Kastration in ihrer Entwicklung gehemmt werden können [PICCO (1936)].

Die bisherigen Untersuchungen lassen annehmen, daß die hormonelle Ansprechbarkeit, die hormonelle Disposition, oder das sog. hormonelle Muster in einem anderen Gen lokalisiert ist, als die genetisch bedingte Ansprechbarkeit verschiedener Mäusezuchtstämme auf das Mammacarcinom-Virus (MTA). Die verschiedenen Untersuchungen von BITTNER und anderen deuten auf verschiedene Merkmale hin, die in verschiedener Weise vererbt werden. Die unterschiedliche Häufigkeit von Tumoren bei verschiedenen Stämmen oder Sublimen, verschiedenem Alter und nach Applikation verschiedener Virusdosen haben BIELKA et al. in ihrem Beitrag ausführlich diskutiert. BITTNER (1956) konnte in Kreuzungsversuchen u. a. nachweisen, daß der genetische Faktor entscheidender ist als die Virusdosis, und daß jüngere Tiere sich für die Tumorenerzeugung durch Viren besser eignen als ältere [BITTNER (1947)]. Das für den hormonellen Faktor entscheidende Gen ist offenbar wesentlich für die Mammatumorenentstehung ausschlaggebend.

Auf die Bedeutung des genetisch bedingten hormonellen Musters haben bereits KAUFMANN, MÜLLER, BUTENANDT und FRIEDRICH-FREKSA (1949) hingewiesen. Sie untersuchten bei verschiedenen Inzuchtstämmen(Bl-H-Stamm, Little-db-Stamm und Bl-C-Stamm) die Einwirkung des Follikelhormons auf die Mammacarcinomentstehung. Den Untersuchern gelang es, eine Oestrogendosis zu bestimmen, die gerade ausreicht, um bei den virginellen Mäusen den physiologischen Proliferationsreiz der Gestation zu ersetzen. Diese Dosis liegt zwischen 2 γ und 30 γ Oestron und bei 1 γ Oestronbenzonat wöchentlich. Geht man über diesen Schwellenwert hinaus, gelingt es zwar, zu einem früheren Zeitpunkt Mammacarcinome zu erzeugen, die Höhe der erzielbaren Tumorrate richtet sich aber ganz nach der Höhe der vorhandenen Tumorbelastung.

Auch das synthetische Stilboestrol zeigte bei gleicher Dosis die gleiche Wirkung (Behandlung bis 20 Monate). Bei beiden Hormonen wurden auch proliferative Änderungen an Uterus und Vagina beobachtet. Auf Grund dieser Tierexperimente wurde angenommen, daß dem Follikelhormon keine cancerogene Wirkung zukommt, man also lediglich von einer Mitwirkung bei vorhandener Krebsanlage sprechen kann. Diese Untersuchungen wurden an einem großen Tiermaterial durchgeführt (5720 Mäuse). Sie zeigen, daß das hormonelle Muster genetisch verankert ist. Der hormonelle Aufbau z. B. der NH-Mäuse scheint nach BITTNER (1953) die Entwicklung der Mammatumoren zu hemmen. Wegen der starken Variation der hormonellen Faktoren auf die Entstehung des Mammacarcinoms und der stark streuenden Angaben einzelner Autoren bei den verschiedenen Tierstämmen ist eine klare Definition des „hormonellen genetischen Musters" nicht möglich.

Ursächlich verantwortlich für die unterschiedliche Tumorhäufigkeit sind offenbar die *Hormone der Schwangerschaft und der Lactation* [SLATTERY (1950)], also ovarielle und hypophysäre Faktoren. Die von BITTNER (1952, 1954, 1958) postulierte hormonelle Empfindlichkeit kann möglicherweise auch mit der veränderten gonadotropen Hormonsekretion zusammenhängen. KORTEWEG (1948) sah beispielsweise bei gering krebsbelasteten Stämmen eine andere Empfänglichkeit gegenüber der Mammatumorenentwicklung als bei stark belasteten Stämmen (DBA), bei denen eine 3mal so starke Oestrondosis zur Erreichung des Schwellenwertes verabreicht werden mußte wie bei den krebsarmen Stämmen [VAN GULLIK und KORTEWEG (1940)]. Es übertrifft die Testosteronproduktion der nicht kastrierten Männchen bei den untersuchten krebsreichen Stämmen (DBA) – nach seiner Ansicht – die der krebsarmen (C 57) um das 3fache. Die relativ hohe Produktion von Oestron beim Weibchen und von Testosteron beim Männchen krebsreicher Stämme ist nach Ansicht von KORTEWEG (1948) ein Beweis für eine hohe Produktion des gonadotropen Hormons. Ähnliche Feststellungen machten SHIMKIN und ANDERVONT (1941, 1942) beim Vergleich des C3H- und C57-Stammes sowie ANDERVONT (1949) und DERINGER, HESTON und ANDERVONT (1945) beim Vergleich des Oestrus virgineller Mäuse des C3H-Stammes und A-Stammes mit hoher und niedriger Tumorrate. Nach KORTEWEG (1948) besteht bei krebsbelasteten Stämmen eine Beziehung zwischen der quantitativen Oestrogenproduktion und der Häufigkeit des Carcinoms. Ein Teil der genetischen Disposition zum Mammacarcinom ist verursacht durch die Überproduktion von Oestrogen, also durch das genetische hormonelle Muster. Von GASS, COATS und GRAHAM (1946) wurde der Versuch unternommen, das Verhältnis zwischen Tumorvorkommen bei Mäusen und der Konzentration von Diethylstilbestrol in der Diät festzustellen. Es wurden intakte C3H Mäuseweibchen und Mäusemännchen und kastrierte Stamm A Mäusemännchen benutzt. Bei C3H Mäuseweibchen verursachten 6,25 Teile per Billion Diethylstilbestrol in der Diät während der ganzen Lebensdauer bedeutend mehr Tumoren als bei den Kontrolltieren. Lineare log. Dosiswirkungskurven mit signifikantem Abfall wurden bei kastrierten Mäusemännchen des A-Stammes (12,5–1000 ppb) und bei C3H Mäuseweibchen (25 bis 500 ppb) gefunden. Das Durchschnittsgewicht der Ovarien eines Musters der

C3H Weibchen ging linear zurück, und zwar zwischen Dosen von 12,5 ppb und 500 ppb.

Schon früher hatten LATHROP und LOEB (1913, 1916) festgestellt, daß die Rate der Mammatumoren bei *Mäusen, die trächtig sind*, zunimmt. Über gleiche Ergebnisse berichten MÜHLBOCK und VAN RIJSSEL (1954), PULLINGER (1955). Bei manchen Stämmen ist eine stärkere Tumorhäufigkeit bei juvenilen Mäusen vorhanden [BITTNER (1952)], BITTNER und HUSEBY (1950), bei anderen dagegen bei weiblichen Mäusen, die schon geworfen haben. SUNTZEFF, KIRTZ, BLUMENTHAL und LOEB (1941) sehen z. B. bei weiblichen C3H-Mäusen nach Oestrogenbehandlung 60% Carcinome, bei Mäusen des A-Stammes 43% (bei Weibchen mit Jungen); bei juvenilen Mäusen betrug die Häufigkeit beim C3H-Stamm nur 19% und beim A-Stamm nur 3%. Bei Tieren mit einem Wurf sahen SHIMKIN und ANDERVONT (1941, 1942) 13% Carcinome und bei Weibchen nach mehreren Würfen 59% Carcinome bei gleicher Behandlung. Nach ihrer Meinung ist aber Voraussetzung die hormonelle Störung bei genetischer Disposition. Bei Kreuzung von juvenilen Fl-hybriden Mäusen wird die spontane Carcinomrate erhöht [BITTNER, HUSEBY (1946)]. Der genetische Faktor ist durch weibliche und männliche Tiere übertragbar.

Ovarektomie bewirkt eine starke Hemmung der Mammacarcinomhäufigkeit [LOEB (1944) u. a.]. Diese Hemmung unterbleibt, wenn bei frühzeitiger Kastration durch eine adenomatöse Hyperplasie der Nebenniere eine weitere Oestrogenproduktion erfolgt [WOOLLEY (1939)]. Wird aber die Gonadektomie erst nach mehreren Monaten vorgenommen, d. h. nachdem das Ovar schon länger seine inkretorische Funktion ausübte, kann die Tumorgenese nicht mehr gehemmt werden. Das Auftreten der Mammacarcinome wird verzögert, die Zahl der spontanen Carcinome vermindert. Nach PILGRIM (1957) tritt das Carcinom dann im höheren Alter auf. Bei weiblichen Mäusen des C3H-Stammes vermindert sich nach SHIMKIN und WYMAN (1945) die Tumorhäufigkeit nach Kastration oder Adrenalektomie von 84% auf 35% und bei gleichzeitiger Adrenalektomie und Kastration auf 9%. Eine Hemmung des Mammatumorwachstums oder Rückgang der Tumoren berichten ebenfalls MARTINEZ und BITTNER (1954) nach Ovarektomie, *Adrenalektomie* und Hypophysektomie und LIEBELT und ECKLES (1957) nach Adrenalektomie.

Für die Entstehung des Mammacarcinoms der Maus bei Follikelhormonbehandlung sind also offenbar folgende Faktoren entscheidend:

Tabelle 4. *Mammacarcinom der Maus, Faktoren bei Entstehung nach Follikelhormonbehandlung*

Voraussetzung:
genetische hormonelle Anfälligkeit

auslösender Faktor
Mammacarcinomvirus bei genetischer Anfälligkeit für das Virus

Fördernde Faktoren
Zunahme der Frequenz oder Tumorrate

Hormonelles Muster = Höhe des Schwellenwertes	Mäuse mit hoher Tumorbelastung haben höhere Follikelhormonsekretion
Zahl der Geburten	Zunahme der Häufigkeit mit der Zahl der Geburten bei bestimmten Stämmen
Mitwirkung anderer hormonaler Faktoren	Förderung des Wachstums durch HVL-Extrakte, Hemmung durch Progesteron und Testosteron
Ernährungsfaktoren	Abnahme der Häufigkeit bei Änderung der Diät
Umweltfaktoren	Änderung der Häufigkeit bei Tieren in Einzel- oder Sammelkäfigen

Silberberg und Silberberg (1949, 1950) konnten durch *Transplantation von Hypophysenvorderlappen und Ovargewebe* besonders bei jungen männlichen Tieren eines Inzuchtstammes, dessen Weibchen spontan Brustkrebs zeigen, häufiger Carcinome der Mamma beobachten. Bei Transplantation auf ältere männliche Tiere traten keine Carcinome auf, es besteht also auch eine Altersabhängigkeit bei der Carcinomentstehung. Auch Ovarimplantation allein erzeugt offenbar über eine verstärkte Produktion des laktotropen Hormons bei kastrierten Stämmen mit Brustkrebsbelastung eine Häufung der Tumorentstehung [Huseby und Bittner (1951)].

Eine Förderung des Mammatumorwachstums nach Ovartransplantation oder HVL-Transplantation bei krebsbelasteten Stämmen sahen außerdem Gardner und White (1942), Loeb, Blumenthal und Kirtz (1944), Loeb und Kirtz (1939), Kunii und Furth (1963).

Mühlbock (1954) nimmt an, daß die Wirkung der Oestrogene auf die Entwicklung des Mammacarcinoms nicht am Tumor angreift, sondern über eine Beeinflussung des Hypophysenvorderlappens das Tumorwachstum gesteigert wird. Er sah nach Implantation von Hypophysenvorderlappengewebe (HVL) eine Steigerung der Mammacarcinomhäufigkeit auch bei Abwesenheit des Milchfaktors. Er beobachtete beim C 57 BL-Stamm nach Transplantation von HVL-Gewebe eine Tumorhäufung des Mammacarcinoms bei einem Stamm, dem der Milchfaktor fehlt und bei dem durch Zusatz des Milchfaktors keine stärkere Häufung von Mammacarcinomen auftritt. Nach Ansicht Mühlbocks (1954) wird unter dem Einfluß von Oestrogen mammatropes Hormon sezerniert, das auch bei Abwesenheit des Milchfaktors dieTumorgenese auslöst; durch den Milchfaktor erfolgt eine Beschleunigung. Nach Boot, Mühlbock, Röpcke und van Ebbenhorst-Tengbergen (1962) wird die Entstehung von Mammatumoren nach Hypophysentransplantation wesentlich durch die im Tier veränderte Prolactin- und Progesteronsekretion bestimmt. Die Wirkung kann aber nur bei Anwesenheit der anderen zirkulierenden Hormone eintreten. Bei MTA-freien Mäusen (♀ O20 × ♂ IF) stieg die Mammacarcinomrate bis 80% an. Heston (1964) sah bei juvenilen weiblichen bei 5 von 21 C57 BL/He Mäusen nach Transplantation von 5 Hypophysen im Verlauf von etwa 20 Monaten Mammatumoren. Bei Weibchen, denen nur eine Hypophyse implantiert wurde und bei kastrierten Weibchen, die mit Diethylstilboestrol und 1–5 Hypophysenimplantaten behandelter, wurden keine Brusttumoren gefunden. Bei männlichen hybriden C3H/A-Mäusen mit einer niederen Spontantumorrate traten nach Hypophysenimplantation bei 27% von 47 Tieren Mammatumoren auf.

Huggins (1965) beschrieb ausführlich die Wirkung der Ovarektomie und der Hypophysektomie auf das Wachstum des durch 7,12-DMBA induzierten Mammacarcinoms der weiblichen Ratte. Eine starke Senkung der Tumorrate sah er bei hypophysektomierten Ratten (10% gegenüber 100% der Kontrollen), eine geringere bei ovarektomierten (80% gegenüber 100%). Nach Huggins sind in den hormonabhängigen Carcinomen die „Hormone von größter Wichtigkeit für die Erhaltung des Lebens der Zellen, da bei ihrer Abwesenheit die Zelle stirbt. Hormonabhängige maligne Tumoren können mit der Zeit unabhängig werden, dabei wird der Grad ihrer Malignität gesteigert".

Hypophysektomie hemmt bzw. verhindert das Brustdrüsenwachstum und die Mammatumorentstehung durch Oestrogene [Gomez, Turner, Gardner und Hill (1937), Lacassagne und Chamorro (1939), Gardner (1942), Gardner und White (1942), Jacobsohn (1954), Martinez und Bittner (1954), Ahren und Jacobsohn (1956), Jacobsohn (1954)]. Wenn gleichzeitig Oestrogene und Progesteron gegeben wurden, war das Wachstum gering [Gardner (1940), Kirkham und Turner (1954)]. Die meisten hyperplastischen Tumoren der Brustdrüse gehen nach Hypophysektomie zurück, nicht aber die schon entwickelten Mammacarcinome [Bern, Nandi, de Ome (1957), Gardner (1942), Lacassagne und Chamorro (1939), Martinez und Bittner (1954), Mühlbock (1958)].

Auch *Umweltfaktoren*, wie z. B. Tierhaltung oder Tierfütterung, können die Mammacarcinomhäufigkeit bei empfindlichen bzw. tumorbelasteten Tierstämmen stark beeinflussen. Eine Verminderung der gesamten Nahrungszufuhr führt nach TANNENBAUM (1953) zu einer Verminderung der Tumorhäufigkeit, ebenso eine cystinarme Diät [WHITE und WHITE (1944)]. Der Nahrungsentzug, der möglicherweise zu einer hormonellen Fehlsteuerung führt, zeigt auch beim Mammacarcinom eine Verminderung der Tumorhäufigkeit, wie dies von der Hypophysektomie bekannt ist. BALL, HUSEBY und VISSCHER (1946) bezeichnen die durch diätetische Faktoren erzeugte Hemmung des Brustdrüsenwachstums und Mammacarcinomentwicklung als Pseudohypophysektomie. Die Änderung des Tumorbefalls bei bestimmten Mäusestämmen während des Krieges führt BITTNER (1954) auf exogene Faktoren (Futterwechsel – offenbar eiweißärmeres Futter) zurück. Über den Einfluß der Diät auf die Häufigkeit des Mammacarcinoms berichten auch KING, CASAS, VISSCHER (1949), CASAS, KING und VISSCHER (1949). MÜHLBOCK (1955) konnte zeigen, daß bei einer Änderung der Tierhaltung die Tumorrate stark variiert. Er verteilte juvenile Tiere aus einem Nest in 4 Typen von Käfigen:

1. Käfige mit 50 Tieren,
2. gleichgroßer Käfig, aber unterteilt in 10 Sektionen mit je 5 Tieren,
3. Glaskäfig mit 5 Tieren,
4. Glasgefäß mit einem Tier.

In den Käfigen mit 50 Tieren war die Tumorfrequenz nur 29%, in den in Sektionen unterteilten Käfigen 56% und bei Einzelglasgefäßen 83%. Bei zusätzlicher Belastung (Käfig mit Laufrad) war die Frequenz gegenüber Kontrollen geringer (43% gegenüber 67%).

Auch bei *Ratten* konnten durch langdauernde Behandlung mit Oestrogen Tumoren der Brustdrüse erzeugt werden. Es entstanden dabei meist Carcinome der Brustdrüse und gleichzeitig häufig Adenome der Hypophyse. Bei diesen Hypophysenadenomen handelt es sich, wie bereits erwähnt, um mammotrope Adenome [FURTH, CLIFTON, GADSDEN und BUFFET (1956)]. Mammatumoren (Carcinome bei der Ratte nach chronischer Oestrogeninjektion oder subcutaner Implantation von Oestrogen-Hormon-Pelotten) wurden von zahlreichen Untersuchern beobachtet.

Gutartige Fibrome und Carcinome der Mamma nach Oestrogenbehandlung sahen MCEUEN (1938), GESCHICKTER (1939, 1940), NOBLE, MCEUEN und COLLIP (1940), MARK und BISKIND (1941), GESCHICKTER und BYRNES (1942), EISEN (1944), NELSON (1944), DUNNING, CURTIS und SEGALOFF (1947, 1948, 1953), DUNNING, CURTIS und MAUN (1949, 1950), DUNNING, CURTIS und MADSEN (1951), DUNNING und CURTIS (1952, 1954, 1956), MACKENZIE (1955), NOBLE und CUTTS (1959).

GESCHICKTER (1939) sah bei einem Inzuchtstamm von Albinoratten ein von der Injektionsdosis abhängiges zeitliches Auftreten der Tumoren. Bei täglichen Injektionen von 30 μg traten die Tumoren nach 600—700 Tagen auf; nach täglichen Injektionen von 200 μg nach 150—200 Tagen. Auch nach Pelotten von 3—10 mg Oestrogen wurden die Tumoren nach 50—200 Tagen beobachtet. Die Tumoren waren oft multipel vorhanden und zeigten Metastasen. CUTTS (1964) sah keine Änderung des Wachstums der bereits gebildeten Tumoren, wenn er mit Hormonpelotten behandelten Ratten zusätzliche Oestrogeninjektionen verabfolgte. Zusätzliche Behandlung mit Testosteron, Progesteron oder STH erhöhte die Latenzperiode bei der Tumorentstehung und zeigte zeitweise Regression der Tumoren. Hormonbehandlung bei hypophysektomierten Tieren zeigte keinen Erfolg.

GESCHICKTER und BYRNES konnten 1958 zeigen, daß die Zeitdauer der Entstehung des Tumors vom Versuchsbeginn an dem Alter der Ratte umgekehrt proportional ist. Bei Ratten von 1 Monat ist eine Behandlung von 293 Tagen nötig, um Tumoren zu entwickeln, bei Ratten im Alter von 20 Monaten eine nur 90 Tage dauernde Behandlung. Tumoren wurden bei kastrierten männlichen und weiblichen Ratten beobachtet. Eine alleinige Behandlung mit Progesteron oder Testosteron erzeugt dagegen keine Mammatumoren.

Nach den Untersuchungen von DUNNING, CURTIS und SEGALOFF (1947, 1948, 1953) ist die Tumorempfänglichkeit bei Oestrogenbehandlung bei den einzelnen Rattenstämmen verschieden. Der August-Stamm 990 zeigte die stärkste Empfänglichkeit gegenüber Mammatumoren. Beim Ax C-Stamm 9935 entwickelten sich bei männlichen 25% und bei weiblichen Tieren 18% Tumoren. Beim Fisher-Stamm 344 waren bei 7% männlichen und bei 16% weiblichen Tieren Tumoren aufgetreten, während der Copenhagen-Stamm 2331 völlig resistent war. Pelotten aus Stilboestrol und Cholesterin waren stärker wirksam als Pelotten mit Oestrogen allein. Die Ax C-Ratten und August-Stammratten zeigten bis 85% Tumoren, die Fisher-Stammratten bis 22% Tumoren, während die Ratten des Copenhagen-Stammes wieder völlig resistent waren. Multiple Tumoren wurden häufiger nach Stilboestrol als nach Oestrogenbehandlung gefunden. Bei Ratten des Copenhagen-Stammes stimuliert Oestrogen das Mammagewebe, erzeugt aber keine Tumoren. NELSON (1944) sah bei Ratten des Long-Evans-Stammes nach Oestrogenbehandlung bis zu 50% Mammacarcinome. Die Unterschiedlichkeit des Auftretens von Mammatumoren bei Ratten findet sich aber nicht nur bei oestrogenbehandelten Ratten. BOYLAND und SYDNOR (1962) sahen z. B. nach Behandlung von weiblichen Sprague-Dawley- oder Wistarratten mit 7,12-Dizuethylbenzoanthracen (DMBA) nach 4 bis 6 Wochen zahlreiche Mammacarcinome. Bei Ratten des Marshallstammes traten bei gleicher Behandlung keine Brustdrüsentumoren auf und bei Ratten des Auguststammes erst nach einer wesentlich längeren Behandlungszeit (Wistar 50 Tage, August 30 Tage). CUTTS und NOBLE (1964) fanden bei Ratten nach Behandlung mit Oestrogen (Pellets von 8–11 mg implantiert bei 30–40 Tage alten weiblichen Ratten) eine große Häufung von Mammatumoren, aber auch eine starke Unterschiedlichkeit bei den einzelnen Tierstämmen.

Stammesunterschiede bei der Empfänglichkeit für die Tumorinduktion durch Oestron

Stamm	Zahl der Ratten	Zahl der Tiere mit Tumoren	Auftreten in %	Latenzzeit (Mittelwert $\pm S$[1])
FISCHER	74	12	16	412 ± 6,27
WISTAR	50	12	24	383 ± 3,19
LEWIS	44	14	32	378 ± 2,88
SPRAGUE-DAWLEY	38	16	42	324 ± 3,04
HOODED	212	182	86	303,5 ± 2,24

[1]) Standardabweichung des Mittelwertes

DUNNING, CURTIS (1954), DUNNING, CURTIS und MAUN (1949, 1950) fanden nach Verminderung der Nahrungszufuhr eine Hemmung der Mammacarcinomentwicklung beim AxC-Stamm. Die Latenzzeit der Mammacarcinomentstehung wurde verlängert, während erhöhte Fettzufuhr die Latenzzeit verringerte. Durch Zugabe von Tryptophan [DUNNING und CURTIS (1954), DUNNING, CURTIS und MAUN (1950)] wurde die Häufigkeit des Tumorbefalls erhöht.

*Progesteron*behandlung vermindert die Mammatumorhäufigkeit bei Mäusen [SYMEONIDIS (1948), MÜHLBOCK (1952), KIRKHAM und TURNER (1954), HEIMAN (1944), LOESER (1941)] ebenso wie Testosteronbehandlung [NATHANSON und ANDERVONT (1939), JONES (1941), HEIMAN (1944)]. Progesteron hemmt auch die Induktion der Mammatumoren durch Carcinogene [JULL (1954)]. Exogene Progesteronzufuhr erhöht nur die Mammatumorrate bei oestrogenbehandelten, kastrierten Mäusen [MOON, SIMPSON, LI und EVANS (1952)], nicht aber bei C3H-

Mäusen ohne oestrogene Behandlung [BURROWS und HOCH-LIGETI (1946)]. Progesteron fördert dagegen die Induktion des Mammacarcinoms nach Behandlung mit Acetaminofluoren bei *Ratten* [CANTAROW (1934), STASNEY und PASCHKIS (1948)].

Progesteronbehandlung hemmt die durch Oestrogengaben induzierte Entstehung von Mammacarcinomen bei Ratten [NOBLE und COLLIP (1941), NOBLE und CUTTS (1959)]. NELSON (1944) sah einen Wachstumsstillstand der Mammatumoren nach Absetzen der Oestrogenzufuhr. HUGGINS (1958) beobachtete auch bei der Ratte eine Verzögerung des Auftretens der Mammacarcinome durch 3-Methylcholanthren und Ovarektomie; während kleine Mengen Oestradiol bei ovarektomierten Tieren das Auftreten beschleunigten, hemmten große Mengen. Die stärkste Beschleunigung sah er bei gleichzeitiger Behandlung von Methylcholanthren und Progesteron.

Eine Hemmung der Mammacarcinomentstehung nach Behandlung mit thyreotropem Hormon sahen CRAMER und HORNING (1938). GROSS und SCHWARTZ (1951) nehmen einen fördernden Einfluß des Thyroxins auf die Mammatumorentstehung an. Fütterung von Thiouracil verhindert die Entwicklung der Milchdrüse und der Mammatumoren bei weiblichen C3H-Mäusen [DUBNIK, MORRIS und DALTON (1950)]. Also widersprechende Resultate.

Eine normale Mammaentwicklung bei hypophysektomierten *Ratten* konnte nur zustande gebracht werden, wenn STH, Prolaktin, Oestrogen und Progesteron in optimalen Dosen gegeben wurden [LYONS, JOHNSTON, COLE und LI (1953), LYONS, LI und JOHNSTON (1956)]; Oestrogen allein zeigt keinen Effekt auf das Brustdrüsenwachstum der Ratte nach Hypophysektomie [GOMEZ und TURNER (1936)]. Das Brustdrüsenwachstum wird gehemmt durch Cortison [JOHNSON und MEITES (1955)], durch Progesteron [DAANE und LYONS (1954), GARDNER und HILL (1936)], durch Testosteron [HEIMANN (1943)] sowie durch *hohe* Dosen Oestrogen [GARDNER (1941)].

Literatur

a) Mammacarcinom

AHREN, K., and D. JACOBSOHN: Mammary growth in hypophysectomized rats injected with ovarian hormones and insulin. Acta physiol. scand. **37**, 190—203 (1956).

ANDERVONT, H. B.: The incidence of mammary tumors in mice of strain C3H and its descendants of fostered strain C. J. nat. Cancer Inst. **10**, 193 (1949).

— Studies on the disappearance of the mammary tumor agent in mice of strains C3H and C. J. nat. Cancer Jnst. **10**, 201 (1949).

—, and T. B. DUNN: Mammary tumors in mice presumably free of the mammary tumor agent. J. nat. Cancer Inst. 8, 227—233 (1948).

— — Attempt to detect a mammary tumor-agent in strain C mice by X-radiation. J. nat. Cancer Inst. **10**, No. 5, 1157 (1950).

— — Influences of heredity and the mammary tumor agent on the occurrence of mammary tumors in hybrid mice. J. nat. Cancer Inst. **14**, No. 2, 317 (1953).

— —, and H. Y. CANTER: Susceptibility of agent-free inbred mice and their F_1 hybrids to estrogen-induced mammary tumors. J. nat. Cancer Inst. **21**, No. 4 (1958).

ARMSTRONG, E. C.: Observations on the nature of the oestrous cycle and on the effect upon it of the milk factor, in mice of two inbred strains, differing in mammary cancer incidence. Brit. J. Cancer **2**, 59 (1948).

BALL, Z. B., R. A. HUSEBY and M. B. VISSCHER: The effect of dietary pseudo-hypophysectomy upon the development of the mammary glands and mammary tumors in mice receiving diethylstilbestrol. Cancer Res. **6**, 493 (1946).

BERN, H. A., S. NANDI and K. B. DEOME: Survival and regression of hyperplastic nodules in the mammary glands of hypophysectomized C3H mice. Proc. Amer. Ass. Cancer Res. **2**, 187 (1957).

BIERICH, R., u. A. ROSENBOHM: Der Einfluß von Follikelhormon und lokaler Disposition auf die Brustkrebsentstehung bei der Maus. Z. Krebsforsch. **53**, Nr. 2, 57 (1942).

BITTNER, J. J.: Possible relationship of the estrogenic hormones, genetic susceptibility and milk influence in the production of mammary cancer in mice. Cancer Res. **2**, 710—721 (1942).

— The mammary tumor milk agent. Ann. N. Y. Acad. Sci. **49**, 69 (1947).

— The causes and control of mammary cancer in mice. Harvey Lect. **13**, 221 (1946—1947).

— The causes of mammary cancer in mice. Acta Un. int. Cancr. **6**, 175 (1948).

— Some enigmas associated with the genesis of mammary cancer in mice. Cancer Res. **8**, 625 (1948).

BITTNER, J. J.: Studies on the inherited susceptibility and inherited hormonal influence in the genesis of mammary cancer in mice. Cancer Res. **12**, 594 (1952).
— Transfer of the agent for mammary cancer in mice by the male. Cancer Res. **12**, 387 (1952).
— The genesis of breast cancer in mice. Tex. Rep. Biol. Med. **10**, No. 1, 160 (1952).
— Inherited hormonal mechanisms and mammary cancer: in NH mice and their hybrids. Cancer Res. **13**, No. 9, 672 (1953).
— Mammary cancer in mice observed in different laboratories and during the war period. J. nat. Cancer Inst. **15**, No .2 (1954).
— Inherited hormonal mechanisms and mammary cancer in CE mice and their hybrids. Cancer Res. **14**, 783 (1954).
— Experimental aspects of mammary cancer in mice. In: E. F. LEWISON, ed., Breast Cancer. S. 75. Baltimore: Williams & Wilkins (1955).
— Mammary cancer in C3H mice of different sublines and their hybrids. J. nat. Cancer Inst. **16**, No. 5 (1956).
— Mammary-cancer-inducing and inhibitory inherited hormonal patterns in mice. J. nat. Cancer Inst. **21**, No. 4 (1958).
—, and M. J. FRANTZ: Spontaneous mammary cancer in mice of the CE stock. Cancer Res. **14**, 81—85 (1954).
—, and R. A. HUSEBY: Relationship of the inherited susceptibility and the inherited hormonal influence to development of mammary cancer in mice. Cancer Res. **6**, 235—239 (1946).
— — Some inherited hormonal factors influencing mammary carcinogenesis in virgin mice. I. Genetic studies, S. 361—368. In: E. S. GORDON (ed.), A Symposium on Steroid Hormones. Madison: Univ. of Wisc. Press 1950.
—, and D. T. IMAGAWA: Effect of the source of the mouse mammary tumor agent (MTA) upon neutralization of the agent with antisera. Cancer Res. **15**, No. 7, 464 (1955).
BONSER, G. M.: Carcinoma of the male breast in mice induced with oestrin: effect of a vitamin-A-deficient diet combined with oestrin treatment. J. Path. Bact. **41**, 33 (1935).
— The effect of oestrone administration on the mammary glands of male mice of two strains differing greatly in their susceptibility to spontaneous mammary carcinoma. J. Path. Bact. **42**, 169 (1936).
— L. H. STICKLAND and K. L. CONNAL: Krebserzeugung durch Oestron bei weiblichen Mäusen eines Stammes, in dem keine Spontanrupturen vorkommen. J. Path. Bact. **45**, 709 (1937); Zbl. allg. Path. path. Anat. **70**, 43 (1938).
BOOT, L. M., and O. MÜHLBOCK: The mammary tumour incidence in the C3H mousestrain with and without the agent (C3H, C3Hf, C3He). Acta Un. int. Cancer, **12**, 569 (1956).
— — G. RÖPCKE, and VAN EBBENHORST TENGBERGEN: Further investigations on induction of mammary cancer in mice by isografts of hypophyseal tissue. Cancer Res. **22**, 713—727 (1962).
BOYLAND, E., and K. L. SYDNOR: The induction of mammary cancer in rats. Brit. J. Cancer **16**, 731 (1962).
BRYAN, W. R.: Some Biological Considerations of Tumor Viruses. Unio internationalis contra cancrum conference on cellular control mechanisms and cancer, p. 338—355. Amsterdam: Elsevier Publishing Company 1964.
BURROWS, H.: The localization of response to oestrogenic compounds in the organs of male mice. J. Path. Bact. **41**, 423 (1936).
— A comparison of the changes induced by some pure oestrogenic compounds in the mammae and testes of mice. J. Path. Bact. **42**, 161 (1936).
— Biological actions of sex hormones. Sec. ed. Cambridge (Engl.): Univ. Press 1949.
—, and C. HOCH-LIGETI: Effect of progesterone on the development of mammary cancer in C3H mice. Cancer Res. **6**, 608—609 (1946).
BUTENANDT, A.: Zur physiologischen Bedeutung des Follikelhormons und der östrogenen Wirkstoffe für die Genese des Brustdrüsenkrebses und die Therapie des Prostata-Carcinoms. Dtsch. med. Wschr. **75**, Nr. 1 (1950).
— Karzinogene Stoffe und Tumorgenese. Verh. dtsch. Ges. Path. **35**, 70 (1952).
CANTAROW, A., J. STASNEY and K. E. PASCHKIS: The influence of sex hormones an mammary tumors induced by 2-acetylaminofluorene. Cancer Res. 8, 412 (1948).
CASAS, C. B., J. T. KING and M. B. VISSCHER: Effects of caloric restriction on the adrenal response of ovariectomized C3H mice. Amer. J. Physiol. **157**, 193—196 (1949).
CORI, C. F.: The influence of ovariectomy on the spontaneous occurrence of mammary carcinomas in mice. J. exp. Med. **45**, 983 (1927).
CRAMER, W., and E. S. HORNING: Über Verhütung des spontanen Brustkrebses der Maus durch thyreotropes Hypophysenhormon. Lancet **234**, 72 (1938); Zbl. allg. Path. path. Anat. **71**, 371 (1939).
CUTTS, J. H.: Estrone-induced mammary tumors in the rat. Cancer Res. **24**, 1124—1130 (1964).
—, and R. L. NOBLE: Estrone-induced mammary tumors in the rat. I. Induction and behavior of tumors. Cancer Res. **24**, 1116—1123 (1964).

DAANE, T. A., and W. R. LYONS: Effect of estrone, progesterone and pituitary mammotropin on the mammary glands of castrated C3H male mice. Endocrinology **55**, 191—199 (1954).
DE OME, K. B.: The role of the mammary tumor virus in mouse mammary nodulligenesis and tumorigenesis in viruses, nucleic acids and cancer, p. 488. Baltimore: The Williams and Wilkins Comp. 1963.
—, L. J. FAULIN, H. A. BERN u. P. B. BLAIR: Cancer Res. **13**, 515 (1959).
DERINGER, M. K., W. E. HESTON and H. B. ANDERVONT: Estrus in virgin strain C3H (high-tumor) and virgin strain A (low-tumor) mice and in reciprocal (AxC3H) F_1 hybrids. J. nat. Cancer Inst. **5**, 403 (1945).
DMOCHOWSKI, L.: Mammary tumour inducing factor and genetic constitution. Brit. J. Cancer **2**, 94 (1948).
— Survival of the milk factor in a transplantable breast tumour in mice. Brit. J. Cancer **3**, 246 (1949).
— Some data on the distribution of the milk factor. Brit. J. Cancer **3**, 525 (1949).
—, and J. W. ORR: Induction of breast cancer by oestrogens and methylcholanthrene in high-and-low breast cancer strain mice. Brit. J. Cancer **3**, 376—383 (1949).
— — Chemically induced breast tumours and the mammary tumour agent. Brit. J. Cancer **3**, 520 (1949).
DUBNIK, C. S., H. P. MORRIS und A. J. DALTON: Verhinderung der Entwicklung der Milchdrüse und der Mammatumoren bei weibl. C3H-Mäusen nach Zuführung von Thiouracil. J. nat. Cancer Inst. **10**, 815 (1950); Arch. Geschwulstforsch. **4**, H. 3, 293 (1952).
DUNNING, W.F., and M.R. CURTIS: The incidence of diethylstilbestrol-induced cancer in reciprocal F_1 hybrids obtained from crosses between rats of inbred lines that are susceptible and resistant to the induction of mammary cancers by this agent. Cancer Res. **12**, 702—706 (1952).
— — Further studies on the relation of dietary tryptophan to the induction of neoplasms in rats. Cancer Res. **14**, 299—302 (1954).
— — The respective roles of longevity and genetic specificity in the occurrence of spontaneous tumors in the hybrids between two inbred lines of rats. Cancer Res. **6**, 61—81 (1956).
— —, and M. E. MADSEN: Diethylstilbestrol-induced mammary gland and bladder cancer in reciprocal F_1 hybrids between two inbred lines of rats. Acta Un. int. Cancr.; Cancer Res. **7**, 238—244 (1951).
— —, and M. E. MAUN: The effect of dietary fat and carbohydrates on diethylstilbestrol-induced mammary cancer in rats. Cancer Res. **9**, 354—361 (1949).
— — — The effect of dietary tryptophane on the occurrence of diethylstilbestrol-induced mammary cancer in rats. Cancer Res. **10**, 319—323 (1950).
— —, and A. SEGALOFF: Strain differences in response to diethyl- stilbestrol and the induction of mammary gland and bladder cancer in the rat. Cancer Res. **7**, 511 (1947).
— — — Strain differences in response to diethylstilbestrol and the induction of mammary gland, adrenal and bladder cancer in the rat. Rev. Acta., No. **1**, Communications du Congrès des St. LOUIS, 1948.
— — — Strain differences in response to estrone and the induction of mammary gland, adrenal and bladder cancer in rats. Cancer Res. **13**, 147—152 (1953).
EISEN, M. J.: The occurrence of benign and malignant mammary lesions in rats treatet with crystalline estrogen. Cancer Res. **2**, 632 (1944).
FISCHER, W., u. J. KÜHL: Geschwülste der Laboratoriumstiere. Dresden, Leipzig: Theodor Steinkopff 1958.
FURTH, J., K. H. CLIFTON, E. L. GADSDEN and R. F. BUFFET: Dependent and autonomous mammatropic pituitary tumors in rats. Their somatotropic features. Cancer Res. **16**, 608 (1956).
GARDNER, W. U.: Growth of the mammary glands in hypophysectomized mice. Proc. Soc. exp. Biol. (N. Y.) **45**, 835—837 (1940).
— The effect of estrogen on the incidence of mammary and pituitary tumors in hybrid mice. Cancer Res. **1**, 345 (1941).
— Inhibition of mammary growth by large amounts of estrogen. Endocrinology **28**, 53 (1941).
— Persistence and growth of spontaneous mammary tumors and hyperplastic nodules in hypophysectomized mice. Cancer Res. **2**, 476—478 (1942).
—, and R. T. HILL: Effect of progestin upon the mammary glands of the mouse. Proc. Soc. exp. Biol. (N. Y.) **34**, 718—720 (1936).
— G. M. SMITH, E. ALLEN and L. C. STRONG: Erzeugung von Brustdrüsenkrebs in männlichen Mäusen durch Oestrin. Arch. Path. (Chicago) **21**, 265 (1936); Zbl. allg. Path. path. Anat. **65**, 335 (1936).
— and L. C. STRONG: Strain-limited development of tumors of the pituitary gland in mice receiving estrogens. Yale J. Biol. Med. **12**, 543—548 (1940).
— —, and G. M. SMITH: The mammary glands of mature female mice of strains varying in susceptibility to spontaneous tumor development. Amer. J. Cancer **37**, 510 (1939).

GARDNER, W. U., and A. WHITE: Mammary growth in hypophysectomized male mice. Anat. Rec. **82**, 414 (1942).
GASS, G. H., D. COATS, and N. GRAHAM: Carcinogenic dose-response curve to oral diethylstilbestrol. J. nat. Cancer Inst. **33**, 971 (1964).
GESCHICKTER, C. F.: Mammary cancer in the rat with metastasis induced by estrogen. Science **89**, 35 (1939).
— Mammary carcinoma in the rat with metastasis induced bei estrogen. Science **89**, 35—37 (1939).
— Estrogenic mammary cancer in the rat. Radiology **33**, 439—448 (1939).
— Mammary cancer in the rat. Acta Un. int. Cancr. **5**, 109 (1940).
—, and E. W. BYRNES: Factors influencing the development and time of appearence of mammary cancer in the rat in response to estrogens. Arch. Path. (Chicago) **33**, 334—356 (1942).
GOMEZ, E. T., and C. W. TURNER: Non-effect of estrogenic hormones on mammary gland of hypophysectomized guinea pig. Proc. Soc. exp. Biol. (N. Y.) **34** (1936).
— — W. U. GARDNER and R. T. HILL: Oestrogenic treatment of hypophysectomized male mice. Proc. Soc. exp. Biol. (N. Y.) **36**, 287—290 (1937).
GRAD, B., J. BERENSON and L. CAPLAN: The influence of hyper- and hypothyroidism on the incidence of lymphogenous leukemia in AKR mice. Proc. Amer. Ass. Cancer Res. **2** (1), 20 (1955).
GRAFFI, A., u. H. BIELKA: Probleme der experimentellen Krebsforschung. Leipzig: Gless & Portig 1959.
GROSS, J., and S. SCHWARTZ: Der Umsatz von Thyroxin in C 57-Mäusen und in C3H-Mäusen mit und ohne Mammatumoren. Cancer Res. **11**, 614 (1951); Arch. Geschwulstforsch. **4**, H. 3, 295 (1952).
VAN GULIK, P. J., and R. KORTEWEG: Susceptibility to follicular hormone and disposition to mammary cancer in female mice. Amer. J. Cancer **38**, 506 (1940).
HAGEN, E. O., and H. E. RAWLINSON: The induction of mammary cancer in male mice by isologous pituitary implants. Cancer Res. **24**, 59—60 (1964).
HEIMAN, J.: Comparative effects of estrogen testosterone and progesterone on benign mammary tumors of the rat. Cancer Res. **3**, 65 (1943).
— Effect of testosterone propionate on the adrenals and on the incidence of mammary cancer in the RIII strain of mice. Cancer Res. **4**, 31 (1944).
— The effect of progesterone and testosterone propionate on the incidence of mammary cancer in mice. Cancer Res. **5**, 426 (1945).
HESTON, W. E.: Genetics of mammary tumors in mice. In "Symposium on mammary tumors in mice". Public. Amer. Ass. Adv. Sci., No. 22 (1945).
— Localization of gene action in the causation of lung and mammary gland tumors in mice. J. nat. Cancer Inst. **15**, 775—783 (1954).
— Induction of mammary gland tumors in strain C57 BL/He. Mice by isografts of hypophyses. J. nat. Cancer Inst. **32**, 947—955 (1964).
— and M.K. DERINGER Occurrence of tumors in agent-free strain C3Hf male mice implanted with estrogencholesterol pellets. Proc. Soc. exp. Biol. (N. Y.) **82**, 731—734 (1953).
— — and T. B. DUNN: Further studies on the relationship between the genotype and the mammary tumor agent in mice. J. nat. Cancer Inst. **16**, No. 6, 1309 (1956).
— — — and W. D. LEVILLAIN: Factors in the development of spontaneous mammary gland tumors in agent-free strain C3H mice. J. nat. Cancer Inst. **10**, 1139—1151 (1950).
— — and W. D. LEVILLAIN: Mammary gland tumors in aline of C3H mice deprived of the milk agent. Cancer Res. **9**, 544 (1949).
—, and G. VLAHAKIS: Influence of the a gene on mammary-gland tumors. Hepatomas, and normal growth in mice. J. nat. Cancer Inst. **26**, 969—983 (1961).
HOWARD, B., B. THELMA and Y. HARRY: Susceptibility of agent-free inbred mice and their F_1 hybrids to estrogen-induced mammary tumors. J. nat. Cancer Inst. **21**, No. 4 (1958).
HUGGINS, CH.: Hormonabhängige Geschwülste — klinisch und experimentell. Klin. Wschr. **36**, H. 23, 1102 (1958).
HUSEBY, R. A., and J. BITTNER: Die Entwicklung von Mammakrebs in Kastraten eines Stammes männlicher Mäuse mit Ovarienimplantaten. Cancer Res. **11**, 450 (1951); Arch. Geschwulstforsch. **4**, H. 3, 291 (1952).
JACOBSOHN, D.: Action of estradiol monobenzoate on the mammary glands of hypophysectomized rabbits. Acta physiol. scand. **32**, 304—313 (1954).
JOHNSON, R. M., and J. MEITES: Effect of cortisone, hydrocortisone and ACTH on mammary growth and pituitary prolactin content of rats. Proc. Soc. exp. Biol. (N. Y.) **89**, 455—458 (1955).
JONES, E. E.: The effect of testosterone propionate on mammary tumors in mice of the C3H strain. Cancer Res. **1**, 787 (1941).

JULL, J. W.: The effects of oestrogens and progesterone on the chemical induction of mammary cancer in mice of the IF strain. J. Path. Bact. **68**, 547—559 (1954).

KAUFMANN, C.: Über die Wirkung fortgesetzter Zufuhr unphysiologischer Mengen Follikelhormon auf das Genitale weiblicher Ratten. Mschr. Geburtsh. Gynäk. **105**, 188 (1937).

—, u. H. A. MÜLLER: Bemerkung zu der Arbeit von A. BUTENANDT. Dtsch. Med. Wsch. 1950, 1409.

— — A. BUTENANDT u. H. FRIEDRICH-FREKSA: Experimentelle Bedeutung des Follikelhormons für die Carcinomentstehung. Z. Krebsforsch. **56**, 482 (1949).

KING, J. T., C. B.CASAS and M. B. VISSCHER: The influence of estrogen on cancer incidence and adrenal changes in ovariectomized mice on caloric restriction. Cancer Res. **9**, 436-437 (1949).

KIRKHAM, W. R., and C. W. TURNER: Induction of mammary growth in rats by estrogen and progesterone. Proc. Soc. exp. Biol. (N. Y.) **87**, 139 (1954).

KIRSCHBAUM, A.: The role of hormones in cancer: laboratory animals. Cancer Res. **17**, 432 (1957).

—, and J. J. BITTNER: Relation of the milk influence to the carcinogenic induction of mammary cancer in mice. Proc. Soc. exp. Biol. (N. Y.) **58**, 18—19 (1945).

KORTEWEG, R.: Genetically determined differences in hormone production, a possible factor influencing the susceptibility to mammary cancer in mice. Brit. J. Cancer **2**, 91 (1948).

KUNII, A., u. J. FURTH: Mammary carcinoma in mice bearing a transplantable mammotropic tumor, carrying the Bittner virus. Proc. Soc. exp. Biol. (N. Y.) **114**, 709—714 (1963).

LACASSAGNE, A.: L' apparition de cancers de la mamelle chez la souris mâle soumis à des injections de folliculine. C. R. Acad. Sci. (Paris) **195**, 630—632 (1932).

— Einfluß eines familiären Faktors auf die Entstehung von Mammakrebsen bei der männlichen Maus mittels Follikulin. C. R. Soc. Biol. (Paris) **114**, No. 31, 427 (1933); Zbl. allg. Path. path. Anat. **60**, 214 (1934).

— Tumeurs malignes apparues au cours d'un traitement hormonal combiné chez des souris appartenant à des lignées réfractaires au cancer spontané. C. R. Soc. Biol. (Paris) **121**, 607 (1936).

— Tentatives pour modifier, par la progestérone ou par la testostérone, l'apparition des adénocarcinomes mammaires provoquées par l'oestrone chez la souris. C. R. Soc. Biol. (Paris) **126**, 385 (1937).

— Statistique des différents cancers constatés dans des lignées selectionnées de souris, après action prolongée d'hormones oestrogènes. Bull. Ass. franç. Cancer **27**, No. 2 (1938).

— Les cancers produits par des substances chimiques endogènes. Paris: Hermann 1950.

— Die hormonell bedingten Krebse. Strahlentherapie **1950**, 83.

— Der Krebs hormonaler Herkunft. Paris méd. **41**, 8: 101, (1951); Dtsch. med. Wschr. **76**, Nr. 23, 786 (1951).

— Endocrine factors concerned in the genesis of experimental mammary carcinoma. J. Endocr. **13**, 9 (1955).

—, et A. CHAMORRO: Conséquences de l'hypophysectomie chez des souris sujettes au carcinome mammaire traitée par hormone oestrogène. C. R. Soc. Biol. (Paris) **131**, 1077 (1939).

LATHROP, A. E. C., and L. LOEB: The influence of pregnancies on the incidence of cancer in mice. Proc. Soc. exp. Biol. (N. Y.) **11**, 38—40 (1913).

— — Further investigations on the origin of tumors in mice. III. On the part played by internal secretion in the spontaneous development of tumors. J. Cancer Res. **1**, 1—19 (1916).

LIEBELT, R. A., and N. E. ECKLES: Effects of castration and adrenalectomy on mammary cancer growth in R III mice. Proc. Amer. Ass. Cancer Res. **2**, 227 (1957).

LIPSCHUTZ, A.: Steroid hormones and tumors. Baltimore: Williams & Wilkins Comp. 1950.

— Steroid homeostasis hypophysis and tumorigenesis. Cambridge: Heffer & Sons, Ltd. 1957.

LOEB, L.: Am. J. med. Res. **8**, 274 (1924).

— The significance of hormones in the origin of cancer. J. nat. Cancer Inst. **1**, 169 (1940).

— H. T. BLUMENTHAL and M. M. KIRTZ: The effectiveness of ovarian and hypophyseal grafts in the production of mammary carcinoma in mice. Science **99**, 230—232 (1944).

—, and M. M. KIRTZ: The effects of transplants of anterior lobes of the hypophysis on the growth of the mammary gland and on the development of mammary gland carcinoma in various strains of mice. Amer. J. Cancer **36**, 56—82 (1939).

LOESER, A. A.: Mammary carcinoma response to implantation of male hormone and progesterone. Lancet **1941, II**, 698.

LYONS, W. R., R. E. JOHNSTON, R. D. COLE and CH. H. LI: Mammary growth and lactation in male rats. In: R. W. SMITH jr., O. H. GAEBLER and C. N. H. LONG (eds.), The Hypophyseal Growth Hormone, Nature and Actions. 401. New York: Mc.Graw-Hill, Broc. Co. Inc. 1953.

— CH. H. LI and R. E. JOHNSTON: Direct action of mammary stimulating hormones. J. clin. Endocr. **16**, 367 (1956).

MacKenzie, I.: The production of mammary cancer in rats using oestrogen. Brit. J. Cancer **9**, 284—299 (1955).
Mark, J., and G. R. Biskind: The effect of long term stimulation of male and female rats with estrone, estradiol benzoate and testosterone proprionate administered in pelled form. Endocrinology **28**, 465 (1941).
Martinez, C., and J. J. Bittner: Effect of ovariectomy, adrenalectomy and hypophysectomy on growth of spontaneous mammary tumors in mice. Proc. Soc. exp. Biol. (N. Y.) **86**, 92—95 (1954).
Moon, H. D., M. E. Simpson, Ch. H. Li and A. M. Evans: Effects of pituitary growth hormone in mice. Cancer Res. **12**, 448 (1952).
Mühlbock, O.: The sensitivity of the mammary gland to oestrone in different strains of mice with and without mammary tumour agent. Acta endocr. (Kbh.) **3**, 105 (1949).
— The effect of steroids on the incidence of mammary tumours in mice. Ciba Found. Coll. Endocr. **1**, 112 (1952).
— Hormonal genesis of mammary cancer in mice. Acta endocr. (Kbh.) **10**, No. 2 (1954).
— Experimentelle Untersuchungen über die Genese des Mamma-Karzinoms. Strahlentherapie **96**, H. 2 (1955).
— Experimentelle Untersuchungen über die Genese des Mamma-Karzinoms. Schweiz. med. Wschr. **85**, Nr. 17, 387 (1955).
— Studies on the hormone dependence of experimental breast tumors in mice. In: A. R. Currie and C. F. W. Illingworth (eds.), Endocrine Aspects of Breast Cancer. 291—296. Edinburgh: E. & S. Livingstone, Ltd. 1958.
—, and T. G. van Rijssel: Studies on mammary tumors in the O_{20} Amsterdam strain of mice. J. nat. Cancer Inst. **15**, 73—98 (1954).
Murray, W. S.: Ovarian secretion and tumor incidence. Science **66**, 600 (1927).
— Amer. J. Cancer **20**, 572 (1934).
Nathanson, I. T., and H. B. Andervont: Effect of testosterone propionate on development and growth of mammary carcinoma in female mice. Proc. Soc. exp. Biol. (N. Y.) **40**, 421 (1939).
Nelson, W. O.: The induction of mammary carcinoma in the rat. Yale. J. Biol. Med. **17**, 217 (1944).
Noble, R. L., and J. P. Collip: Regression of estrogen-induced mammary tumors in female rats following removal of the stimulans. Canad. med. Ass. J. **44**, 1 (1941).
—, and J. H. Cutts: Mammary tumors of the rat. Cancer Res. **19**, 1125 (1959).
— C. S. McEuen, and J. B. Collip: Mammary tumors produced in rats by the action of oestrone tablets. Canad. med. Ass. J. **42**, 413—417 (1940).
—, and J. H. Walters: The effect of hypophysectomy on 9,10-Dimethyl-1-2-benzanthracene-induced carcinogenesis. Proc. Amer. Ass. Cancer Res. **1**, 35 (1954).
Picco, A.: Der Einfluß der Kastration auf die Entwicklung des Fibroadenoma mammae der Ratte. Tumori **22**, 231 (1936); Zbl. allg. Path. path. Anat. **65**, 308 (1936).
Pilgrim, H. I.: A method of evaluating tumor morbidity as applied to the effect of ovariectomy at different ages on the development of mammary tumors in C3H mice. Cancer Res. **17**, 405—408 (1957).
Pullinger, B. D.: The significance of functional differentiation in mammary tumours. Lancet **1949 II**, 823.
— Prevalence of spontaneous benign and malignant mammary tumors in RIIIb mice according to age and parity. Brit. J. Cancer **9**, 613—619 (1955).
Ranadive, K. J.: Relative importance of heredity, hormones and milk borne tumour agent in inducing mammary carcinoma in mice. Indian. J. med. Sci. **7**, No. 10, 545—555 (1953).
—, and V. R. Khanolkar: Effect of foster-nursing on the morphology of mammary glands in mice.Acta Un. int. Cancr. **6**, 155 (1948).
Robson, J. M., and G. M. Bonser: Production of mammary carcinomas in mice in a susceptible strain by the synthetic oestrogen triphenylethylene. Nature (London) **142**, 846 (1938).
Shay, H., M. Gruenstein u. W. B. Kessler: Experimentell erzeugtes Adenoca. der Mamma bei Ratten. J. nat. Cancer Inst. **27**, 503—513 (1961).
Shimkin, M. B.: Hormones and mammary cancer in mice. In "Symp. on Mam. Tum. in Mice." Public. Am. Ass. Adv. Sci. No. 22, Washington 1945.
—, and H. B. Andervont: Effect of foster nursing on the response of mice to estrogens. J. nat. Cancer Inst. **1**, 599 (1941).
— — Effect of foster nursing on the induction of mammary and testicular tumors in mice injected with stilbestrol. J. nat. Cancer Inst. **2**, 611 (1942).
—, and R. S. Wyman: Effect of adrenalectomy and ovariectomy on mammary carcinogenesis in strain C3H mice. J. nat. Cancer Inst. **6**, 187—189 (1945).
— — Mammary tumors in male mice implanted with estrogen-cholesterol pellets. J. nat. Cancer Inst. **7**, 71 (1946).

SILBERBERG, M., and R. SILBERBERG: Mammary growth in orchidectomized mice grafted with anterior lobes of hypophyses and ovaries at various ages. Arch. Path. (Chicago) **49**, 733—751 (1950).
SILBERBERG, R., and M. SILBERBERG: Mammary cancer in castrate male mice receiving ovarian and hypophyseal grafts at different ages. Proc. Soc. exp. Biol. (N. Y.) **70**, 510—513 (1949).
— — Influence of age on mammary growth and involution in male mice treated with estrogen. Arch. Path. (Chicago) **48**, 557 (1949).
SLATTERY, P. A.: Lack of effect of lactogenic hormone on mammary adenocarcinoma in mice. Soc. exp. Biol. (N. Y.) **74**, 539 (1950).
SMITH, F. W.: The relationship of the inherited hormonal influence to the production of adrenal cortical tumors by castration. Cancer Res. **6**, 641 (1948).
SUNTZEFF, V., M. M. KIRTZ, H. T. BLUMENTHAL and L. LOEB: The incidence of mammary gland carcinoma and cancer age in mice injected with estrogen and non-injected mice of different strains. Cancer Res. **1**, 446 (1941).
SYMEONIDIS, A.: Mammary tumor incidence by progesterone in mice. Acta Un. int. Cancr. **6**, 163 (1948).
— The initiation and growth of tumors. Introduction. I. Effects of underfeeding. Amer. J. Cancer **38**, 335 (1940).
TANNENBAUM, A.: Nutrition and cancer. In: F. HOMBURGER and W. H. FISHMAN (eds.), The Physiopathology of Cancer. 392—437. New York: Hoeber-Harper 1953.
TRENTIN, J.: The effect of the presence or absence of the milk faktor and of castration on mammary tumor response to estrogen in male mice of strain of known mammary tumor incidence. Cancer Res. **11**, 286 (1951).
TWOMBLEY, G. H.: Breast cancer produced in male mice of the C57 (Black) strain of little. Proc. Soc. exp. Biol. (N. Y.) **44**, 617—618 (1940).
WHITE, F. R., and J. WHITE: Effect of diethylstilbestrol on mammary tumor formation in strain C3H mice fed a low cystine diet. J. nat. Cancer Inst. **4**, 413—415 (1944).
WOOLLEY, G. W., E. FEKETE and C. C. LITTLE: Mammary tumor development in mice ovariectomized at birth. Proc. nat. Acad. Sci. (Wash.) **25**, 277—279 (1939).
— — — Effect of castration in the dilute brown strain of mice. Endocrinology **28**, 341 (1941).
WRIGHT, A. W., G. H. KLINCK and J. M. WOLFF: Pathologie und Pathogenese spontan auftretender Mammatumoren bei Albany-Ratten. Amer. J. Path. **16**, No. 6 (1940); Zbl. allg. Path. path. Anat. 78, 17 (1942).

b) Hormone und Leukämie, bzw. Geschwülste der lymphatischen Organe

Die Bedeutung der chemischen Carcinogene und der Viren für die Leukämieentstehung wurde in dem Beitrag von BIELKA, BIERWOLF, GRAFFI und SCHRAMM ausführlich besprochen. Die Wirkung der Strahlen wird in dem Beitrag von WRBA erörtert werden. Wir wollen hier nur auf die fördernden und hemmenden Einflüsse der Hormone bei der Leukämieentstehung und bei der Entstehung von Geschwülsten des lymphatischen Gewebes hinweisen.

Verschiedene Agentien bzw. Faktoren können nach KIRSCHBAUM (1951, 1957), KIRSCHBAUM und MIXER (1947) Leukämie erzeugen, so z. B. Viren, Strahlen, Carcinogene und Oestrogene. Die Tatsache, daß bestimmte Mäuseinzuchtstämme eine hohe Rate an Lymphomen (= Lymphosarkome und Leukämien) und andere eine niedere Rate zeigen, wurde als Beweis für den erblichen Einfluß bzw. den Einfluß genetischer Faktoren bei der Entstehung [FURTH, COLE und BOON (1942), FURTH (1946), COLE und FURTH (1941), LAW (1944)] angesehen. Die Spontanrate ist bei weiblichen Tieren höher [LACASSAGNE (1937), MERCIER (1938), GARDNER, DOUGHERTY und WILLIAMS (1944)]. Ausschlaggebend für die Entstehung offenbar neben dem Virus ist die genetische Konstitution der Tierstämme. Diese Leukämien wurden fast ausschließlich bei Mäusen beschrieben. Eine Reihe Untersucher befaßte sich mit den hormonellen Faktoren, die bei der Leukämieentstehung bzw. bei der Tumorentstehung im lymphatischen Gewebe eine Rolle spielen. Über Lymphosarkome bei Mäusen (z. T. in der Thymus) nach langdauernder Behandlung mit Brunsthormon berichtete LACASSAGNE (1937, 1938). Lymphoidtumoren bei Mäusen nach langdauernder *Oestrogenbehandlung* beschrieben 1940 GARDNER, KIRSCHBAUM und STRONG. Eine Oestrogenbehandlung fördert auch das Auftreten von Leukämien nach Röntgenbestrahlung, eine zusätzliche Testosteronbehandlung unterbindet weitgehend den fördernden Effekt des Oestrogens. Nach GARDNER, DOUGHERTY und WILLIAMS (1944) hemmt eine Behandlung mit Testosteronpropionat das Auftreten der durch Oestrogene erzeugten Leukämie bei bestimmten Mäusestämmen.

Bei bestimmten Tieren [KIRSCHBAUM, SHAPIRO und MIXER (1953)] kann Oestrogen als fördernder Faktor bzw. sog. Co-Leukämogen bei der Leukämieerzeugung oder Thymuslymphosarkomentstehung durch Bestrahlung wirken.

Die synergistische Wirkung von Oestrogenen und Strahlen ist besonders am Thymus sichtbar, wo die Oestrogenbehandlung bei BALB-Mäusen die Entstehung von Lymphosarkomen des Thymus durch Bestrahlung beschleunigt. Nach GARDNER und RYGAARD (1954), GARDNER (1950) fördert Oestrogen die genetisch bedingte Leukämiehäufigkeit bzw. Entstehung bei bestimmten Mäusestämmen nach Bestrahlung, während Testosteron diese hemmt.

Die Mäuse werden im Alter von 32—92 Tagen bestrahlt und erhielten wöchentlich vom 6. Bestrahlungstag an 16,6 μg Oestradiol, bzw. 1,25 mg Testosteron. Bestrahlung: 285—380 r, 200 KV, 15 ma, $^1/_2$ mm Cu, 1 mm Al, 38—45 Abstand, 80 r pro Minute.

Ausschlaggebend ist nach den Untersuchungen für die Leukämieentstehung immer der genetische Faktor, während Förderung und Hemmung hormonal gesteuert werden können [KIRSCHBAUM (1957)].

Eine Zunahme von Lymphosarkomen bzw. Lymphoidtumoren nach Oestrogenbehandlung bei belasteten Tierstämmen mit spontaner Tumorrate beschreiben außerdem GARDNER, DOUGHERTY und WILLIAMS (1944), DOUGHERTY (1952), DMOCHOWSKI und HORNING (1952), BISCHOFF, LONG, RUPP und CLARK (1942), ANDERVONT und DUNN (1947), MERCIER und GOSSELIN (1933), COLE und FURTH (1941), KIRSCHBAUM und LIEBELT (1955), KIRSCHBAUM, SHAPIRO und MIXER (1949, 1953), TOCH, HIRSCH, BROWN und KAPLAN (1955).

BISCHOFF, LONG, RUPP und CLARK (1942) beobachteten eine stärkere Wirkung von Oestrogen bei kastrierten als bei nicht kastrierten Tieren und GARDNER, DOUGHERTY und WILLIAMS (1944) und GARDNER (1947) sahen z. B. bei 7 verschiedenen Stämmen mit einer spontanen Belastung von 0—5% nach Oestrogenbehandlung eine Zunahme auf etwa 15%. SILBERBERG und SILBERBERG (1949) fanden auch Lymphoidtumoren bei orchidektomierten Mäusen nach Implantation von Ovar und HVL-Gewebe.

MCENDY, BOON und FURTH (1944) beobachteten nach *Ovarektomie* eine Abnahme der Häufigkeit der Mäuseleukämie von 74% auf 45%. DMOCHOWSKI und HORNING (1952) fanden nach Kastration in der Pubertät eine Zunahme der Lymphome von 59% auf 70%. MURPHY sah 1944 eine Zunahme der Leukämieentstehung bei männlichen Mäusen nach Kastration von 53% auf 97%.

Nach KAPLAN und BROWN (1947, 1951, 1952) hemmt *Testosteron* die Entwicklung von Lymphoidtumoren bei bestrahlten Mäusen, während die Kastration zu einer Steigerung der Häufigkeit führt. Nach KIRSCHBAUM, LIEBELT und FALLS (1955) sind kastrierte Mäuse empfindlicher gegen Leukämieerzeugung durch Methylcholanthren. Testosteron hemmt bei kastrierten Mäusen die Leukämieerzeugung durch das gleiche Carcinogen. Mäuse, die gegen die leukämieerzeugende Wirkung des Methylcholanthren resistent sind, werden wieder empfindlich durch Gonadektomie. Gonadektomie erhöht aber nicht die Empfänglichkeit gegen Leukämieentstehung bei bestrahlten Mäusen. LANNEK (1952) sah eine Hemmung des Wachstums experimentell erzeugter Lymphoidzelltumoren (RPL 19) durch *ACTH* und *Cortisonbehandlung* bei Küken, bei denen die Tumoren durch Transplantation von Tumorzellen erzeugt worden waren.

HEILMAN und KENDALL (1944) fanden eine Hemmung des Wachstums beim transplantierten Lymphosarkom nach Cortisonbehandlung und PEARSON, ELIEL, RAWSON, DOBRINER und RHOADS (1949) nach Cortison und ACTH. Den gleichen Effekt beobachtete WOOLLEY; STURM und MURPHY (1944) sahen eine Förderung der Transplantabilität der Leukämie nach *Adrenalektomie*. Cortisonbehandlung hemmt das Wachstum des transplantierten Lymphosarkoms [WOOLLEY (1951)] und verlängert die Überlebenszeit der an Leukämie erkrankten AKR-Mäuse. Nach STOERK (1950) wird das Wachstum des Lymphosarkoms durch Cortison und Testosteron gehemmt. Nach KAPLAN, BROWN und MARDER (1951) hemmt Cortison das Auftreten von Lymphomen der Thymus nach Bestrahlung, und Adrenalektomie vermindert das Auftreten von Lymphosarkomen der Maus nach Bestrahlung. Über gleiche Beobachtungen berichten LAW, BUNKER und NORRIS (1947). Bei alten Mäusen des C 57-Bl-Stammes treten nach ACTH-Behandlung häufiger maligne Lymphome auf [SILBERBERG und SILBERBERG (1955)]. Nach LAW, BUNKER und MORRIS (1947) hemmt Adrenalektomie das Auftreten der Mäuseleukämie nach Bestrahlung.

Die *Thymektomie* zeigt einen hemmenden Einfluß auf die Lymphoidtumorentstehung nach Bestrahlung [KAPLAN, BROWN und PAULL (1953)] ebenso wie auf das Auftreten der Leukämie [FURTH und BOON (1945)] und die Leukämieerzeugung durch Methylcholanthren [LAW und MILLER (1950)]. Transplantation von Thymusgewebe fördert nach LAW (1952), KAPLAN, HIRSCH und BROWN (1956) bei Mäusen die Leukämieentstehung. Nach LAW (1952) vermindert Thymektomie bei den Mäusestämmen RIL und C 58 das Auftreten spontaner Leukämien. Nach KIRSCHBAUM und LIEBELT (1955) wird das Auftreten der Leukämie nach Behandlung mit Methylcholanthren bei Verminderung der carcinogenen Dosis auf die Hälfte durch Thymektomie gehemmt. Nach KAPLAN, BROWN, HIRSCH und CARNES (1955) stellt transplantiertes, nicht bestrahltes Thymusgewebe einen Focus für die neoplastische Alteration der Lymphocyten nach Bestrahlung dar.

MOON, SIMPSON, LI und EVANS (1950) sahen bei Ratten nach langdauernder Behandlung mit *Wachstumshormon* bei 6 von 15 Tieren Lymphosarkome der Lunge und bei allen Tieren eine Hyperplasie des peribronchialen Lymphgewebes. Die lymphatischen Organe dagegen (Lymphknoten, Milz, Thymus) zeigten keine Veränderungen. Die Malignität dieser Veränderungen ist auf Grund der morphologischen Befunde nicht sicher erkennbar.

NAGAREDA und KAPLAN (1955) beobachteten nach STH-Behandlung eine Proliferation des thymolymphatischen Gewebes bei C 5- und Bl-Mäusen. Hypophysektomie hemmt die Entstehung von Lymphoidtumoren bei C 57-Bl-Mäusen nach Bestrahlung [NAGAREDA und KAPLAN (1955)]. Hemmung der Schilddrüsenfunktion durch Methylthiouracil vermindert die Leukämiehäufigkeit bei AKR-Mäusen [GRAD, BERENSON und CAPLAN (1955)].

Literatur

b) Hormone und Leukämie

ANDERVONT, H. B., and T. B. DUNN: Effect of castration and sex hormones on the induction of tumors in mice with o-aminoazotoluence. J. nat. Cancer Inst. **7**, 455—461 (1947).

BIELSCHOWSKY, F., and E. S. HORNING: Aspects of endocrine carcinogenesis. Brit. med. Bull. **14**, 106 (1958).

BISCHOFF, E., M. L. LONG, J. J. RUPP and G. J. CLARK: Influence of toxic amounts of estrin upon intact and castrated male Marsh-Buffalo mice. Cancer Res. **2**, 198 (1942).

CLIFTON, K. H.: Problems in experimental tumorigenesis of the pituitary gland, gonads, adrenal cortices, and mammary glands: a review. Cancer Res. **19**, 2 (1959).

COLE, R. K., and J. FURTH: Experimental studies on the genetics of spontaneous leukemia in mice. Cancer Res. **1**, 957 (1941).

DMOCHOWSKI, L., and E. S. HORNING: The influence of the male and female sex hormones on the development of lymphoid tumours in mice. Ciba Found. Coll. Endocr. **1**, 24 (1952).

DOUGHERTY, T. F.: Effect of hormones on lymphatic tissue. Physiol. Rev. **32**, 379 (1952).

FURTH, J.: Recent experimental studies on leukemia. Physiol. Rev. **26**, 48 (1946).

—, and M. BOON: The time and site of origin of the leukemic cell. A. A. A. S. Res. Conference on Cancer Am. Assoc. Science Washington D. C. 1945. S. 129.

— R. K. COLE and M. C. BOON: Effect of maternal influence upon spontaneous leukemia of mice. Cancer Res. **2**, 280 (1942).

GARDNER, W. U.: Studies on steroid hormones in experimental carcinogenesis. Recent Progress in Hormone Research. Proc. Laurentian Horm.-Conf. **1**, 217 (1947).

GARDNER, W. U.: Ovarian and lymphoid tumors in female mice subsequent to Roentgen-ray irradiation and hormone treatment. Proc. Soc. exp. Biol. (N. Y.) **75**, 434 (1950).
— T. F. DOUGHERTY and W. L. WILLIAMS: Lymphoid tumors in mice receiving steroid hormones. Cancer Res. **4**, 73—87 (1944).
— A. KIRSCHBAUM and L. C. STRONG: Lymphoid tumors in mice receiving estrogens. Arch. Path. (Chicago) **29**, 1—7 (1940).
—, and J. RYGAARD: Further studies on the incidence of lymphomas in mice exposed to X-rays and given sex hormones. Cancer Res. **14**, 205—209 (1954).
GRAD, B., J. BERENSON and L. CAPLAN: The influence of hyper- and hypothyroidism on the incidence of lymphogenous leukemia in AKR mice. Proc. Amer. Ass. Cancer Res. **2** (1), 20 (1955).
HEILMANN, F., and E. KENDALL: The influence of 11-dehydro-17-hydrocorticosterone on the growth of malignant tumor in mouse. Endocrinology **34**, 416 (1944).
KAPLAN, H. S.: Influence of thymectomie, splenectomie and gonadectomie on incidence of radiation-induced lymphoid tumors in strain C 57 black mice. J. nat. Cancer Inst. **11**, 83 (1950).
—, and M. B. BROWN: Inhibition by testosterone of radiation-induced lymphoid tumors development on intact and castrate adult male mice. Cancer Res. **11**, 706—708 (1951).
— — Inhibition by testosterone of radiation-induced lymphoid tumors development in intact and castrate male mice. Cancer Res. **12**, 262 (1952).
— — Testosterone prevention of post-irradiation lymphomas in C 57 black mice. Cancer Res. **12**, 445 (1952).
— — B. HIRSCH and W. CARNES: Further studies on lymphoma development in non-irradiated thymic implants in thymectomized irradiated C57BL mice. Proc. Amer. Ass. Cancer Res. **2**, 27 (1955).
— —, and S. N. MARDER: Adrenal cortical function and lymphoid tumor incidence in irradiated mice. Cancer Res. **11**, 263 (1951).
— — — Adrenal cortical function and lymphoid tumor incidence in irradiated mice. Cancer Res. **11**, 629—633 (1951).
— —, and J. PAULL: Influence of postirradiation thymectomy and of thymic implants on lymphoid tumor incidence in C57BL mice. Cancer Res. **13**, 677 (1953).
— B. B. HIRSCH and M. B. BROWN: Indirect induction of lymphomas in irradiated mice. IV. Genetic evidence of the origin of tumor cells from the thymic grafts. Cancer Res. **16**, 434—436 (1956).
KIRSCHBAUM, A.: Rodent leukemia: Recent biological studies. A review. Cancer Res. **11**, 741 (1951).
— The role of hormones in cancer: laboratory animals. Cancer Res. **17**, 432 (1957).
— Genetic and nongenetic factors influencing the induction of mouse leukemie. The Leukemias: Etiology, Pathophysiology and Treatment. New York: Academic Press Inc. 1957.
— Etiology of the leukemias: Chemical and hormonal factors in mice. Proc. Cancer Conf. 1957.
— A. G. LIEBELT and N. G. FALLS: Influence of gonadectomy and androgenic hormone on the induction of leukemia by methylcholanthrene in DBA/2 mice. Cancer Res. **15**, 685—688 (1955).
— — Thymus and the carcinogenic induction of mouse leukemia. Cancer Res. **15**, 689 (1955).
—, and H. W. MIXER: Induction of leukemia in eight inbred stocks of mice varying in susceptibility to the spontaneous disease. J. clin. Med. **32**, 720 (1947).
— J. R. SHAPIRO and H. W. MIXER: Synergistic action of estrogenic hormone and X-rays in inducing thymic lymphosarcoma of mice. Proc. Soc. exp. Biol. (N. Y.) **72**, 632 (1949).
— — — Synergistic action of leukemogenic agents. Cancer Res. **13**, 262—268 (1953).
LACASSAGNE, A.: Sarcomes lymphoïdes apparus chez des souris longuement traitées par des hormones oestrogènes. C. R. Soc. Biol. (Paris) **126**, 193 (1937).
— Statistique des différents cancers constatés dans des lignées selectionées de souris après action prolongées d'hormones oestrogènes. Bull. Ass. franç. Cancer **27**, 96 (1938).
— Les cancers produits par des substances chimiques endogènes. Paris: Hermann 1950.
LANNEK, N.: The effect of adrenalcorticotrophic hormone (ACTH), cortisone and hydrocortisone on the growth of experimental lymphoid tumors in chicks. Brit. J. Cancer **6**, 369 (1952).
LAW, L.: Characterization of an influence affecting growth of transplantable leukemias in mice. Cancer Res. **4**, 257 (1944).
— Observations on the effect of thymectomy on spontaneous leukemias in mice of the High-leucemic strains RIL and C58. J. nat. Cancer Inst. **12**, 253 (1952).
— Increase in incidence of leukemia in hybrid mice bearing thymic transplants from High-leukemic strain. J. nat. Cancer Inst. **12**, 789 (1952).
— L. E. BUNKER and B. A. NORRIS: Effect of gonadectomy and adrenalectomy on the appearance and incidence of spontaneous lymphoid leukemia in C58 mice. J. nat. Cancer Inst. **8**, 157—159 (1947).

Law, L., and J. Miller: The influence of thymectomy on the incidence of carcinogen-induced leukemia in strain DBA mice. J. nat. Cancer Inst. **11**, 425 (1950).
Lipschutz, A.: Steroid hormones and tumors. Baltimore: Williams & Wilkins Comp. 1950.
— Steroid homeostasis hypophysis and tumorigenesis. Cambridge: Heffer & Sons, Ltd. 1957.
McEndy, D. P., M. C. Boon and J. Furth: On the role of thymus, spleen, and gonads in the development of leukemia in a high leukemic stock of mice. Cancer Res. **4**, 337—383 (1944).
Mercier, L., et L. Gosselin: Hérédité du lymphosarcome de la souris; hypothèse explicative de cette hérédité. Bull. Acad. Méd. (Paris) **119**, 106 (1933).
— Hérédité du cancer à l'intérieur d'une lignée de souris. Notion de facteur plasmo-chromosomique. C. R. Soc. Biol. (Paris) **127**, 92 (1938).
Moon, H. D., M. E. Simpson, Ch. H. Li and H. M. Evans: Neoplasms in rats treated with pituitary growth hormone. I. Pulmonary and lymphatic tissues. Cancer Res. **10**, 297 (1950).
Murphy, J. B.: The effect of castration, theelin, and testosterone on the incidence of leukemia in a Rockefeller Institute strain of mice. Cancer Res. **4**, 622 (1944).
— and E. Sturm: The adrenals and susceptibility to transplanted leukemia of rats. Science **98**, 568 (1943).
— — The effect of adrenal cortical and pituitary adrenotropic hormones on transplanted leukemia in rats. Science **99**, 303 (1944).
Nagareda, C. S., and H. S. Kaplan: The effect of hypophysectomy and X-irradiation on lymphoid organs and on the induction of lymphoid tumors in C57BL mice. J. nat. Cancer Inst. **16**, 139—152 (1955).
Pearson, O. H., L. P. Eliel, R. W. Rawson, K. Dobriner and C. P. Rhoads: ACTH- and cortisone-induced regression of lymphoid tumors in man. A preliminary report. Cancer (Philad.) **2**, 943 (1949).
Silberberg, M., and R. Silberberg: Malignant lymphoid tumors in orchidectomized mice receiving hypophysial and ovarian grafts at various ages. Proc. Soc. exp. Biol. (N. Y.) **72**, 547 (1949).
— — Leukemogenic action of adreno-corticotrophic hormone (ACTH) in mice of various ages. Cancer Res. **15**, 291 (1955).
Skipper, H.: Partial reversal of the antileukemic activity of A-methopterin by cortisone. Cancer Res. **14**, 86 (1954).
Stoerk, H. C.: Growth retardation of lymphosarcoma implants in pyridoxine-deficient rats by testosterone cortisone. Proc. Soc. exp. Biol. (N. Y.) **74**, 798—800 (1950).
Sturm, E., and J. B. Murphy: The effect of adrenalectomy on the susceptibility of rats to a transplantable leukemia. Cancer Res. **4**, 384 (1944).
Toch, P., B. Hirsch, M. P. Brown and H. S. Kaplan: Lymphoid tumor incidence in C57BL mice treated with estrogen and whole-body X-radiation. Proc. Amer. Ass. Cancer Res. **2** (1), 51 (1955).
Woolley, G. W.: Cortisone, related steroids on transplanted tumors on the mouse. Cancer Res. **11**, 291 (1951).
—, and B. A. Peters: Prolongation of life in high-leukemic AKR mice by cortisone. Proc. Soc. exp. Biol. (N. Y.) **82**, 286—287 (1953).

c, d) Nebennieren- und Hodentumoren

Die nach Hormonbehandlung und nach Störung der hormonellen Korrelation beobachteten malignen Nebennierenrindentumoren (Nebennierencarcinome bzw. maligne Hodenzwischenzelltumoren) haben wir des besseren Verständnisses wegen bei den geschwulstartigen Hyperplasien der Nebenniere und des Hodens abgehandelt. Bei der Entstehung dieser Geschwülste sind genetische Faktoren Voraussetzung, da sie nur bei bestimmten Tierstämmen beobachtet wurden. (Siehe I/A d und g.)

C. Förderung des Geschwulstwachstums durch Hormone im Sinne eines Cocancerogens und Hemmung des Geschwulstwachstums durch Hormone sowie Beeinflussung der Transplantabilität

a) Hypophysenhormone

Bei der Betrachtung der Wirkungsweise der in der Hypophyse gebildeten bzw. von ihr ausgeschiedenen Hormone auf das Krebswachstum oder die Krebsentstehung finden sich außerordentlich unterschiedliche Angaben, die die Problematik dieser Frage sehr deutlich vor Augen führen. Besonders fraglich sind Versuche, bei denen nach Zerstörung oder Röntgenbestrahlung der Hypophyse keine deutlichen Veränderungen des Carcinomwachstums gesehen wurden, da es schwer nachzuweisen ist, ob eine Hypophysektomie exakt durchgeführt wurde. Schon durch die operative Methode ist es außerordentlich schwierig, die ganze Hypophyse zu entfernen; während eine Bestrahlung keine totale Ausschaltung der Hypophysenfunktion sichert.

Hypophysektomie oder Zerstörung der Hypophyse und Wachstum von transplantablen Tumoren

Hayashi (1930) beobachtete bei Kaninchen nach Zerstörung einer Hälfte der Hypophyse ein langsameres Wachstum bei Impfsarkomen. Lacassagne und Nyka (1936) sahen keinen deutlichen Unterschied in der Entwicklung intratestikulärer Transplantate des Brown-Pearce-Tumor bei Tieren, denen die Hypophyse durch Einsetzen einer Tube mit Radon (Radiumemanation) zerstört worden war.

Loefer (1952) beobachtete bei gleichem Alter der Versuchstiere keinen Unterschied beim Anwachsen des Tumors, nur, daß der Tumor beim normalen Tier entsprechend der Körpergewichtszunahme größer war. Der Tumor wuchs, selbst wenn das hypophysektomierte Tier an Gewicht verlor. Auch Funk, Tomashefsky, Ehrlich und Soukup (1950) fanden bei den Kontrollen eine der Körpergewichtszunahme direkt proportionale Zunahme des Tumorgewichtes gegenüber den hypophysektomierten Tieren. Korteweg und Thomas (1949) beobachteten bei deutlicher Wachstumshemmung nach Hypophysektomie ein konstantes Verhältnis zwischen Tumorgewicht und Körpergewichtszunahme.

Über ein langsameres Wachsen des transplantierten Jensen-Sarkoms nach Hypophysektomie berichten Reiss, Druckrey und Hochwald (1933). Eine Verzögerung des Wachstums bei Implantationstumoren nach Hypophysektomie fanden u. a. Samuels und Ball (1933, 1935), Ball und Samuels (1936, 1938), Gardner (1942), McEuen und Thomson (1933), Engel und Murray (1936), Franseen und McTiernan (1936), Talalay, Takano und Huggins (1952), Schrimpf und Willig (1953), Rock und Rabotti (1955). McEuen und Thomson (1933) führen die Hemmung des Tumorwachstums auf eine allgemein schlechtere Ernährung zurück, die durch Hypophysenmangel bedingt ist. Wenn man im bestimmten Verhältnis die Ernährung der Kontrolltiere reduziert, gelingt es nach ihrer Ansicht, das Tumorwachstum bei hypophysektomierten Tieren den Kontrollen anzupassen.

In unseren eigenen Versuchen [Dontenwill (1954, 1955)] sahen wir bei totaler Hypophysektomie eine hochgradige Wachstumshemmung des Walkercarcinoms der Ratte (Kontrollen 100%, Hypophysektomierte 68,7%). Die Wachstumshemmung der Tumoren entsprach der starken Gewichtsabnahme der Tiere (Kontrollen: Zunahme 26,7%, Hypophysektomierte: Abnahme 4,8%). Bei zeitweiligem völligem Nahrungsentzug war die Tumorhemmung noch stärker.

Hypophysektomie hemmt den Einbau von Uracil in die RNS des transplantablen Hepatom (AxC) der Wistar-Ratte; [Cantarow, Williams und Paschkis (1962)] Gaben von STH erzeugten bei jungen Ratten eine Hemmung und bei älteren Ratten eine Förderung des Einbaus. Die Katalaseaktivität des transplantierten Schilddrüsentumors wurde durch Hypophysektomie vermieden [Rechicigl und Wollmyn (1963)].

Beeinflussung der Entstehung von sog. „Reiztumoren" durch Hypophysektomie

Zur Untersuchung der Rolle der Hypophysenhormone bei der Carcinomentstehung schädigten Lacassagne und Nyka (1936) die Hypophyse mittels Einführung von Radon (Radiumemanationseinlage), während des gleichen Zeitraums wurden die Kaninchen im Bereich des Ohres mit Teer oder Benzpyren gepinselt. Die 10 Monate überlebenden Tiere zeigten eine nur langsame Entstehung verhornender Papillome, die Tendenz zu spontaner Rückbildung erkennen ließen. Bei allen Kontrolltieren entwickelten sich Plattenepithelcarcinome. Korteweg und Thomas (1949) beobachteten, daß nach Benzpyrenpinselung bei hypophysektomierten Mäusen seltener und langsamer Papillome auftraten. Heiman (1938) berichtet über gleiche Ergebnisse.

Nach Agate, Antopos, Blaubach, Agate und Graff (1955) ist die Hypophyse zur Entstehung eines Tumors durch 3,4-Benzpyren nicht nötig. Zamurovic (1953) sah keinen zeitlichen Unterschied der Latenzzeit des Benzpyrenkrebses nach Hypophysektomie.

Nach Implantation von Methylcholanthren beobachteten Moon, Simpson und Evans (1952), Moon und Simpson (1955) bei der Ratte nach der Hypophysektomie eine deutliche Hemmung der Carcinogenese (von 15 hypophysektomierten Ratten zeigte nur eine ein Sarkom an der Implantationsstelle). Daniel und Prichard (1963) fanden bei totaler Hypophysektomie eine stärkere Hemmung des durch 3-Methylcholanthren erzeugten Mammatumor als durch Unterbindung des Hypophysenstiel. Nach Zusatz ungereinigten HVL-Extraktes oder STH sahen sie wieder eine den Kontrollen entsprechende Häufigkeit, ACTH hat aber nicht diesen starken Effekt des STH [Moon, Li und Simpson (1950)].

Griffin und Robertson (1953), Richardson (1954), Robertson, O'Neal, Griffin und Richardson (1955), Robertson (1954) fanden nach Hypophysektomie nicht die durch Verfütterung von 3-Methyl-4-Dimethylaminoazobenzol beim Normaltier auftretenden Lebercirrhosen und Leberhepatome. Es wurde beim hypophysektomierten Tier nur vereinzelt eine leichte Lebercirrhose beobachtet [Griffin, Rinfret und Corsigilia (1953) und Richardson und Griffin (1953)].

Simpson und Evans (1959) konnten frühere Beobachtungen, daß die Hypophysektomie bei der Ratte das Intervall zwischen Injektion von 7,12-Dimethylbenzanthracen (DMBA) und Auftreten von Tumoren verlängert oder das Angehen des Tumors beeinflußt, nicht bestätigen. Die Tumoren wuchsen bei hypophysektomierten Ratten langsamer. Bei ihren Untersuchungen konnten sie folgende Beobachtungen machen: Hypophysektomie bei vorhandenen Tumoren verursachte bei normalen Ratten kein Zurückgehen der Tumoren, obgleich die Tumoren langsamer wuchsen. Bei hypophysektomierten Ratten, die mit Wachstumshormon behandelt wurden, war die Tumorentstehung eingeschränkt. Diese Einschränkung war stärker, wenn die Futteraufnahme begrenzt wurde. Eine Kombination von Wachstums-Hormonen, Thyroxin und Hydrocortison, die man hypophysektomierten Ratten nach dem Auftreten von Tumoren in Dosen gab, die den Stoffwechselumsatz erhöhten und die Futteraufnahme über das Normale steigerten, erhöhte die Tumorrate und die Endgröße der Tumoren. Die Nahrungseinschränkung bei unbehandelten Ratten in dem Maß wie bei den hypophysektomierten Tieren, verringerte nicht das endgültige Auftreten von Tumoren, obwohl die Endgröße der Tumoren kleiner war als bei den Kontrolltieren.

Die Wirkung der Hypophysektomie auf die Entwicklung von Spontantumoren

Mäusen mit häufig auftretenden spontanen Mammacarcinomen injizierten Lacassagne und Chamorro (1939) oestrogene Substanzen, um das Auftreten der Tumoren zu beschleunigen. Nachdem (nach 3 Monaten) sog. präcanceröse Stadien (cystische Hypertrophie) entstanden waren, wurde bei gleichzeitiger Weiterbehandlung mit oestrogenen Substanzen die Hypophysektomie vorgenommen. Bei den hypophysektomierten Tieren bildeten sich, im Gegensatz zu den Kontrollen, die Brustdrüsen zurück, es entstanden keine Carcinome. Hatte die hormonale Behandlung mit Oestrogen schon zum Entstehen eines Carcinomknotens vor der Hypophysektomie geführt, änderte die Entfernung der Hypophyse nichts an der weiteren Entwicklung der Carcinome [gleiche Ergebnisse fand Gardner (1942)]. Lacassagne (1949, 1950) sieht darin die Unwirksamkeit der Hypophysektomie auf den Verlauf eines einmal entstandenen Carcinoms.

Nach MARTINEZ und BITTNER (1954), BITTNER (1942) hemmt die Hypophysektomie das spontane Auftreten der Mammacarcinome. Die Entstehung von Nebennieren-Rindentumoren nach Kastration der C3H-Maus wird durch Hypophysektomie verhindert [FERGUSON und VISSCHER (1953)]. HESTON beobachtete (1963) eine totale Hemmung der Entstehung des spontanen Hepatoms bei Mäusen (C3H × YBR)F_1 nach Hypophysektomie.

Wirkung und Substitution einzelner Hypophysenhormone auf das Carcinomwachstum beim hypophysektomierten Tier

REISS, DRUCKREY und HOCHWALD (1933) beobachteten beim hypophysektomierten Tier nach Injektion von ungereinigtem Wachstumshormon eine Steigerung des Carcinomwachstums (transplantable Tumoren), gegenüber den nicht behandelten hypophysektomierten Tieren. FUNK, TOMASHEFSKY, EHRLICH (1950) sahen, daß das Tumorgewicht direkt proportional zum Körpergewicht nach Gaben somatotropen Hormons (STH) zunimmt. Der Einfluß des Wachstumshormons war im allgemeinen gering, ebenfalls bei gleichen Versuchen an hypophysektomierten Tieren. Die Wirkung von Follikelhormonen, gonadotropen Hormon, adrenocorticotropem Hormon oder thyreotropem Hormon zeigt (nach Angaben der gleichen Autoren) einen deutlich stimulierenden Effekt auf das Carcinomwachstum beim hypophysektomierten Tier, der anscheinend stärker war als der auf das Körperwachstum. Bei hypophysektomierten Tieren, die mit 3-Methyl-Dimethylaminoazobenzol zur Erzeugung von Lebertumoren behandelt wurden, konnte durch ACTH die durch die Hypophysektomie hervorgerufene Hemmung der Entstehung von Hepatomen teilweise aufgehoben werden; die Hepatome traten erst nach etwa doppelter Latenzzeit im Vergleich zu den nicht operierten Tieren auf. [ROBERTSON (1954), ROBERTSON, O'NEAL, GRIFFIN und RICHARDSON (1953)]. Auch in unseren Versuchen [DONTENWILL (1954, 1955)] sahen wir nach Substitution von ACTH oder TSH beim hypophysektomierten Tier eine deutlich geringere Tumorwachstumshemmung. Die Versuche zeigen also, daß nicht nur die Substitution von STH, sondern auch von TSH oder ACTH die hemmende Wirkung der Hypophysektomie z. T. ausgleicht. Die bei dieser Substitution nachweisbare Verminderung der Wachstumshemmung der Hypophysektomie geht nicht immer mit einer Zunahme des Körpergewichtes parallel. [Siehe auch SIMPSON und EVANS (1959), MOON, LI und SIMPSON (1956).] Eine kombinierte Behandlung hypophysektomierter Ratten mit STH, Thyroxin und Cortison nach Auftreten von Tumoren bei Behandlung mit 7,12-Dimethylbenz-a-anthracen steigerte die Nahrungsaufnahme und das Tumorwachstum [SIMPSON und EVANS (1959)].

Wirkung der Hypophysenhormone auf das Krebswachstum beim nicht hypophysektomierten Tier

Eine Wachstumssteigerung des Carcinoms durch Applikation von *Wachstumshormon* beobachteten ENGEL (1934), BISCHOFF, MAXWELL und ULLMANN (1934), SCHULMAN und GREENBERG (1949), LI, EVANS und SIMPSON (1945), MCEUEN und THOMSON (1933), REID (1954), MIRAND und HOFFMAN (1957), REISS, DRUCKREY und HOCHWALD (1933) bei Versuchen mit transplantablen Ratten- und Mäusetumoren.

Mit gereinigtem Wachstumshormon (STH) konnten SMITH, SLATTERY, SHIMKIN, LI, LEE, CLARKE und LYONS (1952) eine fast 100%ige Wachstumssteigerung beim transplantablen Adenocarcinom der Mamma an Mäusen des C3H-Stammes feststellen. Eine Förderung des Wachstums sahen beim gleichen Tumor auch SMITH, DAANE, LI, SHIMKIN, LYONS, SPARKS und FURNAS (1954), ARONS, KETCHAM und MANTEL (1961).

LACASSAGNE (1949, 1950) zitiert (ohne Autorenangabe) dagegen Versuche, bei denen eine Hemmung von Teertumoren durch Applikation von Wachstumshormon hervorgerufen wurde. Offenbar handelt es sich dabei um ungereinigte Hormonauszüge des Hypophysenvorderlappens.

WOOD, HOLYOKE, SOMMER und WARREN (1955) sahen bei STH-Behandlung 5 Tage vor der Inoculation eines Mäusesarkoms eine Zunahme der Lungenmetastasen auf das Vierfache, die Tumoren waren außerdem größer. Ein solcher Einfluß war nicht vorhanden, wenn STH nach der Transplantation gegeben wurde.

ROBERT und KLÄRNER (1956) verabreichten Mäusen mit Urethan-Lungentumoren Wachstumshormon und sahen eine Wachstumssteigerung. HAVEN, MAYER und BLOOR (1957) verzeichneten eine Zunahme des Tumor- und Körpergewichtes nach Behandlung mit Wachstumshormon bei Walker-Carcinom tragenden Ratten. Bei kombinierter Behandlung von Prednisolon und Wachstumshormon bei Mäusen, denen ein Adenocarcinom der Mamma transplantiert worden war, trat eine geringere Wachstumshemmung auf als bei alleiniger Prednisolonbehandlung [MCALPIN, BLAIR, GILLIES, LYONS und LI (1958)].

Nach BOOT und MÜHLBOCK (1959) (u. a. siehe Mammacarcinom) kann eine subcutane Transplantation von Hypophysengewebe eine Mammatumorentstehung induzieren (bei verschiedenen Stämmen mit und ohne Milchfaktor). LOEB und KIRTZ beobachteten bereits 1939, daß das Auftreten spontaner Mammacarcinome bei weiblichen Mäusen durch Hypophysenimplantationen von 3% auf 44% gegenüber den Kontrollen gesteigert werden kann. NARIMATSU (1939) konnte diese Befunde bei eigenen Versuchen nicht bestätigen, dies zeigt die von genetischen hormonellen Faktoren abhängige Wirkung bei verschiedenen Tierstämmen.

Das Auftreten von Papillomen nach Benzanthracenbehandlung konnte durch Behandlung mit somatotropem Hormon nach ENGELBRETH-HOLM und JENSEN (1953) nicht wesentlich beeinflußt werden. STH verändert lediglich die Latenzzeit. Bei mit Gesamtextrakten der Hypophyse behandelten Tieren sah HOFBAUER (1952) keinen Einfluß auf das Carcinomwachstum. Behandlung mit Wachstumshormon (10 Wochen 30 γ — 1 mg pro Tier täglich) traten induzierte Knochentumoren bei Wistar-Ratten häufiger auf. Gleichzeitige Gaben von Thyroxin (20—45 g pro Tier täglich) verkürzte die Latenzzeit der Tumorentstehung wesentlich [CATER, BASERGA und LISCO (1959)].

MOON, SIMPSON, LI und EVANS (1950, 1951) und KONEFF, MOON, SIMPSON, LI und EVANS (1951) sahen nach Injektion somatotropen Hormons Lymphosarkome. Die Autoren führen nicht an, ob die Tumoren transplantabel oder ob Metastasen vorhanden waren. Diese Versuchsergebnisse sind schon deswegen umstritten, weil nicht klar erkennbar ist, ob es sich um eine systemartige Veränderung am lymphoreticulären Gewebe oder um einen malignen Tumor handelt. Ebenso umstritten sind die Beobachtungen von WACHTEL (1946, 1949, 1954), der Carcinome und Sarkome bei Mäusen, die mit Hypophysenextrakten behandelt wurden (27,8% der Tiere), nachwies.

CRAMER (1940) sah nach *Hypophysenvorderlappenextraktgaben* bei Mäusen keine spontanen Mammacarcinome bei einem tumorbelasteten Stamm. VIGIER (1953) stellte eine Förderung des Angehens des Rous-Virus-Sarkoms durch HVL-Extrakt fest.

Während FUNK, TOMASHEFSKY, EHRLICH und SOUKUP (1950) nach Gaben von *adrenocorticotropem* Hormon (ACTH) bei der hypophysektomierten Ratte einen deutlich stimulierenden Effekt auf das Carcinomwachstum sahen, beobachteten GOTTSCHALK und GROLLMAN (1952) und VRAT (1951) bei einem transplantierten Mammacarcinom der Maus keinen sicheren Effekt.

STOCK, KARNOFSKY und SUGIURA (1951) und SPARKS, DAANE, HAYASHIDA, COLE, LYONS und LI (1955) konnten bei transplantablen Mäusetumoren eine Wachstumshemmung durch ACTH hervorrufen, BURCHENAL, STOCK und RHOADS (1950) eine Hemmung der transplantierten Leukämie der Maus durch *ACTH* und *Cortison* und LANNECK (1953) bei Lymphoidtumoren (s. auch Leukämie). WILLIG (1954) sah beim Jensen-Sarkom keinen Einfluß des ACTH auf das Wachstum. Auch nach ACTH-Behandlung sahen GOTTSCHALK und GROLLMAN (1952) keine Wirkung auf die Entwicklung des Rous-Sarkoms. Durch Gaben thyreotropen Hormons konnten CRAMER und HORNING (1938) das Auftreten von Mammacarcinomen bei einem Mäusestamm, der häufig spontane Mammatumoren zeigte, verhindern, während, wie schon erwähnt, FUNK, TOMASHEFSKY, EHRLICH und SOUKUP (1950) beim hypophysektomierten Tier eine Wachstumsstimulierung beobachten konnten.

Über den Einfluß des *gonadotropen* Hypophysenhormons (Prolan) auf das Tumorwachstum sind zahlreiche Untersuchungen vorgenommen worden. Eine Hemmung des Tumorwachstums durch Prolan mit gleichzeitig vermindertem O_2-Verbrauch des Tumorgewebes konnten REISS und HOCHWALD (1932) nachweisen.

Über gleiche Ergebnisse (Hemmung) berichten ZONDEK, ZONDEK und HARTOCH (1932), ENGEL (1934), KREHBIEL, HAGENSEN und PLATENGA (1934), LUDWIG und VON RIES (1935), MURPHY und STURM (1934), RAREI und GUMMEL (1938), CRUVEILIER, HAGUENAN, THIEULIN und VIALA (1938), WEISSENFELS (1956). LI MIN-KSIN, HAI-YING, TING-KSIEN und YUNG-SHENG (1962) beobachteten nach Gonadotropingaben bei dem durch Methylcholanthren induzierten Cervixcarcinom der Maus (KM) einen nur geringen Einfluß, während gleichzeitige Oestradiolbehandlung die Entwicklung förderte und Progesteron sie hemmte.

Die Wachstumsenergie wird durch Prolangaben so stark vermindert, daß der Tumor bei der zweiten Tierpassage nicht mehr angeht [ZONDEK u. a. (1932)]. KATZ (1936), der bei Kastrationsversuchen eine gleichzeitig auftretende Wachstumshemmung feststellte, nahm an, daß Prolan direkt an der Zelle angreift. MÖLLER (1933) fand bei ähnlichen Versuchen neben einer Hemmung des Krebswachstums (EHRLICH Adenocarcinom der Maus) eine Verbreiterung der Nebennierenrinde. Nach KATZ (1936) und DRUCKREY (1936, 1937) wird nur die Geschwulstentstehung (beim Teerkrebs), nicht das Geschwulstwachstum, bei dem schon entstandenen Tumor durch die Prolanbehandlung gehemmt. Entsprechend beschrieb GROSS (1933) nach Prolaninjektion beim transplantablen Mäusesarkom keinen Einfluß auf das Tumorwachstum. Nach Angaben einiger Autoren kann Prolan sogar zu einer Steigerung des Tumorwachstums führen [HÜBSCHER (1933), ZEHLENRUST (1935), JULIUS (1934), YANO (1953, 1954), BAATZ (1939)]. Injektionen lactotropen Hormons der Hypophyse zeigten keinen signifikanten Einfluß auf das Wachstum des transplantablen Mammacarcinoms der Maus [SLATTERY, LYONS, SHIMKIN (1950)]. Nach Transplantation des mammatropen Hypophysentumor bei Mäusen (LAF_1) fanden sich bei 9% der Mäuse-Mammatumoren mit Lungenmetastasen in einigen Fällen [HARAN-GHERA (1961)]. Zusätzliche Behandlung mit Methylcholanthren vermehrte die Tumorhäufigkeit auf 35%, wenn die Mamma vorher durch das mammatrope Hormon stimuliert war. Die gleichzeitige Implantation des mammatropen Hypophysentumor MtT/F_4 bei Behandlung der Ratten (Fischer-Stamm) mit einer Diät von 0,016% N-hydroxy-N-2-Fluorenylacetamide erzeugte in der Leber Carcinome nach 13 Wochen. Nach alleiniger Carcinogenbehandlung traten nur praecanceröse Veränderungen auf. Nach Ansicht der Autoren ist dies ein Beweis für die Bedeutung von hypophysären Faktoren bei der Entstehung von Leberkrebs [WEISBURGER, PAI und YAMAMOTO (1964)].

SELYE (1955) untersuchte die Wirkung der *Adaptionshormone* STH und Cortison auf das Wachstum transplantierter Geschwülste. Aus seinen Beobachtungen zieht er den Schluß, daß Stress durch die während der Stress-Situation gebildeten Adaptionshormone auch auf das Tumorwachstum einen großen Einfluß haben kann. Nach seiner Auffassung ist die Geschwulstzelle weitgehend autonom, aber für ihre strukturelle Organisation durch Stroma und für ihre Ernährung durch die Blutgefäße ist sie vom Wirtsorganismus abhängig. In gleicher Weise haben wir [DONTENWILL (1955)] die Wirkung hormoneller Faktoren der Hypophyse auf das Geschwulstwachstum interpretiert, nur haben wir lediglich von der geänderten Stoffzufuhr bzw. Stoffwechselsituation gesprochen, da der Tumor zwar autonom, aber nicht autark und damit von der Nährstoffzufuhr des Wirtsorganismus abhängig ist. Jede Verschlechterung der Stoffzufuhr durch Störung des Stoffwechsels bei Fehlen regulierender Hormone führt, ebenso wie mangelhafte oder fehlende Nahrungszufuhr (Hunger), zu einer Hemmung des Geschwulstwachstums. Die hypophysäre Wachstumsbeeinflussung ist nach unserer

Auffassung im Sinne der allgemeinen Wachstumsregulierung zu verstehen, darf aber nicht mit einer krebsauslösenden Funktion verwechselt werden. Eine carcinogene Eigenschaft ist bisher noch von keinem Hypophysenhormon bewiesen.

Die Empfindlichkeit der Haut gegenüber DMBA ist bei Zwergmäusen wesentlich geringer als bei normalen Mäusen. Während bei ersteren zu 60% Tumoren auftraten, war die Tumorrate bei normalen Tieren 100% [Bielschowsky (1951)].

Nach Robertson, Griffin und Richardson (1954) hemmt Parahydroxypropiophenon durch Beeinflussung der Hypophyse die Entwicklung des Lebercarcinoms durch Azoverbindungen.

Eine Übersicht über die Wirkung der Hypophyse auf das Geschwulstwachstum zeigt Tabelle 5.

Tabelle 5. *Einfluß der Hypophysenhormone auf das Tumorwachstum*

Art der Behandlung	Tumor	Wirkung
Hypophysektomie	Transplantable Tumoren	Hemmung des Wachstums
	Reiztumoren Haut, Leber } durch Carcinogene	Langsameres Wachstum verlängert Intervall zwischen Behandlungsbeginn und Tumorentstehung; verhindert nicht Tumorentstehung. Kein wesentlicher Rückgang schon entstandener Tumoren
	Spontantumoren (Mammacarcinom, Nebennierenrindencarcinom)	Hemmt Auftreten spontaner Tumoren. Kein wesentlicher Einfluß auf bereits entstandene Tumoren
Hypophysektomie und Substitution mit Wachstumshormon (STH) Adrenocorticotropes Hormon (ACTH)	Transplantable und Reiztumoren	STH zeigt stärkste Verminderung der Wachstumshemmung der transplantablen Tumoren und der Reiztumoren, ACTH geringere Verminderung der Hemmung nach Hypophysektomie
STH-Behandlung	Transplantable Tumoren	Wachstumssteigerung
	Reiztumoren	Verkürzung der Latenzzeit
	Spontantumoren	Wachstumssteigerung
ACTH-Behandlung	Transplantable Tumoren Reiztumoren Spontantumoren	Verschiedene Angaben: Förderung und Hemmung, von der Dosis abhängig
TSH	Mammacarcinom	Hemmung
Prolan	Transplantable Tumoren	Hemmung
	Reiztumoren	Hemmung der Entstehung

Rozynek (1950) konnte nachweisen, daß das *Hypophysenhinterlappenhormon* Pitressin keinen Einfluß auf das Carcinomwachstum ausübt. Wachtel (1954) konnte durch Extrakte des Hypophysenhinterlappens das Tumorwachstum hemmen. Der Verfasser spricht daher vom "Cancer checking lipids" des Hypophysenhinterlappens. Aus dem Vorderlappen extrahierte er einen wachstumsfördernden Faktor (Lipoid). Wachtel (1949, 1954) schließt aus dem Vorhandensein carcinomfördernder Vorderlappen- und carcinomhemmender Hinterlappen-Extrakte der Hypophyse, daß das Krebsproblem in einer Störung der Hypophysenfunktion zu suchen ist.

Literatur

C. a) Hypophysenhormone

Agate, F. J., jr., W. Antopos, S. Blaubach, F. Agate and S. Graff: The nonessentiality of the hypophysis for the induction of tumors with 3,4-benzpyrene. Cancer Res. **15**, 6—8 (1955).

Arons, M. S., A. S. Ketcham u. N. Mantel: Die Wirkung von Wachstumshormon und ACTH auf einen transplantierten Tumor. Cancer **14**. 507—511 (1961).

BAATZ, H.: Die Beeinflussung des Spontantumorwachstums der Maus durch Prolan. Z. Geburtsh. Gynäk. **120**, 70 (1939).
BALL, H. A., and L. T. SAMUELS: The relation of the hypophysis to the growth of malignant tumors. III. The effect of hypophysectomy on autogenous tumors. Amer. J. Cancer **26**, 547 (1936).
— — The relation of the hypophysis to the growth of malignant tumors. Amer. J. Cancer **32**, 50 (1938).
BIELSCHOWSKY, F., and M. BIELSCHOWSKY: Carcinogenesis in the pituitary dwarf mouse. The response to dimethylbenzathracene applied to the skin. Brit. J. Cancer **15**, 257 (1951).
—, and E. S. HORNING: Aspects of endocrine carcinogenesis. Brit. med. Bull. **14**, 106 (1958).
BISCHOFF, F., L. MAXWELL and H. ULLMANN: Hormones in cancer; influence of hypophysis. Amer. J. Cancer **21**, 329 (1934).
BITTNER, J.: Possible relationship of the estrogenic hormones genetic susceptibility and milk influence in the production of mammary cancer in mice. Cancer Res. **2**, 710 (1942).
BOOT, L. M., et O. MÜHLBOCK: Mammary gland carcinogenesis by isografts of pituitaries in mice. Acta Un. Cancr. **15**, No. 1 (1959).
BÜNGELER, W., u. W. DONTENWILL: Hormonell ausgelöste geschwulstartige Hyperplasien, hyperplasiogene Geschwülste und ihre Verhaltensweisen. Dtsch. med. Wschr. **1959**, 1885.
BURCHENAL, J. H., C. C. STOCK and C. P. RHOADS: The effects of cortisone and ACTH on transplanted mouse leukemia. Cancer Res. **10**, 209 (1950).
CANTAROW, S., T. L. WILLIAMS, and K. E. PASCHKIS: Hormonal and nutritional influences on the incorporation of uracil into liver and tumor RNA in the rat. Cancer Res. **22**, 1021—1025 (1962).
CATER, D. B., R. BASERGA u. H. LISCO: Studien zur Induktion von Knochen- und Weichteiltumoren durch Y-Strahlen bei Ratten zur Wirkung von Wachstumshormon und Thyroxin. Brit. J. Cancer **13**, 214—227 (1959).
CLIFTON, K. H.: Problems in experimental tumorigenesis of the pituitary gland, gonads, adrenal cortices, and mammary glands: a review. Cancer Res. **19**, 2 (1959).
CRAMER, W.: Verhütung spontanen Mammakrebses bei der Maus durch Hypophysenvorderlappenhormon. Amer. J. Cancer **40**, No. 4 (1940).
—, and E. HORNING: Prevention of spontaneous mammary cancer in mice by the thyrotropic hormone of the pituitary gland. Lancet **1938 I**, 72.
CRUVEILIER, L., J. HAGUENAN, G. THIEULIN et C. VIALA: Influence de l'hormone gonadotrope sur l'évolution de la tumeur de Shope du lapin. C. R. Soc. Biol. (Paris) **127**, 485 (1938).
DANIEL, P. M., and M. M. L. PRICHARD: The response of experimentally induced mammary tumours in rats to hypophysectomy and to pituitary stalk section. Brit. J. Cancer **17**, 446—453 (1963).
DONTENWILL, W.: Die Bedeutung hormonaler Einflüsse für die Enstehung und das Wachstum bösartiger Geschwülste. Habilitationsschrift Kiel 1954.
— Experimentelle Untersuchungen über den Einfluß von Hormonen auf das Walker-Carcinom der Ratte und auf die Entwicklung des Benzpyrentumors der Mäusehaut. Z. Krebsforsch. **60**, 482 (1955).
DRUCKREY, H.: Die Wirkung der Hypophyseninkretion auf Geschwülste. Naunyn-Schmiedeberg's Arch. exp. Path. Pharmak. **180**, H. 4, 367 (1936).
— Hypophysenvorderlappen und Krebs. Z. Krebsforsch. **45**, 352 (1937).
ELSNER, P., u. H. TISCHER: Veränderungen am Ovar bei hormonbehandelten Mammacarcinomen. Arch. Gynäk. **181**, 462 (1952).
ENGEL, P.: Über den Einfluß von Hypophysenvorderlappenhormon und Epiphysenhormon auf das Wachstum von Impftumoren. Z. Krebsforsch. **41**, 281 (1934).
ENGEL, F., and A. MURRAY: Amer. J. Obstet. Gynec. **32**, 593 (1936). Siehe ENGEL, F., Steroid metabolism in cancer. In: F. HOMBURGER and W. H. FISHMAN, eds., Physiopathology of Cancer. London: Cassel & Co. 1953.
ENGELBRETH-HOLM, J., and E. JENSEN: On the mechanism of experimental carcinogenesis. X. Acta path. microbiol. scand. **23**, 257 (1953).
FERGUSON, D. J.: The effect of hypophysectomy on the development of adrenal tumors in C3H mice. Cancer Res. **13**, 405 (1953).
—, and M. B. VISSCHER: The effect of hypophysectomy on the development of adrenal tumors in C3H mice. Cancer Res. **13**, 405 (1953).
FISCHER, W., u. I. KÜHL: Geschwülste der Laboratoriumsnagetiere. Dresden, Leipzig: Theodor Steinkopff 1958.
FRANSEEN, C. C., and C. MCTIERNAN: The effect of hypophysectomy upon the metabolism of grafted tumor tissue. Amer. J. Cancer **26**, 106 (1936).
FUNK, C.: The effect of hormonal factors and the removal of certain organs upon the growth of a transplanted rat tumor. Brit. J. Cancer **5**, 280 (1951); Arch. Geschwulstforsch. **5**, 75 (1953).

FUNK, C.,PH. TOMASHEFSKY, A. EHRLICH and R. SOUKUP: Die Rolle der Hypophysebeim Wachstum eines transplantablen Rattentumors. Proc. Soc. exp. Biol. (N. Y.) **74**, 289 (1950).
GARDNER, W. U.: Persistence and growth of spontaneous mammary tumors and hyperplastic nodules in hypophysectomized mice. Cancer Res. **2**, 476 (1942).
GOTTSCHALK, R. G., and A. GROLLMAN: The action of cortisone and ACTH on transplanted mouse tumors. Cancer Res. **12**, 651 (1952).
GRIFFIN, A. C., A. P. RINFRET and V. F. CORSIGILIA: The inhibition of liver carcinogenesis with 3'-methyl-4-dimethylaminoazobenzene in hypophysectomized rats. Cancer Res. **13**, 77 (1953).
GROSS, L.: Zur Frage des Einflusses der Hypophysenvorderlappengeschlechtshormone auf das Tumorwachstum bei Mäusen. Z. Krebsforsch. **38**, 289 (1933); Zbl. allg. Path. path. Anat. **58**, 208 (1933).
HARAN-GHERA, N.: The role of mammotrophin in mammary tumor induction in mice. Cancer Res. **21**, 790—795 (1961).
HAVEN, F. L., W. D. MAYER and W. R. BLOOR: Growth hormone and tumör phospholipids: effects on tumor and body growth. Cancer Res. **17**, 948—953 (1957).
HAYASHI, T.: Trans. Jap. Path. Soc. **20**, 661 (1930).
HEIMAN, J.: Anterior pituitary gland in tumor-bearing rats. Amer. J. Cancer **33**, 423 (1938).
HESTON, W. E.: Complete inhibition of occurence of spontaneous hepatomas in higly susceptible (C3H × YBR)F_1 male mice by hypophysectomy. J. nat. Cancer Inst. **31**, 467—474 (1963).
HOFBAUER, J.: The interaction of hormone-induced tissue growth and vital inorganic elements in uterine carcinogenesis. Amer. J. Obstet. Gynec. **63**, 136 (1952).
HÜBSCHER, K.: Die biologische Hyperämiebehandlung von Adnexentzündungen mit Hypophysenvorderlappenhormon. Zbl. Gynäk. **57**, 1575 (1933).
HUGGINS, CH.: Functions of the Cancer Cell. Z. Krebsforsch. **67**, 106—112 (1965).
JULIUS, H. W.: Acta brev. neerl. Physiol. **4**, 74 (1934).
KATZ, K.: Hypophysenvorderlappen und Krebs. Z. Krebsforsch. **45**, 139 (1936).
KIRSCHBAUM, A.: The role of hormones in cancer: Laboratory animals. Cancer Res. **17**, 432 (1957).
KLÄRNER, P.: Wirkung von Adaptionshormonen auf Urethan-Lungentumoren der adrenalektomierten Maus. Z. Krebsforsch. **61**, 276 (1956).
KONEFF, A., H. MOON, M. SIMPSON, CH. LI and H. EVANS: Neoplasms in rats treated with pituitary growth hormone. Cancer Res. **11**, 113 (1951).
KORTEWEG, R., and F. THOMAS: Tumor induction and tumor growth in hypophysectomized mice. Amer. J. Cancer **37**, 36—44 (1949).
KREHBIEL, O., C. HAAGENSEN and H. PLANTENGA: Effect of anterior pituitary hormones on growth of mouse sarcoma. Amer. J. Cancer **21**, 346 (1934).
LACASSAGNE, A. Hypophyse und Krebs. Oncologia (Basel) **23**, 3—4 (1949).
— Les cancers produits par des substances chimiques endogènes. Paris: Hermann 1950.
— Hypophyse und Krebs. Strahlentherapie **83**, 429 (1950).
—, et A. CHAMORRO: Conséquences de l'hypophysectomie chez des souris sujettes au carcinome mammaire, traitées par hormone oestrogène. C. R. Soc. Biol. (Paris) **131**, 1077—1078 (1939).
—, et W. NYKA: Einfluß des Hypophysenmangels auf die Geschwulstentwicklung beim Kaninchen. C. R. Soc. Biol. (Paris) **121**, 822 (1936); Zbl. allg. Path. path. Anat. **65**, 332 (1936).
LANNECK, N.: The effect of adrenocorticotrophic hormone (ACTH), cortisone, and hydrocortisone on the growth of experimental lymphoid tumors in chicks. Brit. J. Cancer **6**, 369—376 (1953).
LI, Ch. H., H. M. EVANS and D. I. SIMPSON: J. biol. Chem. **159**, 353 (1945).
LIPSCHUTZ, A.: Steroid hormones and tumors. Baltimore: Williams & Wilkins Comp. 1950.
— Steroid homeostasis hypophysis and tumorigenesis. Cambridge: Heffer & Sons, Ltd. 1957.
LUDWIG, F., u. J. v. RIES: Schweiz. med. Wschr. **1935**, 5.
LOEB, L., and M. M. KIRTZ: The effects of transplants of anterior lobes of the hypophysis on the growth of the mammary gland and the development of mammary gland carcinoma in various strains of mice. Amer. J. Cancer **36**, 56 (1939).
LOEFER, J. B.: Growth of sarcoma in hypophysectomized rats. Cancer (Chic.) **5**, 161 (1952).
MARTINEZ, C., and J. BITTNER: Effect of ovariectomy, adrenalectomy and hypophysectomy on growth of spontaneous mammary tumors in mice. Repr. Proc. Soc. exp. Biol. (N. Y.) **86**, 92—95 (1954).
MCALPIN, R., S. BLAIR, D. GILLIES, W. LYONS and CH. LI: The effects of long term administration of prednisolone and growth hormone on the growth of transplanted mammary adenocarcinoma in C3H mice. Cancer (Chic.) **11**, 731 (1958).
MCEUEN, C., and D. THOMSON: Effect of hypophysectomy on growth of Walker rat tumor. Brit. J. exp. Path. **14**, 384 (1933).

MIN-HSIN, L., T. HAI-YING, CH. TING-HSIEN, and T. YUNG-SHENG: Influence of hormones on carcinogenesis of uterine cervix of mice induced by methylcholanthrene. Chinae med. J. 81, 800—812 (1962).
MIRAND, E. A., and J. G. HOFFMAN: Effect of pituitary growth hormone on transplantable mouse tumors. Proc. Soc. exp. Biol. (N. Y.) 95, 819—824 (1957).
MÖLLER, H.: Die Beziehungen zwischen Hypophysenvorderlappenhormon und Tumorwachstum. Frankfurt. Z. Path. 45, H. 3 (1933); Zbl. allg. Path. path. Anat. 66, 91 (1936/37).
MOON, H. D., CH. H. LI and M. E. SIMPSON: Effect of pituitary hormones on carcinogenesis with 9,10-dimethyl-1,2-dibenzanthracene in hypophysectomized rats. Cancer Res. 16, 111—116 (1956).
—, and M. E. SIMPSON: Effect of hypophysectomy on carcinogenesis: Inhibition of methylcholanthrene carcino-genesis. Cancer Res. 15, 403 (1955).
— —, and H. EVANS: Inhibition of methylcholanthrene carcinogenesis by hypophysectomy. Science 116, 331 (1952).
— —, CH. H. LI and H. M. EVANS: Neoplasms in rats treated with pituitary growth hormone. I. Pulmonary and lymphatic tissues. Cancer Res. 10, 297—308 (1950).
— — — — Neoplasms in rats treated with pituitary growth hormone. II. Adrenal glands. Cancer Res. 10, 364 (1950).
— — — — Neoplasms in rats treated with pituitary growth hormone. III. Reproductive organs. Cancer Res. 10, 549 (1950).
— — — — Neoplasms in rats treated with pituitary growth hormone. V. Absence of neoplasms in hypophysectomized rats. Cancer Res. 11, 535 (1951).
MURPHY, J., and E. STURM: J. exp. Med. 60, 293, 305 (1934).
NARIMATSU, K.: Eine experimentelle Untersuchung über den Einfluß der Hypophysenhormone auf das Wachstum und die Strahlenempfindlichkeit bösartiger Tumoren. Jap. J. Obstet. Gynec. 20, 387 (1939).
RAREI, B., u. H. GUMMEL: Hypophyseninkretion und Geschwulstwachstum. Z. Krebsforsch. 48, 99 (1938); Zbl. allg. Path. path. Anat. 72, 27 (1939).
RECHICIGL, M., and S. H. WOLLMYN: Effect of hypophysectomy on the lowering of organ catalase by a transplanted tumor. J. nat. Cancer Inst. 31, 651—669 (1963).
REID, E.: Growth hormone and adrenocortical hormones in relation to experimental tumors. Cancer Res. 14, 249 (1954).
—, u. A. HOCHWALD: Exper. Beeinflussung des Tumorstoffwechsels am lebenden Tier. Med. Klin. 1932, Nr. 40, 1391; Zbl. allg. Path. path. Anat. 56, 198 (1932/33).
REISS, M., H. DRUCKREY u. A. HOCHWALD: Tumor und Inkretsystem. Z. ges. exp. Med. 90,408 (1933); Klin. Wschr. 12, 1049 (1933).
RICHARDSON, H. L.: The role of hormones in azo-dye induction of liver cancer and the adrenal-lipoid response in hypophysectomized rats. Repr. Cancer 7, No. 5 (1954).
—, and A. C. GRIFFIN: Hypophysectomy and adrenal histologic changes in rats fed the azo-dye 3-methyl-4-dimethylaminoazobenzene. Proc. Amer. Ass. Cancer Res. 1, No. 1 (1953).
ROBERT, A., u. P. KLÄRNER: Wirkung von Adaptationshormonen auf Urethan-Lungentumoren der intakten Maus. Arch. Geschwulstforsch. 12, 28 (1956).
ROBERTSON, C. H.: Further observations on the role of the pituitary and the adrenal gland in azo-dye carcinogenesis. Cancer Res. 14, 549—553 (1954).
— A. C. GRIFFIN and H. L. RICHARDSON: The inhibitory action of p-hydroxypropiophenone on hepatic carcinoma induced by azo-dye. J. nat. Cancer Inst. 15, 519 (1954).
— M. A. O'NEAL, A. C. GRIFFIN and H. L. RICHARDSON: Pituitary and adrenal factors involved in azo-dye liver carcinogenesis. Cancer Res. 13, 776—779 (1953).
ROCK, T., e G. C. RABOTTI: Ricerche sperimentali cuica gli effetti dell' ipofiscetomia sull'attechimento e sulla crescita del tumore transplantabile di Walker de ratto. Tumori 41, 289—306 (1955).
ROZYNEK, W.: Über die Wirkung des Pitressins auf das Wachstum von Benzpyrentumoren. Z. Krebsforsch. 57, 132 (1950); Arch. Geschwulstforsch. 3, 258 (1951).
SAMUELS, L. T., and H. A. BALL: The relation of the hypophysis to the growth of malignant tumors. Amer. J. Cancer 18, No. 2 (1933).
— — Hypophysectomy and tumor growth. Amer. J. Cancer 23, 801 (1935).
SCHRIMPF, H., u. H. WILLIG: Tierexperimentelle Untersuchungen über den Einfluß der Hypophysektomie auf das gesteigerte Geschwulstwachstum des Walker-Carcinoms der Ratte nach dem Wurf. Z. Krebsforsch. 59, 366—370 (1953).
SCHULMAN, M. P., and D. M. GREENBERG: Effect of purified growth hormone on tumor growth. Proc. Soc. exp. Biol. (N. Y.) 72, 676 (1949).
SELYE, H.: Experimentelle Studien über die Wirkung von Adaptationshormonen (STH, Cortisol) auf transplantierbare Geschwülste. Z. Krebsforsch 60, 316—333 (1955).
SIMPSON, M. E., and H. M. EVANS: Effect of pituitary hormones on carcinogenesis induced in rats by 7,12-dimethyl-benzanthracene. Cancer Res. 19, 1096—1104 (1959)

SLATTERY, P. A., W. R. LYONS and M. B. SHIMKIN: Lack of effect of lactogenic hormone on mammary adenocarcinoma in mice. Proc. Soc. exp. Biol. (N. Y.) **74**, 539—540 (1950).

SMITH, M. C., T. A. DAANE, Ch. H. LI, M. B. SHIMKIN, W. R. LYONS, L. L. SPARKS, and D. W. FURNAS: Further studies on the effects of pituitary growth hormone (STH) on C3H mice bearing a transplanted mammary adenocarcinoma. Cancer Res. **14**, 386—390 (1954).

— P. A. SLATTERY, M. B. SHIMKIN, Ch. H. LI, R. LEE, J. C. CLARKE and W. R. LYONS: The effect of pituitary growth hormone (somatotrophin) on the body weight and tumor growth in C3H mice bearing a transplantable mammary adenocarcinoma. Cancer Res. **12**, 59—61 (1952).

SPARKS, L. L., T. A. DAANE, T. HAYASHIDA, R. D. COLE, W. R. LYONS and Ch. H. LI: The effects of pituitary and adrenal hormones on the growth of a transplanted mammary adenocarcinoma in C3H mice. Cancer **8**, 271—284 (1955).

STOCK, C., D. KARNOFSKY and K. SUGIURA: Studies of steroids for inhibition of normal and abnormal growth in experimental animals. In: A. WHITE, Ed., Steroids in Experimental and clinical Practice. Philadelphia: Blaciston Co. 1951.

SYMEONIDIS, A., A. S. MULAY and F. H. BURGOYNE: Liver tumor induction of adrenalectomized and DOCA-treated rats fed with p-dimethyl-aminoazobenzene. Cancer Res. **11**, 285 (1951).

TALALAY, P., G. M. U. TAKANO and C. HUGGINS: Studies on the Walker tumor. II. Effects of adrenalectomy and hypophysectomy on tumor growth in tube-fed rats. Cancer Res. **12**, 838—843 (1952).

VIGIER, P.: Action favorisante de l'extrait antéhypopyraire total sur la réceptivitée de la poule virus du sarcome de Rous. Bull. Ass. franç. Cancer **40**, 59 (1953).

VRAT, V.: Die Wirkungen von adenocorticotropem Hormon (ACTH), Cortison und Arginase auf das Wachstum eines transplantierten Mamma-Adeno-Carcinoms bei C3H Mäusen. Permanente Fdn. med. Bull. **9**, 60—70 (1951); Ber. allg. spez. Path. **16**, H. 3/4, 145 (1953).

WACHTEL, H.: Carcinogenic substances from pituitary glands of cattle. Science **103**, 556 (1946).

— Krebs und Hypophyse. Experientia (Basel) **6**, 474 (1950).

— Therapeutic studies with pituitary lipids on cancer; preliminary report. Persönl. Mitt. (1954).

WEISBURGER, J. H., S. H. PAI, and R. S. YAMAMOTO: Pituitary hormones and liver carcinogenesis with N-Hydroxy-N-2-Fluorenylacetamide. J. nat. Cancer Inst. **32**, 881—904 (1964).

WEISSENFELS, N.: Über die hemmende Wirkung von Progynon B auf die Entwicklung experimentell induzierter Hauttumoren. Z. Krebsforsch. **61**, 320 (1956).

WILLIG, H.: Tierexperimentelle Untersuchungen über den Einfluß der Hypophysektomie auf das gesteigerte Geschwulstwachstum des Walker-Carcinoms der Ratte nach dem Wurf. Z. Krebsforsch. **59**, 366—370 (1953).

— Tierexperimentelle Untersuchungen über den Einfluß von ACTH auf das Geschwulstwachstum des Jensen-Sarkoms bei Ratten. Ärztl. Forsch. **8**, 1 (1954).

WOOD, J. S., jr., E. D. HOLYOKE, S. C. SOMMER and S. WARREN: Influence of pituitary growth hormone on growth and metastasis formation of a transplantable mouse sarcoma. Bull. Johns Hopk. Hosp. **96**, 93—100 (1955).

YANO, Y.: Acta derm. (Kyoto) **22**, 140 (1953); **23**, 328 (1954).

ZAMUROVIC, D. A.: Sarkomi kod hipofizektomiranih pacova izazvani 3 : 4 benzpyren- om. Acta med. iugosl. **7**, Fas. 3 (1953).

— Période latente dans la carcinogénèse chimique chez les rats hypophysectomisés. Oncologia (Basel) **6**, 180 (1953).

— Les sarcomes chez les rats hypophysectomisés provoqués par 3 : 4-benzopyrène. Acta med. iugosl. **7**, 208 (1953).

ZEHLENRUST, J.: Acta brev. neerl. Physiol. **4**, 182 (1935).

ZONDEK, H., B. ZONDEK u. W. HARTOCH: Prolan und Tumorwachstum. Klin. Wschr. **1932**, Nr. 43; Zbl. allg. Path. path. Anat. **57**, 35 (1933).

b) Epiphysenhormon

Bei einem transplantablen Osteoidsarkom der Ratte sah VECCHI (1932) nach Entfernung der Epiphyse keine Beeinflussung des Sarkomwachstums. Nach ENGEL (1934) vermögen Epiphysenextrakte die krebsfördernde Wirkung des Hypophysenwachstumshormons aufzuheben. Nach Injektion des Epiphysenhormons bei der Ratte sah er eine Hemmung des Carcinomwachstums. RODIN (1963) beobachtete bei pinealektomierten Sprague Dawley-Ratten eine Beschleunigung des Tumorwachstums (Walker-Carcinom). Die Tumoren waren größer, die Metastasen häufiger und die Überlebenszeit kürzer.

Literatur

C. b) Epiphysenhormon

ENGEL, P.: Über den Einfluß von Hypophysenvorderlappenhormonen und Epiphysenhormon auf das Wachstum von Impftumoren. Z. Krebsforsch. **41**, 281 (1934); Zbl. allg. Path. path. Anat. **62**, 159 (1935).

RODIN, A. E.: The growth and spread of walker 256 carcinoma in pinealectomized rats. Cancer Res. **23**, 1545—1548 (1963).

VECCHI, G.: Blastomverpflanzung auf epiphysektomisierte Ratten. Cancro **3**, 122 (1932); Zbl. allg. Path. path. Anat. **57**, 412 (1933).

c) Schilddrüsenhormon

REISS und BALINT (1934) (Jensensarkom) und YANO (1954) (Jensensarkom) sahen nach Thyreoidektomie eine Hemmung des Wachstums des Jensensarkoms im Tierexperiment, das durch Thyroxingaben wieder eine geringe Steigerung erfuhr. Nach SPENCER (1954) hemmt eine Unterfunktion der Schilddrüse das Carcinomwachstum. Die Behandlung mit Thyroxin verhindert die Entstehung von Lebertumoren durch Buttergelb [BATHER und FRANKS (1952)] und das Wachstum des Walker-Carcinoms [HERBUT, KRAEMER und JACKSON (1950)]. Durch Benzpyren induzierte Hauttumoren entstehen nach Schilddrüsenhormonbehandlung nicht wesentlich früher [SILVERSTONE und TANNENBAUM (1949)] Dies zeigt nach Ansicht der Autoren, daß erhöhter Stoffwechsel und Grundumsatz nur dann mit einer Beeinflussung des Tumorenwachstums einhergeht, wenn ein Körpergewichtsverlust eintritt (50% Grundumsatzsteigerung der Tiere).

Nach CRAMER und HORNING (1938) und HAAGENSEN, RANDALL und AUCHINCLOSS (1940) hemmt TSH das Auftreten des spontanen Mammacarcinoms der Maus. Die Wirkung des TSH, des Thyroxin und Thiouracil auf das Mammacarcinom der Maus ist nach BURROWS und HORNING (1952) eine Folge der veränderten Ovarfunktion. GROSS und SCHWARTZ (1951) sahen einen fördernden Einfluß des Thyroxins auf die Mammatumorentstehung. Das Wachstum des transplantablen Mammacarcinoms bei weiblichen C3H/HeN-Mäusen wurde nach Angaben von WILKINS und MORTON (1963) durch Schilddrüsenhormongaben nicht beeinflußt. Das durch 3-Methylcholanthen induzierte Mammacarcinom der Sprague-Dawley-Ratte wird in seiner Entstehung durch Gaben von Thyroxin (0,5 mg) im Wachstum gefördert, durch Schilddrüsenentfernung, ebenso wie durch Ovarektomie gehemmt [JULL und HUGGINS (1960)].

Nach SLOVITER (1951) zeigt die vollständige Abtragung der Schilddrüse durch radioaktives Jod keine Wirkung auf das transplantable Fibrosarkom der Maus. Thyreoidektomie vor der Anwendung von 2-Aminofluorenen verhindert die Entwicklung von Lebertumoren; Thyreoidektomie nach der Entwicklung von Lebertumoren, ändert nicht die Carcinogenese [BIELSCHOWSKY und HALL (1953)]. Nach BARKER (1953) hat die Thyreoidektomie keinen Einfluß auf das transplantierte Fibrosarkom der Ratte. Eine totale Thyreoidektomie fördert nach DARGENT, VIALLIER-REYNARD und GUINET (1949, 1951) das Wachstum des transplantablen Rattenmammacarcinoms.

Nach GILLMAN, GILBERT und SPENCER (1955) hemmt eine Unterfunktion der Schilddrüse die Entstehung eines induzierten Reticulosarkoms.

MORRIS und DUBNIK und DALTON (1946) sahen eine Hemmung der Entwicklung der Milchdrüse und der Mammatumoren bei C3H-Mäusen nach Hemmung der Thyroxinsynthese durch *Thiouracil*. Es traten nur 17% Mammacarcinome gegenüber 94% bei den Kontrollen auf. Propylthiouracil hemmt bei gleichzeitigem Gewichtsverlust das Wachstum des transplantierten Mammacarcinoms bei C3H-Mäusen [JACOBS und HUSEBY (1959)]. Die Brustdrüsenentwicklung sistiert bei

Behandlung mit Thiouracil vollständig [DUBNIK, MORRIS und DALTON (1950). Brustdrüsengeschwülste treten beim C3H-Stamm nur bei 19% der Tiere gegenüber 32% bei den Kontrollen auf. Außerdem verzögert sich das Auftreten um 2 Monate. Die gleichzeitig beobachtete Schilddrüsenvergrößerung wird auf vermehrte Sekretion von TSH zurückgeführt.

Thiouracil zeigt nach BATHER und FRANKS (1952) eine Förderung der Tumorentstehung der Haut nach 1-2-5-6-Dibenzanthracenpinselung, verhütet aber auch nach PASCHKIS, CANTAROW und STASNY (1948, 1951), ebenso wie die Thyreoidektomie [BIELSCHOWSKY und HALL (1953)], die Carcinomentstehung in der Leber durch Acetaminofluoren.

Literatur

C. c) Schilddrüsenhormon

BARKER, S. B.: Effect of thyroid function on tissue metabolism of tumor-bearing rats. Cancer Res. **13**, 817 (1953).

BATHER, R., and W. FRANKS: Further studies on the role of thyroxine in chemical carcinogenesis. Cancer Res. **12**, 247 (1952).

BIELSCHOWSKY, F., and W. H. HALL: Carcinogenesis in the thyroidectomized rat. Brit. J. Cancer **7**, 358—366 (1953).

—, and E. S. HORNING: Aspects of endocrine carcinogenesis. Brit. med. Bull. **14**, 106 (1958).

BURROWS, H., and E. S. HORNING: Oestrogens and neoplasia. Oxford: 1952.

CRAMER, W., and E. S. HORNING: Prevention of spontaneous mammary cancer in mice by the thyrotropic hormone of the pituitary gland. Lancet **1938**, **1**, 72.

DARGENT, M., J. VIALLIER et E. GUINET: Influence de la secretion thyreoïdienne sur la croissance des tumeurs. II. Action de la thyreoïdectomie sur la croissance du cancer experimental greffe du rat blanc (souche T. de Guerin). Ann. Inst. Pasteur **76**, 539 (1949); **81**, 357 (1951).

DUBNIK, C. S., H. P. MORRIS u. A. I. DALTON: Die Wachstumshemmung der Brustdrüse und ihrer Geschwülste bei weiblichen C_3H-Mäusen nach Thiouracil-Behandlung. J. nat. Cancer Inst. **10**, 815—841 (1950).

GILLMAN, J., C. GILBERT and J. SPENCER: The prevention of experimentally induced reticulosarcoma by hypothyroidism. Experientia (Basel) **11**, 157—158 (1955).

GROSS, J., and S. SCHWARTZ: Der Umsatz von Thyroxin in C57-Mäusen und in C3H-Mäusen mit und ohne Mammatumoren. Cancer Res. **11**, 614 (1951).

HAAGENSEN, C. D., H. T. RANDALL and R. AUCHINCLOSS: Failure of thyrotropic pituitary hormone to prevent spontaneous mammary cancer in mice. Proc. Soc. exp. Biol. (N. Y.) **45**, 820 (1940).

HERBUT, P. A., W. H. KRAEMER and J. JACKSON: Effect of hepbisul (heptyl aldehyde - sodium bisulfite addition compound) and thyroxin on Walker carcinoma. Cancer Res. **10**, 224 (1950).

JACOBS, B. B., u. R. A. HUSEBY: Hormonale Einflüsse auf das Wachstum transplantierbarer Mamma-Adenocarcinome in C_3H-Mäusen. J. nat. Cancer Inst. **23**, 1107—1121 (1959).

JULL, J. W., u. CH. HUGGINS: Der Einfluß der Über- und Unterfunktion der Schilddrüse auf experimentelle Mammacarcinome. Nature (Lond.) 188, 73 (1960).

MORRIS, H. P., C. S. DUBNIK and A. J. DALTON: Effect of prolonged ingestion of thiourea on mammary glands and appearance of mammary tumors in adult C3H mice. J. nat. Cancer Inst. **7**, 159—169 (1946).

PASCHKIS, K. E., A. CANTAROW and J. STASNY: Influence of thiouracil on carcinoma induced by 2-acetaminofluorene. Cancer Res. 8, 257—263 (1948).

— — — Competitive action of 2-thiouracil and uracil in AAF-induced cancer. Science **114**, 264 (1951).

REISS, N., u. J. BALINT: Thyreoidektomie und Tumorwachstum. Med. Klin. **1934**, No. 21, 706; Zbl. allg. Path. path. Anat. **61**, 359 (1934/35).

— A. HOCHWALD u. H. DRUCKREY: Thyreotroper Wirkstoff des Hypophysenvorderlappens und Gewebsstoffwechsel. Med. Klin. **29**, 1112 (1933).

SILVERSTONE, H., u. A. TANNENBAUM: Der Einfluß des Schilddrüsenhormons auf die Entwicklung induzierter Hauttumoren bei der Maus. Cancer Res. **9**, 684—688 (1949).

SLOVITER, H. A.: The effect of complete ablation of thyroid tissue by radioactive iodine on the survival of tumor-bearing mice. Cancer Res. **11**, 447—449 (1951).

SPENCER, J. G. C.: The influence of the thyroid in malignant disease. Brit. J. Cancer 8, 393—411 (1954).

WILKINS, R. H., and D. L. MORTON: The influence of thyroid hormone analogues on an isotransplanted spontaneous mammary adenocarcinoma in mice. Cancer **16**, 558—563 (1963).
YANO, Y.: Acta derm. (Kyoto) **23**, 328 (1954).

d) Nebennierenhormone

Adrenalektomie

Eine starke Hemmung des Tumorwachstums nach Adrenalektomie beobachteten SHIMKIN und WYMAN (1945) beim Mammacarcinom der Maus; FUNK, TOMASHEFSKY, SOUKUP und EHRLICH (1951), DONTENWILL (1954, 1955) beim Walker-Carcinom (Tab. 6). BISCHOFF und MAXWELL (1953) dagegen glauben, daß die Adrenalektomie das Wachstum des Walkercarcinoms nicht deutlich beeinflußt.

JOANNOVICS (1916) und KUTSCHERENKO und MAISLISCH (1935) sahen eine Wachstumshemmung bei Sarkomen und Chondromen. Beim transplantierten Rattencarcinom wurden sie festgestellt von INGLE und BAKER (1951), TALATAY, TAKANO und HUGGINS (1952), ROFFO (1930) und LACLAU (1914). Nach WILLIG (1953) ist das Wachstum des Jensen-Sarkoms bei den Kontrollen dreimal stärker als bei den epinephrektomierten Tieren, die unter einer Erhaltungsdosis von 2 mg Cortison standen. Die Wachstumssteigerung des Walker-Carcinoms der Ratte nach dem Wurf wurde nach WILLIG (1953) durch Adrenalektomie nicht beeinflußt.

AGATE und AGATE (1952) sahen bei Hamstern nach Adrenalektomie eine leichtere Transplantierbarkeit des Mäusesarkoms, das sich bei 90% der adrenalektomierten Tiere und nur bei 10% der Kontrollen übertragen ließ.

Nach MURPHY und STURM (1943, 1944), STURM und MURPHY (1944) sinkt die Resistenz gegen die transplantable Leukämie der Ratte nach Adrenalektomie, während Cortison das Wachstum hemmt. Nach STASNEY, PASCHKIS und CANTAROW (1951) fördert Adrenalektomie das Wachstum des transplantierten Lymphosarkoms der Ratte.

HERSCH (1932) beobachtete eine Hemmung der Epithelproliferation nach Teerpinselung bei adrenalektomierten Tieren und SYMEONIDIS, MULAY und BURGOYNE (1954) sahen keine Hepatome bei adrenalektomierten Tieren und bei normalen Tieren nach Behandlung mit Desoxycorticosteron-Acetat (DOCA) nach Einwirkung von p-Dimethylaminoazobenzol. SCHOBER (1953) beobachtete eine verstärkte fibroepitheliale Wachstumsleistung nach Adrenalektomie bei gleichzeitiger Benzpyrenpinselung. BENTON (1963) beobachtete nach Adrenalektomie eine Regression des durch 3,4-9-10-Dibenzpyren induzierten Hauttumors um etwa 43%.

Wirkung von Glucocorticoiden und Mineralocorticoiden auf das Krebswachstum

Glucocorticoide. Besonders bei hochdosierter Behandlung von tumortragenden Tieren wurde von vielen Untersuchern meist eine Hemmung des Wachstums nach Cortisonbehandlung beobachtet.

Nach MACALPIN, BLAIR, GILLIES, LYONS und LI (1958) hemmt Prednisolon das Wachstum des transplantierten Mammacarcinoms der C3H-Maus.

NEUKOMM (1952) sah nach Cortisonbehandlung eine Hemmung des Wachstums des transplantierten Osteosarkoms und Lymphosarkoms der Maus, und BURCHENAL, STOCK und RHOADS (1950) beobachteten nach Cortison- und ACTH-Behandlung eine Hemmung der transplantablen Mäuseleukämie. Nach ROBERT und KLÄRNER (1956) hemmt Cortison das Wachstum der durch Urethan erzeugten Lungentumoren der Maus. Die beim transplantierten Tumor mit dem Körpergewicht parallel gehende Gewichtsabnahme nach Behandlung mit ACTH und Cortison wird nach DAANE u. Mitarb. (1954) und REID (1955) durch gleichzeitige Gabe von STH ausgeglichen, nicht aber die Hemmwirkung des Cortisons auf den Tumor. SELYE (1955) konnte eine Hemmung des Wachstums des transplantierten Walker-Carcinoms nach Cortisonbehandlung nachweisen, und BLOOM (1952) beschreibt eine Hemmung des Mastocytomwachstums beim Hund, DILLER, BECK und BLAUCH (1937, 1948) beim transplantierten Mäusesarkom. NANDI und BERN (1958) fanden nach Cortisonbehandlung eine dosisabhängige Hemmung beim transplantierten Fibrosarkom der Maus, KALISS, BORGES und DAY (1954) beim Mäusesarkom, BASERGA und SHUBIK (1954) beim transplantablen Adenocarcinom der Maus. Eine Hemmung oder Rückbildung vorwiegend transplantabler Tumorarten durch Glucocorticoidbehandlung (Cortison) beobachteten HIGGINS, WOODS und BENNET (1950), PEARSON, ELIEL, RAWSON, DOBRINER und RHOADS (1949), SUGIURA, STOCK, DOBRINER und RHOADS (1950). VRAT (1951), GOTTSCHALK und GROLLMAN (1952), INGLE und NEZAMIS (1951), INGLE, PRESTRUD und RICE (1950), TOOLAN, CRABB und KELDALL (1953), BOUTWELL und RUSCH (1953), HEILMAN und KENDALL (1956). POMEROY (1954) berichtet über eine hemmende Wirkung auf die

Metastasierung des Adenocarcinoms bei der Maus und GOTTSCHALK und GROLLMAN (1952) beim transplantierten Mammacarcinom.

BAKER (1950) beobachtete nach Cortisonbehandlung bei einem durch Methylcholanthren hervorgerufenen Carcinom eine Wachstumsverzögerung. SCHOBER (1953) beobachtete eine vollständige Verhinderung der normalerweise durch Benzpyrenbehandlung entstandenen proliferativen Hautveränderungen. ENGELBRETH-HOLM und ASBOE-HANSEN (1953) und wir [DONTENWILL (1954, 1955)] beobachteten nur eine Hemmung, keine Verhinderung der durch Benzpyren entstehenden Papillome (Tab. 7).

Tabelle 6. *Wachstumsbeeinflussung des Walkercarcinoms durch verschiedene hormonelle Korrelationsstörungen im Vergleich zum Körpergewicht*

Versuchsart	Tumorwachstum %	Körpergewicht zunahme + abnahme — %
Kontrollen (Mittelwerte aller Ko.)	100	+ 12
Hypophysektomierte ohne	29,8	— 9,4
Hypophysektomierte + ACTH	58,7	—20,0
Hypophysektomierte + TSH	41,5	—15,4
Adrenalektomierte ohne	34,2	+ 2,9
Adrenalektomierte + Cortison	34,6	— 9,9
Adrenalektomierte + DOCA	38,8	— 4,9
Normale Ratten + Cortison	51,0	— 8,0
Hungertiere	18,5	—27,2

Tabelle 7. *Einwirkung verschiedener Hormone auf die Wirkung des Benzpyrentumors der Mäusehaut*

Versuchsart	Epitheldicke der Haut Flächenmaß	Milz ‰	Aktivierung des RES der Milz
Benzpyrenpinselung ohne 42 Tg.	1,131	1,09	stark
Benzpyrenpinselung + Cortison 32 Tg.	0,806	0,27	keine (Atrophie)
Benzpyrenpinselung + Percorten 42 Tg.	1,421	1,06	sehr stark
Benzpyrenpinselung + STH 42 Tg.	1,093	1,17	sehr stark
Normale Mäusehaut	0,315	0,55	—

Bei anderen Tumorarten wurde dagegen von einigen Untersuchern kein oder nur ein unwesentlicher Einfluß auf das Wachstum gesehen [DILLER, BECK, BLAUCH (1948), SUGIURA (1931), PICCAGLI (1955)]. SULZBERGER, HERRMANN, PICCAGLI, FRANK (1953) und SPAIN, MOLOMUT und NOVIKOFF (1956) konnten eine Zunahme der Hauttumoren bei gleichzeitiger Behandlung mit Benzpyren bzw. Methylcholanthren und Cortison nachweisen. SULZBERGER u. Mitarb. (1953) fanden bei Pinselung mit Methylcholanthren 48% Papillome und bei zusätzlicher Cortisonbehandlung 69% Papillome. GORSKI (1959) fand bei Behandlung von Mäusen im Bereich des Pankreas mit Methylcholanthren bei 21 Tieren 10 Sarkome, bei zusätzlicher Behandlung mit Cortison bei 36 Tieren 15 maligne Tumoren.

DILLER, BECK, BLAUCH (1948), BARONI, COMSIA und BARONI (1938), ZACHARIAE und ASBOE-HANSEN (1954) sahen bei örtlicher Behandlung mit Hydrocortison eine Rückbildung bei den durch 9-10-Dimethyl 1-2-Benzanthrazen (DMBA) erzeugten Hauttumoren der Maus. Nach ZACHARIAE und ASBOE-HANSEN (1958) hemmt Cortison nur in den ersten 8—11 Wochen die durch DMBA erzeugte Tumorentstehung. Nach der 11. Woche tritt erneutes Tumorwachstum auf.

Rosenkilde, Küchmeister, Herzberg und Lange-Cordes (1955) berichten über ein früheres Auftreten von Hauttumoren nach Pinselung mit DMBA und Cortison. Read und McGovern (1953) führen an, daß eine Implantation von Nebennierengewebe in die Milz ohne Einfluß auf die Carcinogenese in der Leber durch 2-Acetaminofluoren bleibt. Ritchie (1953) fand ebenfalls eine Hemmung der Epithelproliferation der Haut nach DMBA wie nach Crotonöl bei gleichzeitiger Behandlung mit Cortison. Baserga und Shubik (1954) sahen keinen Einfluß der Cortisonbehandlung auf das durch Methylcholanthren ausgelöste Tumorwachstum der Haut bei Mäusen und auf das Adenocarcinom der Maus.

Transplantation

Nach Greene und Whiteley (1952, 1953) wachsen auf Ratten übertragene Sarkome von einem differenten Tierstamm mit stark regressivem Wachstum wieder progressiv, wenn man die Tiere mit Cortison behandelt; die Tiere selbst gehen dabei zugrunde. Durch Cortisonbehandlung vor und nach *Transplantation* kann man sogar maligne Tumoren von der Ratte auf die Maus übertragen, insbesondere dann, wenn man zu dem Transplantat zusätzlich Cortison hinzufügt. Ebenso gelingt mittels dieser Technik die Übertragung der Tumoren von Hühnern auf Tauben und von Menschen auf Mäuse. Diese Abschwächung der homologen und heterologen Immunität gegen Tumorwachstum zeigt besonders deutlich die allgemein immunitätsmindernden Eigenschaften des Cortisons.

Eine Förderung der Heterotransplantation durch Cortison fanden Koch und Uebel (1954) bei der Transplantation von Mäuse-Ehrlich-Carcinom auf Ratten, Agate und Agate (1952) beim Mäusesarkom 180 auf Hamster, Boucher, Syverton und Bittner (1956) beim Adenocarcinom der Maus, sowie Greene (1946, 1949) und Foley und Silverstein (1951) bei anderen transplantablen Tiertumoren.

Patterson, Chute, Sommers (1954) transplantierten menschliche Tumoren auf cortisonvorbehandelte Hamster. Eine Förderung der Heterotransplantation durch Cortison bei menschlichen Tumoren beobachteten Greene (1942, 1946), Greene und Lund (1944), Jones, Hale, Dambach (1946), Eichwald (1948), Hovenanian und Deming (1948), Toolan (1953, 1954), Handler und Foley (1956), Handler, Davis, Sommers (1956), Buttle, Arcy, Howard und Kelett (1953), Gallagher und Korson (1959). Kaliss, Borges und Day (1954) sahen durch Cortison eine Förderung der Homologen-Transplantation. Nach ihrer Ansicht ist dies verständlicher, wenn man den Einfluß des Cortisons auf die Zellteilung berücksichtigt.

Keinen wesentlichen Einfluß auf die *Metastasierung* nach Cortisonbehandlung fanden Agosin, Christen, Badinez, Gasic, Neghme, Pizarro und Jarpa (1952).

Skipper, Mitchell, Bennet, Newton, Simpson und Eidson (1951) beobachteten eine Hemmung der *Nucleinsäuresynthese* nach Cortisongaben (gleiche Ergebnisse bei Kaliumarsenit, Urethan und Senfgas); Veränderungen der Nucleinsäureverteilung sahen auch Pirozynski und von Bertalauffy (1953).

Cagianut (1951, 1952) konnte zeigen, daß die Hormone der Nebennierenrinde eine für die ungesättigten Steroide typische Wachstumsstörung aufweisen. Er fand bei den Zellen ähnliche Teilungsstörungen wie sie durch cancerogene Kohlenwasserstoffe und Steroide (Foll. H.) hervorgerufen wurden. Nach seiner Ansicht wird im wesentlichen das Cytoplasma in Mitleidenschaft gezogen. Dadurch wird die Teilungsbereitschaft herabgesetzt. Studer (1953) fand an der Haut nach Cortisonbehandlung eine Hemmung der Mitoseaktivität, die auch nach vorausgegangener mitosesteigernder Testosteronwirkung eintritt. Diese Hemmungswirkung ist aber nur auf einzelne Gewebsarten (Haut) beschränkt. Zu ähnlichen Ergebnissen gelangten Teir und Isolato (1953). Auf die Nebennierenrindenhormone, ihren Einfluß auf Stoffwechselvorgänge (Eiweiß, Kohlehydratstoffwechsel) und ihre möglichen Zusammenhänge mit dem Tumorwachstum werden wir später eingehen.

Erwähnenswert wären hier noch die Arbeiten von RITCHIE, SHUBIK, LANE, LEROY (1953), die eine deutliche Hemmung der Crotonölwirkung durch Cortison an der Haut sahen, und die Befunde von FAWCETT und DEANE (1951), die nachweisen konnten, daß die durch Oestradiol hervorgerufenen muskulären Hyperplasien durch Cortison gehemmt werden.

Mineralocorticoide

STRAIT und DE OME (1947) beobachteten trotz Mineralocorticoidgaben (Desoxycorticosteron) kein Auftreten von Mammacarcinomen bei der männlichen Maus. Sie glauben deshalb, daß dem Desoxycorticosteron keine oestrogene oder cancerogene Wirkung zukommt. Desoxycorticosteron zeigte in unseren Versuchen [DONTENWILL (1954, 1955)] keinen signifikanten Einfluß auf die Epithelproliferation nach Benzpyrenpinselung der Haut. FIRMINGER und REUBER (1962) fanden nach Behandlung mit N-2-fluorenyldiacetamid bei AxC-Ratten eine hohe Rate von Lebercirrhose und Lebercarcinomen bei männlichen Tieren. Desoxycorticosteron-acetatbehandlung vermindert sowohl die cirrhogene als auch die cancerogene Wirkung. Kastration hemmt nur die cirrhogene. Testosteron fördert ebenso wie Noräthandrolon die Entstehung der Cirrhose und der Lebercarcinome.

HOUSSAY, HIGGINS und BENNET (1951) beobachteten eine Hemmung der Nebennierentumor-(Carcinom)entwicklung bei der kastrierten Maus nach Behandlung mit Desoxycorticosteron. Während häufig Nebennierencarcinome auftraten, sah man nach DOCA-Behandlung nur knotige Hyperplasien. MADDOLINO (1940) fand eine wachstumsfördernde Wirkung des Desoxycorticosterons auf das Adenocarcinom (EHRLICH). Der Verfasser glaubt, daß die Wirkung auf der Blutcholesterinzunahme beruht. Über einen hemmenden Einfluß der Fibromyomentstehung des Uterus durch Desoxycorticosteron haben wir bereits eingangs (Uterus) berichtet.

Die sehr unterschiedliche Wirkung besonders der Glucocorticoide auf Entstehung und Wachstum von transplantablen und induzierten Tumoren ist sicher durch die sehr unterschiedliche Dosierung bedingt. Hohe Dosen hemmen celluläre und humorale Abwehr und fördern die Transplantierbarkeit, schädigen aber auch den Stoffwechsel, hemmen die Zellteilung und beeinflussen damit wachsende transplantierte und spontane Tumoren. Bei der Wirkung des Cortisons muß zwischen dem lymphoklastischen Effekt, der antianabolen Wirkung auf den Stoffwechsel und der Beeinflussung der humoralen und cellulären Abwehr unterschieden werden. Bei der Wirkung der Adrenalektomie ist nur dann ein Effekt zu erzielen, wenn keine Nebennierenrindenreste in der Bauchhöhle zurückbleiben. Bei der Wirkung der Adrenalektomie ist ausschlaggebend der zeitliche Abstand zwischen Nebennierenentfernung und Tumortransplantation.

Literatur

C. d) Nebennierenhormone

AGATE, F. J., and F. E. AGATE: Wachstum von Mäusesarkom 180 beim nebennierenektomierten erwachsenen Hamster (Mesocricetus auratus). Cancer Res. **12**, 243 (1952); Arch. Geschwulstforsch. **5**, 162 (1953).

AGOSIN, M., R. CHRISTEN, O. BADINEZ, G. GASIC, A. NEGHME, O. PIZARRO and A. JARPA: Cortisone-induced metastases of adenocarcinoma in mice. Proc. Soc. exp. Biol. (N. Y.) **80**, 128—131 (1952).

BAKER, W. J.: Endocrinology (Amer.), 234 (1950).

BARONI, V., COMSIA and E. BARONI: Versuche über das Verhältnis zwischen einigen endokrinen Drüsen und Tumortransplantaten. (Rumänisch.) Endocr. gynec. obstet. (Cluj) **3**, 131 (1938).

BASERGA, R., and P. SHUBIK: The action of cortisone on transplanted and induced tumors in mice. Cancer Res. **14**, 12—16 (1954).

BENTON, D. A.: Die Wirkungen von Adrenalektomie und Pyridoxinmangel auf das Wachstum von durch 3.4.9.10-Dibenzpyren induzierten Tumoren. Cancer Res. **23**, 1016—1020 (1963).

BISCHOFF, F., and G. C. MAXWELL: Amer. J. Cancer Res. **20**, 647 (1953).

BLOOM, F.: Effect of cortisone on mast cell tumors (mastocytoma) of the dog. Proc. Soc. exp. Biol. (N. Y.) **79**, 651—654 (1952).

BOUCHER, N. E., jr., J. T. SYVERTON and J. J. BITTNER: Effects of radiophosphorus and cortisone on transplanted mammary adenocarcinomas in susceptible and resistant mice. Cancer Res. **16**, 22 (1956).
BOUTWELL, R. K., and H. P. RUSCH: The effect of cortisone on the development of tumors. Proc. Amer. Ass. Cancer Res. **1**, 9 (1953).
BURCHENAL, J. H., C. C. STOCK and C. P. RHOADS: The effects of cortisone and ACTH on transplanted mouse leukemia. Cancer Res. **10**, 209 (1950).
BUTTLE, G. A. H., P. F. ARCY, E. M. HOWARD u. D. N. KELETT: Faktoren, welche das Wachstum von menschl. Sarkomen bei Ratten und Hamstern beeinflussen. Arch. exp. Path. Pharmak. **236**, 272—274 (1959).
CAGIANUT, B.: Fortgesetzte Untersuchungen über den Einfluß von Steroiden auf das Wachstum. Die Wirkung der Hormone der Nebennierenrinde. Schweiz. Z. allg. Path. **14**, Fasc. 6 (1951).
— Steroide und Wachstum. Die Wirkung der natürlich vorkommenden Gallensäuren. Schweiz. Z. allg. Path. **15**, Fasc. 2 (1952).
CASTOR, WILLIAM C., and BURTON L. BAKER: The local action of adrenocortical steroids on epidermis and connective tissue of the skin. Endocrinology **47**, 234—241 (1950).
CLIFTON, K. H.: Problems in experimental tumorigenesis of the pituitary gland, gonads, adrenal cortices, and mammary glands: a review. Cancer Res. **19**, 2 (1959).
DAANE, T. A., L. L. SPARKS, W. R. LYONS, CH. H. LI, R. D. COLE and T. HAYASHIDA: Inhibition of mammary tumours during lactation induced in virgin mice. Nature (London) **173**, 1035 (1954).
DILLER, I. C., L. V. BECK and B. BLAUCH: Effect of adrenal cortical extract on the growth of certain mouse tumors. Cancer Res. **8**, 581 (1948).
DRUCKREY, H.: Mitosegiftwirkung von Oestrogenen. Naturwissenschaften **39**, H. 16 (1952).
EICHWALD, E. J.: Heterologous transplantation of cancer of childhood. Cancer Res. **8**, 273 (1948).
ENGELBRETH-HOLM, J., and G. ASBOE-HANSEN: Effect of cortisone on skin carcinogenesis in mice. Acta path. microbiol. scand. **32**, 560—564 (1953).
DONTENWILL, W.: Experimentelle Untersuchungen über den Einfluß von Hormonen auf das Walker-Carcinom der Ratte und auf die Entwicklung des Benzpyrentumors der Mäusehaut. Z. Krebsforsch. **60**, 482 (1955).
FAWCETT, D. W., and H. W. DEANE: Quarterly J. micr. Sci. **92**, 385 (1951).
FIRMINGER, H. I., u. M. D. REUBER: Einfluß von Nebennierenrinden-androgenen und anabolen Hormonen auf die Entwicklung von Lebercarcinomen und -cirrhosen nach Verfütterung von N-2-fluorenyldiacetamid bei Ax C-Ratten. J. nat. Cancer Inst. **27**, 559—595 (1961).
FOLEY, E. J.: Effect of cortisone acetate on growth of strain specific tumors in alien strains of mice. Proc. Soc. exp. Biol. (N. Y.) **80**, 669—671 (1952).
—, and R. SILVERSTEIN: Progressive growth of C3H mouse lymphosarcoma in CF mice treated with cortisone acetate. Proc. Soc. exp. Biol. (N. Y.) **77**, 713 (1951).
FRANK, L.: Incidence of epidermal methylcholanthrene tumors in mice after administration of cortisone. Proc. Soc. exp. Biol. (N. Y.) **82**, 673—675 (1953).
FUNK, C., P. TOMASHEFSKY, R. SOUKUP and A. EHRLICH: The effect of hormonal factors and the removal of certain organs upon the growth of transplanted rat tumors. Brit. J. Cancer **5**, 280 (1951).
GALLAGHER, F. W., u. R. KORSON: Wachstum von menschlichem Krebs in normalen Ratten. Proc. Soc. exp. Biol. (N. Y.) **100**, 805—810 (1959).
GORSKI, T.: Pankreascarcinom bei Mäusen durch kombinierte Einwirkung von Methylcholanthren und Cortison hervorgerufen. Bull. Acad. pol. Sci. Sér. Sci. biol. **7**, 101—104 (1959).
GOTTSCHALK, R. G., and A. GROLLMAN: The action of cortisone and ACTH on transplanted mouse tumors. Cancer Res. **12**, 651—653 (1952).
GREENE, H. S. N.: Heterologous transplantation of a human fibrosarcoma. Cancer Res. **2**, 649 (1942).
— The heterologous transplantation of mouse tumors induced in vitro. Cancer Res. **6**, 396 (1946).
— The use of heterologous transplants as an aid to the diagnoses and classification of human tumors. Cancer. Res. **6**, 502 (1946).
— Heterologous transplantation of the Brown-Pearce Tumor. Cancer Res. **9**, 728 (1949).
—, and P. K. LUND: The hetorologous transplantation of human cancers. Cancer Res. **4**, 352 (1944).
—, and H. J. WHITELEY: Cortisone and tumour growth. Brit. J. Med. **2**, 538 (1952); ref. Dtsch. med. Wschr. **78**, 114 (1953).

Handler, A. H., S. Davis and S. S. Sommers: Heterotransplantation experiments with human cancers. Cancer Res. **16**, 32—36 (1956).
—, and G. E. Foley: Growth of human epidermoid carcinoms (Strains KB and HeLa) in hamsters from tissue culture inocula. Proc. Soc. exp. Biol. (N. Y.) **91**, 237—240 (1956).
Heilman, F. R., and E. C. Kendall: The influence of 11-dehydro-17-hydroxycorticosterone (compound E) on the growth of a malignant tumor in the mouse. Endocrinology **34**, 416—420 (1944).
— — The influence of the hormones of the adrenal cortex, compounds A, B, and E on deposition of fat in the mouse. Proc. Mayo Clin. **31**, 454—458 (1956).
Hersch, M.: Tierversuche zur endokrinen Beleuchtung des Krebsproblems. Gyógyszerész (ung.) **3**, (1932); Zbl. allg. Path. path. Anat. **58**, 329 (1933).
Higgins, G. M., K. A. Woods and W. A. Bennet: The influence of cortisone (compound E) upon the growth of a transplanted Rhabdomyosarcoma in C3H mice. Cancer Res. **10**, 203 (1950).
Houssay, A., G. M. Higgins and W. A. Bennett: Der durch Desoxycorticosteronacetat verursachte Einfluß auf die Erzeugung von Nebennierentumoren bei kastrierten Mäusen. Cancer Res. **11**, 297 (1951); Arch. Geschwulstforsch. **3**, 348 (1951).
Hovenanian, M. S., and C. L. Deming: The heterologous growth of cancer of the human prostate. Surg. Gynec. Obstet. **86**, 29 (1948).
Ingle, D. J., and B. L. Baker: The effect of adrenalectomy in the rat upon the rate of growth of transplanted tumors. Endocrinology **48**, 313—315 (1951).
—, and J. E. Nezamis: Effect of cortisone acetate upon growth of a lymphosarcoma in the rat. Endocrinology **48**, 484—485 (1951).
— M. C. Prestrud and K. L. Rice: The effect of cortisone acetate upon the growth of the Walker rat carcinoma and upon urinary nonprotein nitrogen, sodium chloride and potassium. Endocrinology **46**, 510—513 (1950).
Isolato, A.: Influence of cortisone on mitosis. Annales Med. exp. Fenn. **31**, Fasc. 3 (1953).
Joannovics, G.: Über das Wachstum der transplantablen Mäusetumoren in kastrierten und in epinephrektomierten Tieren. Beitr. path. Anat. **62**, 194 (1916).
Jones, E. G., W. Hale and B. Dambach: Heterologous transplantation of human malignant ovarian tumor. Amer. J. Obstet. Gynec. **51**, 893 (1946).
Kaliss, N.: The fate of mouse tumor homografts in mice that have been pretreated with lyophilized tissue and cortisone. Amer. Ass. Cancer Res. **1**, No. 1 (1953).
— P. R. F. Borges and E. D. Day: The survival and metastatic spread of homografts of mouse tumors in mice pretreated with lyophilized tissue and cortisone. Cancer Res. **14**, 210 (1954).
Kirschbaum, A.: The role of hormones in cancer laboratory animals. Cancer Res. **17**, 432 (1957).
Koch, F., u. H. Uebel: Experimenteller Beitrag zur Frage der Heterotransplantation des Ehrlichschen Mäusecarcinoms unter Cortisonwirkung. Z. Krebsforsch. **60**, 239 (1954).
Kutscherenko, P., and M. Maislisch: Die anatomische Insuffizienz der gl. parathyroidea und Anzeichen von Spasmophylie bei Blastomkranken. Acta med. scand. **85**, 89 (1935).
Laclau, N.: La croissance des tumeurs chez les rats blancs privés de capsules surrénales. C. R. Soc. Biol. (Paris) **106**, 146 (1931).
MacAlpin, R. N., S. M. Blair, D. R. Gillies, W. R. Lyons and Ch. H. Li: The effects of long term administration of prednisolone and growth hormone on the growth of transplanted mammary adenocarcinoma in C3H mice. Cancer (Chic.) **11**, 731 (1958).
Maddolino, F.: Corticosterone und experimentelle Geschwülste. Rass. Oncol. **14**, 151 (1940); Zbl. allg. Path. path. Anat. **78**, 25 (1942).
Martinez, C., and J. J. Bittner: Effect of cortisone on lung metastasis production by a transplanted mammary adenocarcinoma in mice. Proc. Soc. exp. Biol. (N. Y.) **89**, 569 (1955).
Murphy, J. B., and E. Sturm: The adrenals and susceptibility to transplanted leukemia of rats. Science **98**, 568 (1943).
— — The effect of adrenal cortical and pituitary adrenotropic hormones on transplanted leukemia in rats. Science **99**, 303 (1944).
Nandi, J., and H. A. Bern: The effect of cortisol on the growth of a transplantable mouse fibrosarcoma. Cancer Res. **18**, No. 7 (1958).
Neukomm, S.: Hormones stéroides et cancer. Brux. méd. **32**, 2539 (1952).
Patterson, W. B., R. N. Chute and S. C. Sommers: Transplantation of human tumors into cortisone-treated hamsters. Cancer Res. **14**, 656 (1954).
Pearson, O., L. Eliel, R. Rawson, K. Dobriner and C. Rhoads: ACTH and cortisone-induced regression of lymphoid tumors in man. A preliminary report. Cancer (Chic.) **2**, 943 (1949).
Piccagli, R. W.: Über die Entwicklung epidermaler Methylcholanthren-Tumoren bei Mäusen unter Cortisonbehandlung. Berichte **26**, 12 (1955).

PIROZYNSKI, W., and L. VON BERTALAUFFY: Effect of hormones on distribution of ribonucleic acid in liver cells. Changes following administration of cortisone, desoxycorticosterone acetate and thyroxine. Acta anat. (Basel) **19**, 7 (1953).
POMEROY, T. C.: Studies on the mechanism of cortisone-induced metastases of transplantable mouse tumors. Cancer Res. **14**, 201 (1954).
READ, G., and V. MCGOVERN: The influence of steroids on the carcinogenic action of 2-acetylaminofluorene. Aust. J. exp. Biol. med. Sci. **31**, 66 (1953).
REID, E.: Growth hormone and adrenocortical hormones in relation to experimental tumors: a review. Cancer Res. **14**, 249 (1954).
RITCHIE, A. C., PH. SHUBIK, M. LANE and E. P. LEROY: The effect of cortisone on the hyperplasia produced in mouse skin by croton oil. Cancer Res. **13**, 45 (1953).
ROBERT, A., u. P. KLÄRNER: Wirkung von Adaptationshormonenauf Urethan-Lungentumoren der intakten Maus. Arch. Geschwulstforsch. **12**, 28 (1956).
ROFFO, A.: Der Einfluß der Nebenniere auf die Entwicklung der Geschwülste von Tieren, welchen die Nebenniere weggenommen wurde, und von Tieren, welche mit den Nebennierenprodukten behandelt wurden. Bol. Inst. Med. exp. Cancer (B. Aires) **7**, 1174 (1930).
ROSENKILDE, H., H. KÜCHMEISTER, J. J. HERZBERG u. E. LANGE-CORDES: Der Einfluß von Cortison auf das Wachstum chemisch erzeugter Hauttumoren. Klin. Wschr. **33**, 582—586 (1955).
SCHOBER, R.: Die Beziehungen der Nebennierenrindenhormone zu exper. Geschwulstwachstum. Z. Krebsforsch. **59**, 28 (1953).
SELYE, H.: The effect of antiphlogistic-corticoid conditioning (the A-CC effect) upon the Walker tumor. Cancer Res. **15**, 26—30 (1955).
— Experimentelle Studien über die Wirkung von Adaptationshormonen (STH, Cortisol) auf transplantierbare Geschwülste. Z. Krebsforsch. **60**, 316—333 (1955).
SHIMKIN, M., and R. WYMAN: Effect of adrenalectomy and ovarectomy on mammary carcinogenesis in strain C3H mice. J. nat. Cancer Inst. **6**, 187 (1945).
SKIPPER, H. E., J. H. MITCHELL, jr., L. L. BENNET, jr., M. A. NEWTON, L. SIMPSON and M. EIDSON: Beobachtungen über Hemmung der Nukleinsäuresynthese als Folge der Behandlung mit Senfgas, Urethan, Colchinin, 2,6-Diaminopurin, 8-Azoguanin, Kaliumarsenit und Cortison. Cancer Res. **11**, 145 (1951); Arch. Geschwulstforsch. **3**, 337 (1951).
SPAIN, D. M., N. MOLOMUT and A. B. NOVIKOFF: Cortisone and carcinogenesis in mouse skin. I. Effect of cortisone during multiple paintings with methylcholanthrene. Cancer Res. **16**, 138—141 (1956).
STASNEY, F., K. F. PASCHKIS and A. CANTAROW: The influence of adrenalectomy on the growth of transplanted rat lymphosarkoma. Cancer Res. **11**, 283 (1951).
STRAIT, L. A., and K. B. DE OME: Desoxycorticosteronacetat, Milchdrüsenwachstum und Krebsentstehung bei Mäusen. Cancer Res. **7**, 310—311 (1947).
STUDER, A.: Zur Frage der Angriffsorte von Compound E (Cortison). Z. ges. exp. Med. **121**, 287 (1953).
STURM, E., and J. B. MURPHY: The effect of adrenalectomy on susceptibility of rats to a transplantable leukemia. Cancer Res. **4**, 384—388 (1944).
SUGIURA, K.: Amer J. Cancer **15**, 707 (1931).
— C. C. STOCK, K. DOBRINER and C. P. RHOADS: The effect of cortisone and other steroids on experimental tumors. Cancer Res. **10**, 244—245 (1950).
SULZBERGER, M. B., F. HERRMAN, R. PICCAGLI and L. FRANK: Incidence of epidermal methylcholanthrene tumors in mice after administration of cortisone. Proc. Soc. exp. Biol. (N. Y.) **82**, 673—675 (1953).
SYMEONIDIS, A., A. S. MULAY and F. H. BURGOYNE: Liver tumor induction of adrenalectomized and DOCA-treated rats fed with p-dimethylaminoazobenzene. Cancer Res. **11**, 285 (1951).
— — — Effect of adrenalectomy and of desoxycorticosterone acetate on the formation of liver lesions in rats fed p-dimethylaminoazobenzene. J. nat. Cancer Inst. **14**, 805—817 (1954).
TALATAY, P., G. M. V. TAKANO and CH. HUGGINS: Studies on the Walkertumor. II. Effects of adrenalectomy and hypophysectomy on tumor growth in tube-fed-rats. Cancer Res. **12**, 838 (1952).
TEIR, H., and A. ISOLATO: Influence of cortisone on mitosis. Ann. Med. exp. Fenn. **31**, Fasc. 2 (1953).
TOOLAN, H.: Transplantable human neoplasms maintained in cortisone-treated laboratory animals. Cancer Res. **14**, 660 (1954).
— C. CRABB and A. KELDALL: Growth of human tumors in cortisone-treated laboratory animals. The possibility of obtaining permanently transplantable human tumors Cancer Res. **13**, 389—394 (1953).
VRAT, V.: Effects of adrenocorticotropic hormone (ACTH), cortisone, and arginase on growth of transplanted mammary adenocarcinoma in C3H mice. Permanente Fdn. med. Bull. **9**, 60 (1951).

WILLIG, H.: Tierexperimentelle Untersuchungen über den Einfluß der Nebennierenexstirpation auf das gesteigerte Geschwulstwachstum des Walker-Carcinoms der Ratte nach dem Wurf. Z. Krebsforsch. 59, 533 (1953).
— Tierexperimentelle Untersuchungen über den Einfluß der Nebennierenexstirpation auf das Wachstum des Jensen-Sarkoms bei Ratten. Klin. Wschr. 31, 758 (1953).
ZACHARIAE, L., and G. ASBOE-HANSEN: Regression of experimental skin tumor in mice following local injection of 17-hydroxycorticosterone-21 acetate. Cancer Res. 14, 488—489 (1954).
— — Reversibility of hydrocortisone-effected regression of induced skin carcinomas in mice. Cancer Res. 18, 822 (1958).

e) Geschlechtshormone

Eine Hemmung des Tumorwachstums nach Transplantation durch *Kastration* wurde beim Mammacarcinom u. a. von BAATZ und SCHOLZ (1941) beobachtet. Kastration hemmt auch das Wachstum von Transplantationstumoren [ROSENBOHM (1941), FUNK, TOMASCHEFSKY, SOUKUP, EHRLICH (1951), PRIBRAM (1933), KING, CASAS, VISSCHER (1949), BROWNING, WHITE und SADLER (1959)] und von Virustumoren [RAREI und GUMMEL (1938)]. Nach HERSCH (1932) hemmt die Kastration ebenso wie die Nebennierenentfernung die Entwicklung von Teercarcinomen.

Nach BIELSCHOWSKY (1944) findet sich nach Kastration von Ratten eine Zunahme von Hepatomen nach Acetaminofluoren bei beiden Geschlechtern. Der Geschlechtsunterschied der Tumorhäufigkeit bei einem Lebertumor erzeugenden Carcinogen wird durch Kastration ausgeglichen [GORER (1940), KIRBY (1947), LEATHEM (1951), RUMSFELD, MILLER und BAUMANN (1951), ANDERVONT (1950), MORRIS und FIRMINGER (1956)]. Ovarektomie senkt die durch Behandlung mit DMBA erzielte lokale Vaginaltumorhäufigkeit bei Ratten (Sarkome + Carcinome). Oestrogenbehandlung erhöht sie nur leicht [CHERRY und GLUCKSMANN (1960)]. Kastration vermindert die Häufigkeit von Spontantumoren verschiedenen Ursprungs bei Hamstern [FORTNER (1961)]. Mammacarcinome bei unbehandelten Hamstern sind exzessiv selten. Bei Behandlung weiblicher Hamster mit DMBA (10 × 2 mg in 0,4% Öl mittels Magensonde) traten nach DELLA PORTA (1963) bei 22,4% der Tiere Mammacarcinome auf. Eine zusätzliche Oestrogenbehandlung (Pellets à 20 mg) steigerte die Tumorhäufigkeit erheblich. Wenn die Oestrogenbehandlung im Alter von 50 Tagen und die DMBA-Behandlung am 50. bis 60. Tag begonnen wurde, betrug die Mammacarcinomhäufigkeit 60%. Wurde die DMBA-Behandlung am 50. bis 60. Tag begonnen und die Oestrogenbehandlung am 70. Tag, fanden sich 100% Mammacarcinome.

Follikelhormonbehandlung hemmt das Wachstum des transplantierten Mammacarcinoms bei C57 BL-Mäusen [SHAPIRO (1952)]. Eine Oestrogenbehandlung zeigt dagegen nach MOLNAR (1932) keinen Einfluß auf Impfcarcinome. FOULDS (1949) sah eine Förderung im Angehen transplantierter Mammacarcinome der Ratte durch Oestrogenbehandlung. Auf den spontanen transplantablen Granulosazelltumor der Ratte zeigen Oestrogene und Testosteron eine fördernde Wirkung [IGLESIAS und MARDONES (1954, 1956)]. Oestradiol hemmt stärker als Testosteron das Wachstum von Hela-Zellen in vitro [BIMES, PLANEL und DAVID (1961)].

Nach GRAFFI und GUMMEL (1952) ist die Co-carcinogene Wirkung des Follikelhormons bedeutend geringer als die des Crotonöls, also geringer als die des chronischen Reizes (FISCHER-WASELS). Nach Ansicht der Verfasser sind die Steroidhormone nicht in der Lage, den die Cancerogenese einleitenden Initialvorgang (Tumorkeimanlagebildung) auszulösen. Wie widerspruchsvoll die Resultate bei Anwendung der Oestrogene sind, zeigen die folgenden in der Literatur zu findenden Resultate.

GILMOUR sah 1937 eine Steigerung des Wachstums der durch Benzpyren erzeugten Hauttumoren bei Behandlung mit Oestrogen. Das Auftreten der durch Benzpyren ausgelösten Hauttumoren erfolgte dabei zeitlich früher.

Oestrogenbehandlung hemmt nach HORNING (1958) die durch Carcinogene (Dimethylbenzanthracen) hervorgerufene Melanomentstehung beim Hamster möglicherweise über eine Beeinflussung der Melanogenese des Hypophysenmittellappens. Nach LI und TSAI (1963) fördern Oestrogene die Entstehung von Cervixcarcinomen durch Methylcholanthren. LAFFARGUE, SAMSO, LUSCAN und FRANCOIS (1963) behandelten kastrierte weibliche Mäuse (C3H) mit Methylcholanthren im Bereich der Cervix und gleichzeitig mit Oestrogen (8—10 mg). Die

Carcinome traten bei kastrierten Tieren ohne Oestrogenbehandlung häufiger und schneller auf (39,3%) als bei kastrierten mit Hormonbehandlung (20%).

Intrauterine Implantation von 20-Methylcholanthren (I) und 9,10-Dimethyl-1,2-benzanthracen erzeugt bei unreifen, intakten Mäusen (Stamm WLL und Strong A) Carcinome und Sarkome, eine solche von 3,4-Benzpyren und Dibenz-(1,2:5,6)-anthracen nur Carcinome. Methylcholanthren wirkte am stärksten carcinogen. Der Strong-A-Stamm war empfindlicher als der WLL-Stamm. Methylcholanthren induzierte bei reifen und unreifen ovariektomierten CBA-Mäusen Carcinome und Sarkome. Die Latenzphase beider Tumorarten wurde bei unreifen Mäusen durch Oestradiolgaben vermindert. Progesteron und Testosteron unterdrückten bei ausgewachsenen Tieren die Bildung von Tumoren [KASLARIS und JULL (1962)].

Die Mammatumorentstehung durch Methylcholanthren bzw. Benzanthracen wird durch gleichzeitige Behandlung mit Oestrogen gefördert [SHAY, HARRIS und GRUENSTEIN (1952), GEYER, BRYANT, BLEISCH, PIERCE, STARE (1954)].

Die Häufigkeit von Mammacarcinomen durch perorale Gaben von Methylcholanthren (etwa 200 mg MC in Dosen zu 10 mg/ml) ist bei den einzelnen Tierstämmen unterschiedlich [ENGELBART und GERICKE (1964)]. Die Tumorrate lag bei Sprague-Dawley-Ratten immer höher. Nach JÖCHLE (1961) ist die Mammatumorinduktion bei jungen weiblichen Sprague-Dawley-Ratten durch Methylcholanthren nicht nur ein stammspezifisches, sondern darüber hinaus ein bislang nur auf eine Zucht beschränktes Phänomen (Madison-Zucht).

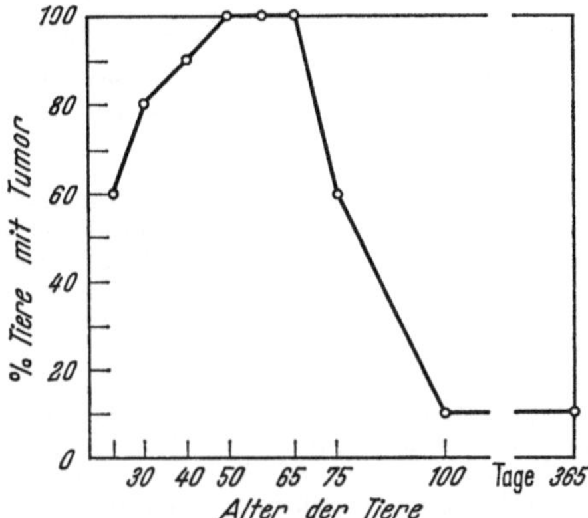

Abb. 44. Abhängigkeit der Enstehung von Mammatumoren vom Alter der Tiere. Einmalige Fütterung mit Methylcholanthren an weiblichen Ratten. [Nach C. HUGGINS, L. C. GRAND, und F. P. BRILLANTES: Nature (Lond.) 189, 204 (1961)].

Ovarektomie hemmt nach HUGGINS, BRIZIARELLI und SUTTON (1959) das Angehen der Tumoren ebenso wie Hypophysektomie und Testosteronbehandlung. Das Auftreten der Mammacarcinome nach einmaliger Verfütterung von Methylcholanthren ist weitgehend von dem Zeitpunkt der Behandlung abhängig. Die Tumoren entstehen fast nur, wenn MC im Alter von 25—100 Tagen appliziert wird (Maximum bei 50—65 Tagen). Bei Applikation nach 100 Tagen entstehen nur wenige Tumoren (Abb. 44) [HUGGINS, GRAND und BRILLANTES (1961)]. Entfernt man den Tieren vor Behandlung mit MC die Ovarien, entstehen keine Tumoren. Die maximale Tumorhäufigkeit fällt bei den Tieren in die Zeit der Brustdrüsenentwicklung.

SHAY, GRULLENSTEIN und KESSLER (1952) sahen eine Verminderung der Mammatumorhäufigkeit nach Verfütterung von Methylcholanthren (2—10 mg) bei weiblichen Ratten nach Oestradiolbehandlung und nach Ovarektomie. Eine Behandlung mit Ovartransplantaten bei kastrierten Mäusen, die mit Methylcholanthren behandelt wurden, ändert nicht das negative Resultat der Behandlung; es traten keine Tumoren auf [MARCHANT (1961)]. MARCHANT (1963) verglich die Tumorhäufigkeit von Weibchen nach Behandlung mit MC (C57 Bl × IF), die mit vasektomierten Männchen gehalten wurden. Bei diesen Weibchen erfolgte die Tumorentstehung früher. Eine Änderung des Vaginalsmearbefundes trat nicht auf.

ARAGONA und PANUCCIO (1949) beobachteten zwar nach Oestrogenbehandlung keine Neubildung in der Leber, aber nach Schädigung der Leber eine Begünstigung der Tumorentstehung durch carcinogene Kohlenwasserstoffe im Bindegewebe (Sarkome). SHELTON (1955) sah eine

Stimulierung der Lebercarcinomentstehung durch o-Aminoazobenzol bei gleichzeitiger Behandlung mit Stilboestrol. Eine Oestrogenbehandlung bei kastrierten Tieren hemmt die Entwicklung von bösartigen Lebertumoren [LACASSAGNE, HURST, ZAJDELA und ROYE (1953)]. Nach GLÜCK (1957) begünstigt langandauernde Anwendung von Oestrogen die tumorerzeugende Wirkung von Acetaminofluoren. Injektionen von homologen Sexualhormonen führten zu einer Vermehrung der Lebertumoren, erzeugt durch 2-Acetaminofluoren bei männlichen und weiblichen Ratten. Die Empfindlichkeit gegenüber einem Lebertumor erzeugenden Carcinogen ist wesentlich niedriger als bei Männchen.

Nach MÖLLENDORFF (1941), TÖNDURY (1947), DEBRUNNER (1953), CAGIANUT (1948, 1951), LETTRÉ (1949), DRUCKREY (1952) können Steroidhormone den *Mitosenablauf* vorwiegend in der Gewebekultur beeinflussen. Oestrogene sind dabei stark wirksam, z. T. ähnlich wie Mitosegifte.

Progesteron zeigt nach SYMEONIDIS (1948), CANTAROW, STASNEY und PASCHKIS (1948), GEYER, BLEISCH, BRYANT, PIERCE und STARE (1953), JULL (1954) eine fördernde Wirkung auf die Induktion des Mammacarcinoms durch Carcinogene bei der Ratte und Maus. Progesteron senkt die Häufigkeit des spontanen Mammacarcinoms beim R 3-Stamm von 54% auf 17% [HEIMAN (1945)], zeigt aber beim Marsh-Buffalo-Stamm [BISCHOFF und RUPP (1946)] und beim C3H-Stamm [BURROWS und HOCH-LIGETI (1946)] keine solche Wirkung.

BEGG (1951) sah keine Wirkung auf das Walker-Carcinom der Ratte nach *Testosteronbehandlung*. Testosteron hemmt das Wachstum des Adenocarcinoms der Maus [LACASSAGNE und RAYNAUD (1939), NATHANSON und ANDERVONT (1939), LOESER (1941)], verringert bei weiblichen Mäusen das Auftreten von spontanen Hepatomen, noch stärker wirkt Oestrogen bei männlichen Tieren [AGNEW und GARDNER (1952)].

TOMITA (1938, 1940) sah eine Beschleunigung der Hepatomentstehung nach Acetaminoazotoluol durch Testosteron und Kastration, während SUKEHARU (1939) einen stimulierenden Effekt durch die Kastration bei Weibchen beobachtete. Testosteron hemmt das Wachstum des Mammacarcinoms in vitro [PARSONS (1965)]. Die Entwicklung von Hautcarcinomen nach Behandlung mit Benzpyren wird durch Testosteron gehemmt, ebenfalls die Entstehung von Sarkomen durch Methylcholanthren und die Entstehung spontaner Mammacarcinome [FLAKS (1948)]. Nach Testeronbehandlung bei kastrierten Ratten beider Geschlechter kommt es zu einer Zunahme von Hepatomen. Nach CANTAROW, WILLIAMS, MELNICK und PASCHKIS (1958) fördert Testosteron und STH den Einbau von Uracil-2-C 14 in die Ribonucleinsäure der Leberzellen und damit die Regeneration. Die Regenerationsfähigkeit nach Leberschädigung mit Acetaminofluoren wird dagegen durch Hemmung der Schilddrüsenfunktion (Thiouracil oder J 131) gemindert.

Veränderungen der Prostata

DE JONGH (1935) sah auch bei kombinierter Oestrogen- und Androgenbehandlung keine Tumoren der *Prostata* der Maus. HORNING (1949, 1952) beobachtet eine Rückbildung bzw. Hemmung der Tumorentstehung in der Prostata durch Methylcholanthren bei gleichzeitiger Kastration und Follikelhormonbehandlung. Kombinierte Behandlung von Stilboestrol und Methylcholanthren beschleunigt bei jungen Mäusen die Carcinogenese [HORNING (1949)]. LASNITZKI (1954) beobachtete nach Einwirkung von Oestrogen auf Prostatagewebekulturen alter Mäuse Hyperplasie und Metaplasie des Epithels bei niederen Dosen, bei hohen Dosen Hemmung der Hyperplasie. Die hohen Dosen hemmen auch die Methylcholanthrenwirkung auf das Prostatagewebe. In der Gewebekultur stimuliert Testosteron das Wachstum von Prostatagewebe. Oestrogen hemmt dagegen das Wachstum [FRANKS (1959)].

Literatur

C. e) Geschlechtshormone

AGNEW, L. R. C., and W. U. GARDNER: The incidence of spontaneous hepatomas in C3H (Low Milk Factor) and CBA mice and the effect of estrogen and androgen on the occurrence of these tumors in C3H mice. Cancer Res. 12, 757 (1952).

ANDERVONT, H. B.: Studies on the occurrence of spontaneous hepatomas in mice of strains C3H and CBA. J. nat. Cancer Inst. **11**, 581—592 (1950).

ARAGONA, F., e P. PANUCCIO: La capacità oncogena degli ormoni sessuali. I. Effetto delle sostanze estrogene iniettate in animali con fegato leso. Ist. di Anat. e Istol. Pat., Univ., Osp. Piemonte, Messina. Arch. De Vecchi Anat. pat. **13**, 123—156 (1949).

BAATZ, H.: Carcinomwachstum und inkretorisches Kräftefeld. Exper. Ergebnisse an Spontan- und Impftumoren. Z. Krebsforsch. **50**, 481 (1940).

—, u. E. SCHOLZ: Der Einfluß der Kastration auf das Krebswachstum. Z. Krebsforsch. **51**, 451 (1941); Zbl. allg. Path. path. Anat. **79**, 290 (1942).

BEGG, R. W.: Steroid-Hormone und Beziehungen zu Tumorträgern. Cancer Res. **11**, 407 (1951); Arch. Geschwulstforsch. **4**, 289 (1952).

BIELSCHOWSKY, F.: Distant tumours produced by 2-amino and 2-acetylamino-fluorene. Brit. J. exp. Path. **25**, 1 (1944).

BIMES, C., u. J. F. DAVID: Vergleichende Untersuchungen der Oestradiol- und Testosteron-Wirkung auf den Carcinom-Stamm Hela, auf Fibroblasten und auf Korpusschleimhautepithelzellen in der Gewebskultur. Path. Biol. **9**, 604—609 (1961).

BISCHOFF, F., and J. J. RUPP: The production of a carcinogenetic agent in the degradation of cholesterol to progesterone. Cancer Res. **6**, 403 (1946).

BROWNING, H. C., W. D. WHITE u. W. A. SADLER: Wachstumshemmung eines transplantierten Nebenrindentumors durch Geschlechtssteroide. Cancer Res. **19**, 819—823 (1959).

BURROWS, H., and A. HOCH-LIGETI: Effect of progesterone on the development of mammary cancer in C3H mice. Cancer Res. **6**, 608 (1946).

CAGIANUT, B.: Zur Wirkung von Sexualhormonen auf das Wachstum. Schweiz. Z. Path. **11**, 598 (1948).

— Fortgesetzte Untersuchungen über den Einfluß von Steroiden auf das Wachstum. Schweiz. Z. Path. **14**, 667 (1951).

CANTAROW, A., K. E. PASCHKIS, J. STASNEY and M. S. ROTHENBERG: The influence of sex hormones upon the hepatic lesions produced by 2-acetaminofluorene. Cancer Res. **6**, 610—616 (1946).

—, J. STASNEY and K. E. PASCHKIS: The influence of sex hormones on mammary tumors induced by 2-acetylaminofluorene. Cancer Res. **8**, 412 (1948).

— T. L. WILLIAMS, I. MELNICK and K. E. PASCHKIS: Influence of acetylaminofluorene, growth hormone testosterone and hypothyroidism on incorporation of uracil-2-C^{14} in liver RNA in the rat. Cancer Res. **18**, 818 (1958).

CHERRY, C. P., u. A. GLUCKSMANN: Wirkung von endokrinen Veränderungen, von Bestrahlung und von zusätzlicher Behandlung der Haut auf die Entstehung von Tumoren im weiblichen Genitaltrakt von Ratten durch chemische Cancerogene. Brit. J. Cancer **14**, 489—501 (1960).

DEBRUNNER, H. U.: Zur Wirkung von Sexualhormonen auf die Mitose. Schweiz. Z. allg. Path. **16**, No. 4 (1953).

DELLA PORTA, G.: Mammary Carcinogenesis in the Hamster. S. 305—309. Unio internationalis contra cancrum conference on cellular control mechanisms and cancer. Amsterdam: Elsevier Publishing Company 1964.

DÖRNER, G.: Der Einfluß des Hypophysen-Keimdrüsensystems auf das Ehrlich Ascites-Carcinom. Z. Krebsforsch. **62**, 125 (1957).

DRUCKREY, H.: Mitosegiftwirkung von Oestrogenen. Naturwissenschaften **39**, 381 (1952).

ENGELBART, K., u. D. GERICKE: Vergleichende Untersuchung über die Induktion von Mammacarcinomen bei Wistar- und Sprague-Dawley-Ratten durch perorale Gaben von Methylcholanthren. Z. Krebsforsch. **66**, 59—64 (1964).

FLAKS, J.: Der Einfluß von Testosteronproprionat auf die Erzeugung subcutaner Tumoren durch 20-Methylcholanthren. Brit. J. Cancer **2**, 386—394 (1948).

FORTNER, J. G.: The influence of castration on spontaneous tumorigenesis in the syrian (golden) hamster. Cancer Res. **21**, 1491—1498 (1961).

FOULDS, L.: Mammary tumours in hybrid mice: Hormone-responses of transplanted tumours. Brit. J. Cancer **3**, 240—246 (1949).

FRANKS, L. M.: Der Einfluß des Alters auf die Struktur und die Oestrogen- und Testosteronempfindlichkeit der Prostata der Maus in Organkulturen. Brit. J. Cancer **13**, 59—68 (1959).

FUNK, C., P. TOMASCHEWSKY, R. SOUKUP and A. EHRLICH: Der Effekt hormonaler Faktoren und der Entfernung gewisser Organe auf das Wachstum eines Rattentransplantationstumors. Brit. J. Cancer **5**, 280 (1951); Arch. Geschwulstforsch. **5**, 75 (1953).

GEYER, R. P., J. E. BRYANT, V. R. BLEISCH, E. M. PIERCE and F. J. STARE: Effect of dose and hormones on tumor production in rats given emulsifed 9,10-dimethyl-1-2-benzanthracene intravenously. Cancer Res. **13**, 503 (1953).

— — — — — Effect of dose and hormones on tumor production in rats given emulsified 9,10-dimethyl-1,2-benzanthracene intravenously. Cancer Res. **13**, 503—506 (1954).

GILMOUR, M. D.: Der Einfluß von Oestron auf Wachstum und Entstehung bösartiger Geschwulstzellen. J. Path. Bact. **45**, 179 (1937); Zbl. allg. Path. path. Anat. **69**, 41 (1937).
GLÜCK, E.: Influence des hormones sexuelles sur les tumeurs hépatiques expérimentales du rat provoquées par l'acéthylaminofluorène. Ann. anat. path. **2**, 77 (1957).
GORER, P. A.: Incidence of tumors of liver and other organs in pure line of mice (Strong's CBA strain). J. Path. Bact. **50**, 17—24 (1940).
GRAFFI, A., u. H. GUMMEL: Zur Frage der cancerogenen Wirkung der steroiden Geschlechtshormone. Dtsch. Gesundh.-Wes. **7**, 1250 (1952).
GRIFFIN, A. C., H. L. RICHARDSON, C. H. ROBERTSON, M. A. O'NEAL and J. D. SPAIN: The role of hormones in liver carcinogenesis. J. nat. Cancer Inst. (Suppl.) **15**, 1623—1628 (1955).
HEIMAN, J.: The effect of progesterone and testosterone propionate on the incidence of mammary cancer in mice. Cancer Res. **5**, 426 (1945).
HERSCH, M.: Tierversuche zur endokrinen Beleuchtung des Krebsproblems. Gyógyászat (ung.) **1932**, 3; Zbl. allg. Path. path. Anat. **58**, 329 (1933).
HORNING, E. S.: The effects of castration and stilbestrol on prostate tumors in mice. Brit. J. Cancer **3**, 211—230 (1949).
— The local action 20-methylcholanthrene and sex hormones on prostatic grafts. Brit. J. Cancer **6**, 80—88 (1952).
— Induction of pituitary tumours and melanomas in the golden hamster. Ciba Fdn. Coll. Endocr. **12**, 22 (1958).
HORNING, S.: Über die Wirkung von Kastration und Behandlung mit Stilboestrol auf Prostatatumoren der Mäuse. Brit. J. Cancer **3**, 211—230 (1949).
HUGGINS, CH., G. BRIZIARELLI u. H. SUTTON jr.: Schnelle Induktion des Mammacarcinoms der Ratte und der Einfluß von Hormonen auf den Tumor. J. exp. Med. **109**, 25—42 (1959).
IGLESIAS, R., and E. MARDONES: Evolution of the functional spontaneous transplantable ovarian tumor of the rat. The influence of the gonads and steroid hormones on the growth of the tumor. Third Panamer. Congr., Endocrinol. (Santiago) 32 (1954).
— — On the influence of gonadal steroids on the growth of the spontaneous and transplantable ovarian tumor in AXC rats. Cancer Res. **16**, 756 (1956).
JÖCHLE, W.: Zur experimentellen Erzeugung von Mammatumoren bei Ratten. Naturwissenschaften **48**, 481—482 (1961).
DE JONGH, S. E.: Der Einfluß von Geschlechtshormonen auf die Prostata und ihre Umgebung bei der Maus. Acta brev. neerl. Physiol. **5**, 28 (1935).
JULL, J. W.: The effects of oestrogens and progesterone on the chemical induction of mammary cancer in mice of the If strain. J. Path. Bact. **68**, 547 (1954).
KASLARIS, E., u. J. W. JULL: Die Induzierung von Tumoren nach direkter Implantation von vier chemischen Carcinogenen in den Uterus von Mäusen und die Wirkung von Stamm und Hormonen hierauf. Brit. J. Cancer **16**, 479—483 (1962).
KING, J. T., C. B. CASAS and M. B. VISSCHER: Der Einfluß von Oestrogenen auf Krebsentstehung und Nebennierenveränderungen bei ovariektomierten, unterernährten Mäusen. Cancer Res. **9**, 436—437 (1949).
KIRBY, A. H. M.: The combined action of 2-acetylaminofluorene and sex hormones in the wistar rat. Brit. J. Cancer **1**, 68—79 (1947).
KREKELS, A.: Einfluß hoher Follikelhormondosen auf chronisch arsenvergiftete Mäuse. Frankfurt. Z. Path. **49**, H. 3 (1936); Zbl. allg. Path. path. Anat. **66**, 160 (1936/37).
LACASSAGNE, A., L. HURST, F. ZAJDELA et R. ROYE: Influence des hormones sexuelles sur la production du cancer du foie chez le rat. Acta physiol. lat.-amer. **3**, 136 (1953).
—, et A. RAYNAUD: Effects, sur la souris, d'injections longtemps répétées de propionate de testosterone. C. R. Soc. Biol. (Paris) **130**, 689 (1939).
LAFFARGUE, P., A. SAMSO, R. LUSCAN et H. FRANÇOIS: Cancer expérimental du col utérin de la souris et son conditionnement par les oestrogènes. Ann. Anat. path. 8, 85—108 (1963).
LASNITZKI, I.: The effect of estrone alone and combined with 20-methylcholanthrene on mouse prostate. Glands grown in vitro. Cancer Res. **14**, 632—639 (1954).
LEATHEM, J. H.: Influence of sex on 2-acetylamino-fluorene-induced liver tumors in rats and mice. Cancer Res. **11**, 266 (1951).
LETTRÉ, H.: Beeinflussung der Zellteilung durch Vitamine und Hormone. Angew. Chem. **61**, 258 (1949).
LI, and TSAI: Influence of hormones on carcinogenesis of uterine cervix of mice induced by methyl cholanthrene. Chin. med. J. 800 (1962).
LOESER, A. A.: Mammary carcinoma response to implantation of male hormone and progesterone. Lancet **1941 II**, 698.
MARCHANT, J.: Failure of methylcholanthrene to induce breast tumours in male of mice when administered before stimulation of the breast tissue by ovarian secretion. Brit. J. Cancer **15**, 133—137 (1961).

MARCHANT, J.: The influence of pseudopregnancy on breast tumour induction by methylcholanthrene in IF or F_1 hybrid (C57Bl × IF) mice. Brit. J. Cancer **17**, 495—503 (1963).
MÖLLENDORFF, W. VON: Mitosenschädigung durch Geschlechtshormone und das Tumorproblem. Schweiz. med. Wschr. 329 (1941); Zbl. allg. Path. path. Anat. **79**, 277 (1942).
— Wachstumsschädigung durch Steroide und hormon-spezifische Wirksamkeit. Ausblick auf das Problem des Spontantumors. Schweiz. med. Wschr. **51**, 1573 (1941).
MOLNAR, K.: Über die Beeinflußbarkeit des Angehens und Wachstums von Impftumoren durch östrogene Substanzen. Z. Krebsforsch. **38**, 188 (1932); Zbl. allg. Path. path. Anat. **59**, 340 (1933/34).
MORRIS, H. P., and H. I. FIRMINGER: Influence of sex and sex hormones on development of hepatomas and other hepatic lesions on strain AXC rats ingesting 2-diacetylaminofluorene. J. nat. Cancer Inst. **16**, 927—950 (1956).
MOSINGER, M.: Über die mit oestrogenen Substanzen und mit Dimethyl-Benzanthracen erzeugten Tumoren bei der Ratte und dem Meerschweinchen. C. R. Ass. Anat. **55**, 285—291 (1949).
NATHANSON, I. T., and H. B. ANDERVONT: Effect of testosterone propionate on development and growth of mammary carcinoma in female mice. Proc. Soc. exp. Biol. (N. Y.) **40**, 421 (1939).
PARSONS, J. C.: Inhibitory action of testosterone on mouse mammary tumours in vitro. Nature (Lond.) **206**, 717 (1965).
PRIBRAM, E.: Studie zur Geschwulstimmunität. 14. Mitt. Weitere Versuche zur Frage der Bedeutung der Geschlechtsdrüsenfunktion für das Geschwulstwachstum bei der weißen Maus. Z. Krebsforsch. **39**, 399 (1933); Zbl. allg. Path. path. Anat. **59**, 342 (1933/34).
RAREI, B., u. H. GUMMEL: Hypophyseninkretion und Geschwulstwachstum. Z. Krebsforsch. **48**, 99 (1938); Zbl. allg. Path. path. Anat. **72**, 27 (1939).
ROSENBOHM, A.: Der Einfluß der Kastration auf das Wachstum von Transplantattumoren. Z. Krebsforsch. **51**, 164 (1941); Zbl. allg. Path. path. Anat. **79**, 290 (1942).
RUMSFELD, H. W., W. L. MILLER and C. A. BAUMANN: A sex difference in the development of liver tumors in rats fed 3-methyl-4-dimethyl-aminoazobenzene or 4-fluoro-4-dimethylaminoazobenzene. Cancer Res. **11**, 814—819 (1951).
SELIGER, H.: Über den Wirkungsmechanismus des Hypophysenvorderlappen-Nebennierenrinden-Hormons bei malignen Tumoren und dessen klinische Bedeutung. Dtsch. Med. Journ. **4**, Heft 13/14 (1949).
SHAPIRO, D.: Combination chemotherapy with 8-azoguanine and sex hormones on a mouse mammary carcinoma. Cancer Res. **12**, 713 (1952).
SHAY, H., C. HARRIS and M. GRUENSTEIN: Influence of sex hormones on the incidence and form of tumors produced in male or female rats by gastric instillation of methylcholanthrene. J. nat. Cancer Inst. **13**, 307—331 (1952).
SHELTON, J.: Hepatomas in mice; factors affecting rapid induction of high incidence of hepatomas by o-aminoazotoluene. J. nat. Cancer Inst. **16**, 107 (1955).
STASNEY, J., K. E. PASCHKIS, A. CANTAROW and M. S. ROTHENBERG: Neoplasms in rats treated with 2-acetaminofluorene and sex hormones. II. Cancer Res. **7**, 356—362 (1947).
SUKEHARU, J.: Gann **33**, 453 (1939).
SYMEONIDIS, A.: Zitiert bei LIPSCHUTZ, A.: Steroid homeostasis hypophysis and tumorigenesis. Cambridge: Heffer and Sons. Ltf. 1957.
TÖNDURY, G.: Acta anat. (Basel) **4**, 269 (1947).
TOMITA, T.: Gann **32**, 258 (1938); **34**, 182 (1940).

f) Thymus, Placenta, u. a.

Wegen eines möglichen Zusammenhangs zwischen Thymus und Krebswachstum wurden um die Jahrhundertwende (1904) Untersuchungen vorgenommen, die meist ein negatives Resultat zeigten [FOULERTON (1904), HANSON (1930)].

FREUND und KAMINER (1925) konnten eine cytolytische Wirkung von Thymusgewebe auch in großer Verdünnung feststellen. Auch die von FICHERA (1934) hergestellten krebshemmenden Extrakte enthielten neben anderen Stoffen Thymusextrakt.

KARNICKI (1932) beobachtete eine Rückbildung bereits entwickelter Teergeschwülste durch Injektion von Thymusextrakten. KORPASSY (1937, 1939) versuchte an Ratten, „die Epithelmetaplasie fördernde Wirkung“ des Follikelhormons durchThymusextraktgaben auszuschalten. Durch Transplantation von Hunde-

und Rattenthymus gelang es Murray (1939), das Wachstum des Rattenbrustcarcinoms zu verhindern.

Hirschfeld und Stark (1937) isolierten aus Thymus und Knochenmark einen Stoff, den sie „Blasthormon" nannten; unter seiner Einwirkung verfielen die Carcinomzellen einer regressiven Metamorphose, während die Bindegewebszellen nicht beeinflußt wurden. Auch den Sarkomzellen gegenüber war die Substanz nicht wirksam. Molnar und Kovács (1953), Molnar, Kovács, Tiboldi, Kürtösi und Vavady (1953) konnten durch Thymusextraktgaben beim Brown-Pearce-Carcinom des Kaninchens „eine Malignitätserhöhung" feststellen (mehr Milzmetastasen). Eine direkte Wirkung auf das Tumorgewebe konnte durch morphologische Untersuchungen von ihnen nicht nachgewiesen werden.

Nach Miller, Grant und Roe (1965) wird die Empfindlichkeit von Mäusen gegenüber 3,4 Benzpyren durch Thymektomie erhöht. Nach 100 Tagen zeigten 50% der thymektomierten Mäuse Papillome, die Kontrollen nur in 5%. Bei längerer Zeitdauer der Applikation wurde der Unterschied wesentlich geringer. Bei C3H-Mäusen zeigte der transplantable Mastzelltumor keine Veränderung des Wachstums bei thymektomierten Tieren [Ross und Best (1963)]. Die Wirkung der Thymektomie auf die Häufigkeit des Mammacarcinoms, wurde von Martinez untersucht. Er sah gegenüber den Kontrollen (94,5%, C3H Bi) eine Verminderung der Mammacarcinomrate auf 54,6%, bei thymektomierten Tieren. Auch Money (1965) fand ein langsameres Wachstum des thiouracil-induzierten Schilddrüsentumors bei Transplantation auf thymektomierte Ratten.

Eine Wachstumshemmung durch Behandlung mit Placentarextrakten sahen Cramer (1955) beim Walkercarcinom und Profitlich (1955) und Eschbach (1955) beim Ehrlich-Ascitestumor der Maus.

Eine Wachstumshemmung des transplantablen Hepatoms durch Zerstörung der Inseln des Pankreas *(Alloxanvergiftung)* beschreiben Goranson, Botham und Willms (1954).

Jehl, Mayer und McKee (1955) beobachteten keinen starken Einfluß auf das Ehrlich-Ascites-Carcinom. Salzberg und Griffin (1952) sahen bei der alloxan-diabetischen Ratte eine Hemmung der Carcinogenese durch Azoverbindungen. Das Sarkom 37 ließ bei alloxandiabetischen Ratten keine Änderung im Wachstum erkennen [Carrie und Ham (1949)]. Die Induktion eines Sarkoms durch Benzpyren bei Ratten nach Alloxanvergiftung zeigte keinen wesentlichen Unterschied [Dunning, Curtis und Friedgood (1949)].

Literatur

C. f) Thymus usw.

Carrie, A. W., and A. W. Ham: An experimental study of the effects of malignancy and diabetes on each other. Cancer Res. **9**, 629—630 (1949).

Cramer, H.: Wachstumshemmung des Walker-Carcinoms bei Ratten durch Placentaextrakt. Med. Klin. **1955**, 161.

Dunning, W. F., M. R. Curtis and C. Friedgood: The incidence of benzpyrene-induced sarcomas in diabetic and alloxan refractive rats of three strains. Cancer Res. **9**, 546 (1949).

Eschbach, W.: Wachstumshemmung des Walker-Ca. bei Ratten und des Ehrlichschen Mäuseascites-Ca. durch Placentaextrakt. Med. Klin. **50**, 1530—1531 (1955).

Fichera, G.: Organotherapie der malignen Geschwülste. Z. Krebsforsch. **41**, 151 (1934).

Foulerton, E.: Arch. Middx. Hosp. **2**, 143 (1904).

Freund, E., u. G. Kaminer: Biologische Grundlagen der Disposition für Karzinom. Wien: 1925.

Goranson, E. S., F. Botham and M. Willms: Inhibition of growth of transplanted hepatomas in alloxanized wistar rats. Cancer Res. **14**, 730 — 733 (1954).

—, and G. J. Tilser: Studies on the relationship of alloxan-Diabetes and tumor growth. Cancer Res. **15**, 626 (1955).

Hanson, A. M.: Minn. Med. **13**, 65 (1930).

Hirschfeld, A., u. G. Stark: Beiträge zu einer hormonalen Krebspathologie und Krebstherapie. Wien. med. Wschr. **87**, 405—410 (1937).

Jehl, J., G. Mayer and R. W. Mc Kee: Influence of the hereditary obese-hyperglycemia syndrome and of alloxan diabetes on the survival of mice with Ehrlich Ascites Carcinoma. Cancer Res. **15**, 341—343 (1955).

KARNICKI, W.: Über den Einfluß der endokrinen Drüsen auf das Entstehen und Verhalten der experimentellen Krebserkrankungen. Z. Krebsforsch. **35**, 523 (1932).
KORPASSY, B.: Verhandl. d. Ges. ung. Pathol., 1939; zit. bei MOLNAR und KOVÁCS.
MARTINEZ, C.: Effect of early thymectomy on development of mammary tumours in mice. Nature (Lond.) **203**, 1188 (1964).
MILLER, J. F. A. P., G. A. GRANT, and F. J. C. ROE: Effect of thymectomy on the induction of skin tumours by 3,4-Benzopyrene. Nature (Lond.) **199**, 920—922 (1963).
MOLNAR, P., u. K. KOVÁCS: Die Wirkung eines Thymusextraktes auf das Brown-Pearce-Carcinom des Kaninchens. Arch. Geschwulstforsch. **5**, 33 (1953).
— — T. TIBOLDI, L. KÜRTÖSI u. I. VAVADY: Weitere Untersuchungen über die malignitätsfördernde Wirkung des Thymusextraktes und anderer Organextrakte beim Brown-Pearce-Carcinom. Arch. Geschwulstforsch. **5**, 365 (1953).
MONEY, W. L.: The growth and function of thiouracil-induced thyroid tumors transplanted into non-inbred rats thymectomized at birth. Cancer Res. **25**, 423 (1965).
MURRAY, M.: Effect of thymus transplants on tumor growth. J. Lab. clin. Med. **24**, 1247—1250 (1939).
PROFITLICH, H.: Über die Wirkung von Placentainhaltsstoffen auf den Ascitestumor der Maus. Z. Krebsforsch. **60**, 390—398 (1955).
ROSS, P. W., P. V. BEST, and M. G. MCENTEGART: Growth of the mast-cell tumour P. 815 in thymectomised mice. Lancet (1963), 611—612.
SALZBERG, D. A., and C. A. GRIFFIN: Inhibition of azo-dye carcinogenesis in the alloxan-diabetic rat. Cancer Res. **12**, 294 (1952).

Zusammenfassung

Aufgabe der vorstehenden Abhandlung war es, einen Überblick über die bekannten Methoden der Geschwulsterzeugung, hervorgerufen durch hormonelle Faktoren, zu geben. In der Einleitung haben wir die Gründe dargelegt, die uns veranlaßt haben, nach dem vorliegenden Einteilungsprinzip die hormonell erzeugtenGeschwülste abzuhandeln, und wir wollen am Ende der Besprechung noch einmal erläutern, weshalb wir einzelne Geschwulstgruppen nach ihrem biologischen Verhalten bei der Besprechung der Wirkungsweise der verschiedenen Hormone in bezug auf ihre krebsauslösende oder krebsfördernde Wirkung abgegrenzt haben.

Als geschwulstartige Hyperplasien im Sinne BÜNGELERs, d. h. als Anpassungsvorgang eines bestimmten Organs an einen erhöhten Bedarf oder als regulierten Wachstumsvorgang durch eine verstärkte Stimulierung eines Organs oder Gewebes, sind fast alle im ersten Kapitel abgehandelten Geschwülste anzusehen. Wir haben bei der Besprechung der Ovartumoren, der Hypophysen-Nebennieren- und Schilddrüsenveränderungen im Sinne von Hyperplasien ausführlich dargelegt, daß die beobachteten Hyperplasien der genannten endokrinen Drüsen fast immer ihre Ursache in einer vermehrten tropen Stimulierung, d. h. in einer gestörten hormonellen Korrelation haben. Diese Hyperplasien sind den Regulationseinrichtungen des Körpers noch weitgehend unterworfen und zeigen eine meist vollständige Abhängigkeit des Wachstums von einem stimulierenden, hormonellen Wachstumsfaktor. Wenn wir im ersten Kapitel des besseren Verständnisses wegen z. B. die Schilddrüsencarcinome nach Thiouracilbehandlung miterwähnt haben, so haben wir auch gleichzeitig angeführt, wie umstritten gerade bei diesen Befunden der Begriff Carcinom oder „maligne" ist, der sich hier fast ausschließlich auf morphologische Kriterien und nicht auf die biologischen Verhaltensweisen stützt. Bei den übrigen im ersten Abschnitt referierten Arbeiten über Tumoren, z. B. der Nebenniere und der Hodenzwischenzellen, müssen wir in Rechnung setzen, daß diese z. T. als bösartig zu bezeichnenden Tumoren nur bei bestimmten Tierstämmen auftreten, die Entstehung gerade der malignen Tumoren also an genetische Faktoren gebunden ist. Wenn wir eine vielleicht etwas starre Einteilung der hormonell erzeugten Geschwülste treffen, so kommen wir damit gleichzeitig dem Bedürfnis des Klinikers entgegen, der nicht nur Bindendes über die Ätiologie, sondern auch über die Prognose und Therapie wissen will.

MOSINGER (1946, 1947) hat z. B. die nach Follikelhormonbehandlung beim Meerschweinchen auftretenden, z. T. invasiv wachsenden Fibrome als Spindelzellsarkome bezeichnet, obwohl sie nicht metastasieren und nicht transplantierbar sind. Gründe, die LIPSCHUTZ (1950) veranlaßten, die Anschauungen MOSINGERs als falsch zu bezeichnen. Dieses Beispiel zeigt, daß bei der Beurteilung nicht allein morphologische Kriterien gewertet werden dürfen. Bei der Besprechung der Schilddrüsengeschwülste haben wir erwähnt, daß Einbrüche in Lymphbahnen und starke Polymorphie auch bei stark proliferierenden Schilddrüsengeschwülsten vorkommen können, was aber kein absolutes Kriterium der Malignität darstellt; bei der Besprechung der Uterus- und Portioveränderungen haben wir z. B. gesehen, wie tief Drüsen- bzw. Schleimhautgewebe manchmal einwächst, ohne daß daraus je einmal echte Carcinome entstehen. Daraus geht auch hervor, wie umstritten der Begriff „präcancerös" im morphologischen Sinne ist. Wenn wir eine Veränderung „präcancerös" nennen, so müssen wir mit großer Wahrscheinlichkeit annehmen, daß die gefundenen Veränderungen gesetzmäßig in ein Carcinom übergehen [BÜNGELER und DONTENWILL (1954), DONTENWILL (1965)], dies ist aber keineswegs der Fall bei zahlreichen am Uterus als „präcancerös" bezeichneten Veränderungen. Es ist nach unserer Ansicht also durchaus berechtigt, bei den Tumoren eine Abgrenzung vorwiegend nach dem biologischen und nicht nach dem morphologischen Verhalten vorzunehmen, wenn dies auch von vielen, vorwiegend amerikanischen Autoren, abgelehnt wird. In der Klinik bzw. Praxis können wir nicht alle durch hormonelle Faktoren auslösbare Gewebswucherungen bzw. Tumoren gleich behandeln und bewerten. Wir richten auch hier nach der aus den morphologischen Befunden und der Erfahrung über das biologische Verhalten gewonnenen Erkenntnis unsere Entscheidung über die notwendige Therapie und unsere Aussage über die Prognose.

Eine metastasierende Struma (GIERKE), ein Parotismischtumor mit oft starkem destruktivem Wachstum, ein atypisches proliferierendes Portioepithel, eine Endometriose oder ein in die Tiefe wachsendes Carcinoid sind eben nach unseren Erfahrungen, trotz der bei ihnen nachweisbaren morphologischen oder biologischen Veränderungen, die im einzelnen — Metastasierung, infiltratives und destruktives Wachstum — für Malignität verdächtig sind, keine bösartigen Geschwülste im Sinne von Sarkomen und Carninomen. Wenn wir z. B. ein Schilddrüsenadenom, ein Myom oder ein Nebennierenrindenadenom oder eine andere obenangeführte proliferierende Gewebswucherung entfernt haben, so ist damit meist eine genügende Therapie durchgeführt, und wir können eine andere, meist bessere Prognose stellen als bei den echten, metastasierenden malignen Tumoren.

Die durch hormonelle Fehlsteuerung entstandenen Hyperplasien sind in der Regel nicht nur klinisch und biologisch gutartig, sie zeigen auch eine meist durch die heutigen Kenntnisse der Endokrinologie verständliche Entstehungsursache, was bei den meisten bösartigen Geschwülsten keineswegs der Fall ist. Wir bestreiten nicht, daß bei einer verstärkten Proliferation in Geweben, wie dies bei verstärkter hormoneller Stimulierung der Fall ist, auch aus den gutartigen Proliferationen maligne Neubildungen entstehen können und haben dies am Beispiel der Schilddrüsencarcinome schon früher erläutert [BÜNGELER und DONTENWILL (1954)]. So ist die Zahl der Schilddrüsencarcinome unter allen Carcinomen beider Geschlechter in Kropfgegenden wesentlich höher als in kropffreien Gegenden, aber die relative Häufigkeit der Schilddrüsencarcinome unter den gutartigen Kropfbildungen ist in kropfreichen und kropfarmen Gegenden gleich: d. h. also, je häufiger Strumen entstehen, desto häufiger kommt es aus noch unbekannten Ursachen zu einer malignen Entartung des proliferierenden Schilddrüsengewebes. Damit ist aber der Proliferationsreiz durch das thyreotrope Hormon nicht als carcinogener Reiz oder Noxe zu werten, ebenso wenig wie die chronische Entzündung beim Magen- oder Hautulcus als alleinige carcinogene Noxe aufzufassen ist, denn bei beiden Veränderungen liegen zahlenmäßig gleiche Verhältnisse vor. Gerade die Tatsache, daß Nebennierencarcinome und Hodencarcinome bei einer hormonellen Korrelationsstörung nur bei bestimmten Tierstämmen auftreten, zeigt, daß nicht der hormonelle Faktor, der bei allen Tieren eigentlich im wesentlichen der gleiche sein müßte, ausschlaggebend ist, sondern, daß dieser nur bei einer bestimmten genetischen Bereitschaft des Organs, d. h. bei einer bestimmten Disposition zum Krebs führt. Ob noch andere Faktoren, die nicht genetisch gebunden sind, eine Rolle spielen, ist noch unbekannt.

Die genetisch bedingte Ansprechbarkeit der Organe auf Hormone oder das genetisch bedingte oder festgelegte „Hormonmuster“ [LIPSCHUTZ (1957), DONTENWILL (1961)] sind wesentliche Faktoren für die Entstehung von Geschwülsten in endokrinen Organen oder endokrin gesteuerten Geweben. Diese Tatsache wird uns am besten klar, wenn wir die Mamma-, Uterus- oder Hodenveränderungen nach gleichartiger Hormonbehandlung bei verschiedenen Tierarten vergleichen und sehen, daß bei einem Rattenstamm keine Mammacarcinome, beim anderen eine große Zahl entstehen, daß beim Meerschweinchen keine Mammatumoren, aber Fibrome des Uterus gefunden werden, und daß z. B. der Hamster bei der gleichen Behandlung nur Nierentumoren zeigt. Das genetisch festgelegte hormonelle Muster zeigt sich auch bei der Untersuchung des Hormonstoffwechsels und insbesondere des Hormonabbaus, der bei den einzelnen Tieren verschieden ist; bei Ratte, Maus und Meerschweinchen entstehen durch den Abbau des Follikelhormons in der Leber aus dem transplantierten Ovar in der Milz Geschwülste. Beim Affen dagegen, der das Follikelhormon in der Leber nicht abbaut, ist die zu dieser Tumorentstehung notwendige Vorbedingung nicht vorhanden. Nicht nur die hormonelle Sekretion und der Hormonabbau sind bei den einzelnen Tieren verschieden, sondern auch die hormonelle Ansprechbarkeit der Gewebe. So zeigen z. B. Hamster bei Follikelhormonbehandlung nicht das gesteigerte Brustdrüsenwachstum wie die Maus und Ratte. Vergleichen wir die Entstehung eines Hypophysen-Nebennierenrinden- oder Schilddrüsenadenoms bei gestörter hormoneller Korrelation oder bei hormoneller Imbalance, Disturbance oder Homeostase der Hypophyse (LIPSCHUTZ) mit einem Tumor, der durch die Wirkung eines Carcinogens, wie z. B. Benzpyren, Benzanthracen oder Buttergelb, entsteht, sehen wir nach der Einwirkung dieser Stoffe (cancerogene Kohlenwasserstoffe) Geschwülste, die schrankenlos wachsen und metastasieren und bei Wachstum und Transplantation von keinem stimulierenden Wachstumsprinzip abhängig sind, Tumoren, deren Autonomie durch die Cancerisierung der Zelle entstanden ist, behalten die Eigengesetzlichkeit auch bei Übertragung einer Einzelzelle. Das Verhalten dieser Zellen ist völlig von dem der Hyperplasien verschieden und die manchmal bei einzelnen Tieren beobachtete, offenbar genetisch bedingte Anfälligkeit einzelner Organe gegenüber bestimmten Carcinogenen ist lediglich in dem Sinne zu verstehen, daß in diesen Organen leichter Carcinome entstehen, aber die Cancerisierung beim Tier nicht von dem genetischen Faktor abhängig, dieser also nicht Vorbedingung ist [s. b. GRAFFI und BIELKA (1959)].

Bei genauem Studium der vorliegenden Ausführungen wird es verständlich, weshalb wir das von BÜNGELER (1951) postulierte Einteilungsprinzip gewählt haben und immer wieder versuchen alle Kriterien abzuwägen, die für oder gegen eigengesetzliches oder ein reguliertes überschüssiges Wachstum sprechen. Gerade der Nierentumor des Goldhamsters, der nur bei einer dauernden Follikelhormonstimulierung wächst und transplantierbar ist, zeigt den wesentlichen Unterschied zwischen einer hormonell erzeugten Geschwulst und einem durch ein Carcinogen erzeugten Tumor. Der Nierentumor des Goldhamsters entsteht erst nach langdauernder kontinuierlicher Hormonbehandlung, das Wachstum sistiert bei Absetzen der Hormonzufuhr. Der Tumor wächst nur bei dauernder hormoneller Stimulierung nach der Transplantation, d. h. sein Wachstum ist von einer dauernden hormonellen Stimulierung, seine Entstehung von einer bestimmten hormonellen Ausgangslage abhängig, es handelt sich also um einen hormonabhängigen oder „dependent Tumor". Das von uns durch Benzpyren erzeugte Nierensarkom des Goldhamsters dagegen zeigt eine völlige Unabhängigkeit von der Cancerogenzufuhr bei der Transplantation. Die nach einmaliger Benzpyreninjektion cancerisierten Zellen zeigten ein völlig eigengesetzliches, nicht von den Regulationseinrichtungen des Körpers abhängiges Wachstum.

Bei der Besprechung des Mammacarcinoms haben wir ausführlich die Mitwirkung genetischer Faktoren und der Viren bei der Geschwulstentstehung erwähnt und dargelegt, daß die von BUTENANDT aufgestellte Behauptung der bedingt krebsauslösenden und nicht vollcarcinogenen Wirkung des Follikelhormons für das Mammacarcinom heute mehr denn je besteht. Das Follikelhormon als Carcinogen im Sinne eines carcinogenen Kohlenwasserstoffes zu bezeichnen, ist sicher nicht berechtigt. Die syncancerogene Wirkung des Follikelhormons bei genetischer Disposition eines Organs oder Gewebes bei der Carcinomentstehung ist durch den am Gewebe ansetzenden dauernden Proliferationsreiz verständlich, da gerade die Dauerstimulierung wesentlich ausschlaggebend ist für die carcinomauslösende Wirkung des Hormons bei vorhandener genetischer Disposition. Der wesentliche Faktor bleibt bei der hormonell bedingten Entstehung des Mammacarcinoms der genetische Faktor, bei dessen Fehlen eine Carcinomentstehung nicht möglich ist (s. Mamma).

Daß die hormonelle Wirkung eine andere ist als die eines Cancerogens, zeigt schon die gegenseitige Beeinflußbarkeit der einzelnen Hormone bei der Tumorentstehung. Die hormonelle Wirkung z. B. des Follikelhormons auf das Mammacarcinom kann durch Progesteron gehemmt werden, weil Progesteron die Wirkung des Follikelhormons hemmt, alleinige Progesteronbehandlung fördert dagegen die Wirkung eines Vollcarcinogen an der Mamma, das direkt schädigend an der Zelle angreift, also nicht im wesentlichen über Störungen der Wachstumskorrelation zur Gewebswucherung führt.

Auch FURTH verneint die carcinogene Eigenschaft der Hormone. Nach seiner Ansicht [FURTH, KIM und CLIFTON (1959)] „werden die Hormone am besten als Regulatoren des Zellwachstums aufgefaßt und nicht als Carcinogene. Die Hormone fördern die Bereitschaft zur krebsigen Umwandlung der Zellen, weil sie die Zellen zur Vermehrung anregen". Nach seiner Ansicht fördert die hormonelle Wachstumsbeeinflussung die Bereitschaft zur autonomen Umwandlung der Zellen, während eine Ruhigstellung der Zellen die Umwandlung hemmt. Wenn Zellen schon in Umwandlung zum autonomen Wachstum begriffen sind, so bestimmen sekundäre Stimulatoren den eigentlichen Beginn der autonomen Transformation. FURTH (1959) ist auch der Meinung, daß der Begriff der Autonomie oft verwirrend gebraucht wird. Er versteht unter Autonomie die Fähigkeit von Zellen, im normalen isologen Wirtstier hemmungslos (unrestrainedly) zu proliferieren. Unsere eigene Auffassung von den Begriffen der Autonomie und der carcinogenen Eigenschaft bestimmter Stoffe stimmt weitgehend mit denen von FURTH überein.

Beim Mammacarcinom (Abb. 45) und bei anderen bösartigen durch Hormonbehandlung oder hormonelle Korrelationsstörung ausgelösten Geschwülsten können wir annehmen, daß bestimmte genetisch festgelegte Bedingungen zur Entstehung unbedingte Notwendigkeit oder Voraussetzung sind. Die genetische Tumoranfälligkeit ist also Voraussetzung zur Entstehung von malignen Tumoren durch hormonelle Beeinflussung, wobei die verschiedene Ansprechbarkeit einzelner Stämme von ihrem genetisch verschiedenen hormonellen Muster (Höhe der Follikelhormonsekretion) abhängig sein kann (s. Mamma).

Die hormonelle Wirkung auf die Geschwulstentstehung und das Geschwulstwachstum (Abb. 46), die wir im dritten Kapitel abgehandelt haben, zeigt wiederum eindeutig die cocancerogene oder wachstumsbegünstigende Wirkung der Hormone. Die Bedeutung der Hypophyse und Nebenniere ist für die Aufrechterhaltung des Geschwulstwachstums schon deswegen größer, weil in der Geschwulst ein gesteigerter Stoffwechsel durch die dauernde Zellvermehrung vorhanden ist und weil gerade dieses sich stark vermehrende Gewebe zur Regulierung des Stoffwechsels und zum Zellaufbau genügend Nährstoffe braucht, die nach Hypophysektomie oder Adrenalektomie sicher nicht mehr in gleicher Weise zur Verfügung stehen. Das beweist schon die starke Gewichtsabnahme der Tiere nach diesen Eingriffen.

Wir haben schon früher hervorgehoben, daß der bösartige Tumor auf seiner Eigengesetzlichkeit zwar autonom, aber nicht autark ist, d. h. er braucht vom Körper Nährstoffe, vor allem Kohlehydrate und Eiweiß zum Zellaufbau, ohne die er auch in der Gewebekultur nicht leben kann. Bei gestörtem Körperstoffwechsel, z. B. nach Hypophysektomie, sind diese Nährstoffe nicht genügend vorhanden, und daraus resultiert eine veränderte Wachstumsgeschwindigkeit. Die Wirkung einzelner Hormone kann auch als Störung der Hypophysenhormonsekretion aufgefaßt werden, wobei einzelne Hormone auch über eine allgemeine stoffwechselsteigernde Wirkung wachstumsanregend sind. Die Glucocorticoide und andere Steroide in hoher Dosis können aber, wie wir ausgeführt haben, auch als Mitosegifte wirken, sie sind außerdem wie das Cortison in der Lage, durch Störung der humoralen und cellulären Abwehrvorgänge auf das Tumorwachstum einzuwirken.

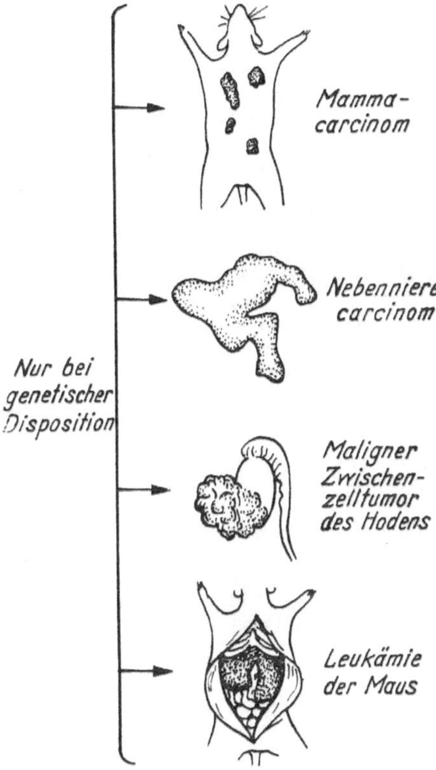

Abb. 45. Bedingt carcinogene Wirkung des Follikelhormons bei verschiedenen Tumoren

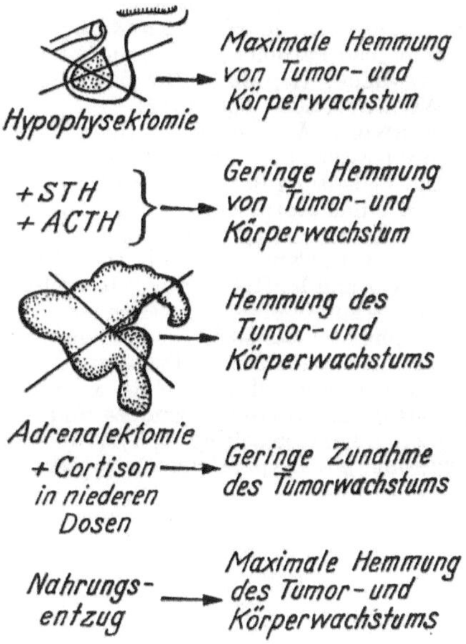

Abb. 46. Hormonale Beeinflussung transplantabler Tumoren im Experiment

Die Wirkung der Hormone ist im wesentlichen eine Wirkung über den allgemeinen Stoffwechsel und den Zellstoffwechsel, wobei die einzelnen Hormone verschiedene Angriffspunkte bei verschiedenen Tieren und Tierstämmen zeigen. Die normalen Hormone sind aber nach den heutigen Untersuchungen nicht als Vollcarcinogene anzusehen, d. h. nicht mit den cancerogenen Kohlenwasserstoffen in ihrer Wirkung vergleichbar. Diese Tatsache rechtfertigt die von uns im Sinne Büngelers vorgenommene Einteilung in gut- und bösartige Geschwülste.

Literatur

Zusammenfassung

Büngeler, W.: Geschwülste und regulierte abhängige Wachstumsstörungen (Hyperplasien) im Rahmen der Cellular- und Relationspathologie. Z. Krebsforsch. **58**, 72 (1951).

—, u. W. Dontenwill: Über den Begriff der Praecancerose unter besonderer Berücksichtigung der Mastopathie und des atypischen Portioepithels. Med. Klin. **1954**, 1589.

— — Hormonell ausgelöste geschwulstartige Hyperplasien, hyperplasiogene Geschwülste und ihre Verhaltensweisen. Dtsch. med. Wschr. **84**, 1885—1894 (1959).

— Das Problem der gutartigen Geschwülste. Münchn. med. Wschr. **105**, 121—129 (1963).

Butenandt, A., u. H. Dannenberg: Die Biochemie der Geschwülste. Handbuch der allgemeinen Pathologie. Berlin-Göttingen-Heidelberg: Springer 1956.

Dannenberg, H.: Zum Wirkungsmechanismus krebserzeugender Faktoren. Dtsch. med. Wschr. 88, 605—616 (1963).

Dontenwill, W.: Die endokrinen Regulationen hyperplastischer und maligner Gewebsproliferationen. S. 74. Verh. dtsch. Ges. Path. 45. Tag. Münster 1961.

— Die Bedeutung der Hormone für die Geschwulstentstehung. Zbl. Gynäk. **83**, 1704 (1961).

— Krebs und Hormone. Hippokrates **36**, 89—94 (1965).

Furth, J.: A meeting of ways in Cancer Research: Thoughts on the evolution and nature of neoplasms. Cancer Res. **19**, 241 (1959).

— U. Kim and K. H. Clifton: On evolution of the neoplastic state; progression from dependence to autonomy. Symposium on Normal and Abnormal Differentiation and Development. National Cancer Institute Monograph, Nr. 2, 1959.

Graffi, A., u. H. Bielka: Probleme der experimentellen Krebsforschung. Leipzig: Akademische Verlagsgesellschaft Gless & Portig 1959.

Lipschutz, A.: Steroid hormones and tumors. Baltimore: Williams & Wilkins Comp. 1950.

— Steroid homeostasis hypophysis and tumorigenesis. Cambridge: Heffer & Sons, Ltd. 1957.

Mosinger, M.: Le problème du cancer et son évolution récente. Paris: Masson & Cie. 1946.

Namenverzeichnis

Die *kursiven* Seitenzahlen beziehen sich auf die Literatur

Sachverzeichnis